A Professional Guide to Nursing

A Professional Guide to Nursing

Veronica Sutton

MURPHY & MOORE
www.murphy-moorepublishing.com

A Professional Guide to Nursing
Veronica Sutton
ISBN: 978-1-63987-005-9 (Hardback)

MURPHY & MOORE

Published by Murphy & Moore Publishing,
1 Rockefeller Plaza,
New York City, NY 10020, USA

Cataloging-in-Publication Data

A professional guide to nursing / Veronica Sutton.
p. cm.
Includes bibliographical references and index.
ISBN 978-1-63987-005-9
1. Nursing--Vocational guidance. 2. Care of the sick--Vocational guidance.
I. Sutton, Veronica.
RT42 .P76 2022
610.73--dc23

For more information regarding Murphy & Moore Publishing and its products, please visit the publisher's website www.murphy-moorepublishing.com

Table of Contents

Preface VII

Chapter 1 Understanding the Profession of Nursing 1
- Nursing 1
- How to know if Nursing is for you 3
- How to be a Nurse 7
- How to become a Nurse Practitioner 18
- How to become a Registered Nurse 27
- How to become a CNA (Certified Nursing Assistant) 34

Chapter 2 Preparing for Nursing School 40
- How to Prepare for Nursing School 40
- How to Prepare for the Nursing School Entrance Exams 49
- How to get into Nursing School 58
- How to Pay for Nursing School 64

Chapter 3 Developing Nursing Skills 72
- How to be a Good Nurse 72
- How to Talk to Patients 82
- How to Deal with the Elderly 92
- How to be Patient with Kids 104
- How to Develop Emotional Intelligence 110
- How to Empathize 118

Chapter 4 Basic Nursing Tasks 127
- How to take Blood Pressure Manually 127
- How to take a Temperature 137
- How to use a Glucometer 144
- How to give a Sponge Bath 150
- How to Change Sheets in an Occupied Bed 158
- How to Position a Bedpan 164
- How to Perform a Full Physical Exam 177

Chapter 5 Developing a Career in Nursing 183
- How to become a Nurse Anesthetist 183
- How to become a Maternity Nurse 187
- How to become a Pediatric Nurse 194
- How to become a Psychiatric Nurse 200
- How to become a Nurse Practitioner 204
- How to become a Nursing Consultant 212
- How to become a Neonatal Nurse 220

Permissions

Index

Preface

A nurse is a health care professional who specializes in the care and well-being of individuals and communities so that they obtain and maintain optimum health. Nurses often work in tandem with physicians, therapists and other health care professionals so that the best of care is provided for the patient. They also implement a care plan by assessing the needs and possible outcomes of a patient. Activities of daily living assistance (ADL) is an important part of the nurse's profession. This book studies, analyses and upholds the pillars of nursing and its utmost significance in modern times. The topics covered in this book offer the readers new insights into this field.

A foreword of all Chapters of the book is provided below:

Chapter 1- Nursing is a health care profession that is involved with the optimum well-being and quality of life of people. Care and treatment is provided for patients until their recovery is complete. This is an introductory chapter which will introduce briefly all the significant aspects of nursing; **Chapter 2-** Nursing is a significances expounding professional. To become a professional nurse, an individual needs training in order to acquire a license. Professional nursing is best understood in confluence with the major topics listed in the following chapter; **Chapter 3-** Nurses nurture and treat a person who requires care. They provide physical and mental care to persons in order to improve their health and quality of life. Talking to patients, assessing their health, having the ability to empathize, etc. are some of the qualities of a good nurse. The aspects elucidated in this chapter are of vital importance and provide a better understanding of nursing; **Chapter 4-** Tasks such as checking an individual's temperature and blood pressure, providing patients with bedpans, sponge baths, clean linen are basic nursing skills. It also includes ensuring that the patients have their medication in time. The major nursing tasks are discussed in this chapter; **Chapter 5-** Professional nursing has many specializations. These include maternity nurse, pediatric nurse, nurse anesthetist, psychiatric nurse, neonatal nurse, nursing consultant, etc. The topics discussed in the chapter are of great importance to broaden the existing knowledge on professional nursing.

I would like to thank the entire editorial team who made sincere efforts for this book and my family who supported me in my efforts of working on this book. I take this opportunity to thank all those who have been a guiding force throughout my life.

Veronica Sutton

Chapter 1

Understanding the Profession of Nursing

Nursing is a health care profession that is involved with the optimum well-being and quality of life of people. Care and treatment is provided for patients until their recovery is complete. This is an introductory chapter which will introduce briefly all the significant aspects of nursing.

Nursing

Nursing is a profession within the health care sector focused on the care of individuals, families, and communities so they may attain, maintain, or recover optimal health and quality of life. Nurses may be differentiated from other health care providers by their approach to patient care, training, and scope of practice. Nurses practice in many specialties with differing levels of prescription authority. Many nurses provide care within the ordering scope of physicians, and this traditional role has shaped the public image of nurses as care providers. However, nurses are permitted by most jurisdictions to practice independently in a variety of settings depending on training level. In the postwar period, nurse education has undergone a process of diversification towards advanced and specialized credentials, and many of the traditional regulations and provider roles are changing.

Nurses develop a plan of care, working collaboratively with physicians, therapists, the patient, the patient's family and other team members, that focuses on treating illness to improve quality of life. In the United States and the United Kingdom, advanced practice nurses, such as clinical nurse specialists and nurse practitioners, diagnose health problems and prescribe medications and other therapies, depending on individual state regulations. Nurses may help coordinate the patient care performed by other members of a multidisciplinary health care team such as therapists, medical practitioners and dietitians. Nurses provide care both interdependently, for example, with physicians, and independently as nursing professionals.

Definition

Although nursing practice varies both through its various specialties and countries, these nursing organizations offer the following definitions:

Nursing encompasses autonomous and collaborative care of individuals of all ages, families, groups and communities, sick or well and in all settings. Nursing includes the promotion of health, prevention of illness, and the care of ill, disabled and dying people. Advocacy, promotion of a safe environment, research, participation in shaping health policy and in patient and health systems management, and education are also key nursing roles.

—International Council of Nurses

The use of clinical judgment in the provision of care to enable people to improve, maintain, or recover health, to cope with health problems, and to achieve the best possible quality of life, whatever their disease or disability, until death.

—*Royal College of Nursing* (2003)

Nursing is the protection, promotion, and optimization of health and abilities; prevention of illness and injury; alleviation of suffering through the diagnosis and treatment of human responses; and advocacy in health care for individuals, families, communities, and populations.

—*American Nurses Association*

The unique function of the nurse is to assist the individual, sick or well, in the performance of those activities contributing to health or its recovery (or to peaceful death) that he would perform unaided if he had the necessary strength, will or knowledge.

— *Virginia Avenel Henderson*

As a Profession

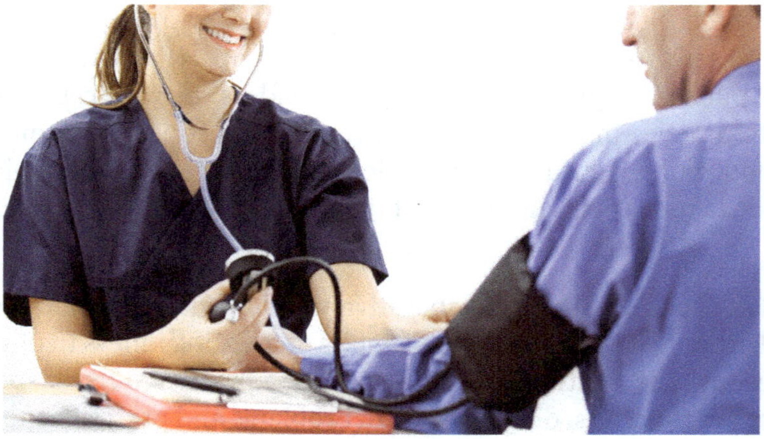

A nurse examining a patient

The authority for the practice of nursing is based upon a social contract that delineates professional rights and responsibilities as well as mechanisms for public accountability. In almost all countries, nursing practice is defined and governed by law, and entrance to the profession is regulated at the national or state level.

The aim of the nursing community worldwide is for its professionals to ensure quality care for all, while maintaining their credentials, code of ethics, standards, and competencies, and continuing their education. There are a number of educational paths to becoming a professional nurse, which vary greatly worldwide; all involve extensive study of nursing theory and practice as well as training in clinical skills.

Nurses care for individuals of all ages and cultural backgrounds who are healthy and ill in a holistic manner based on the individual's physical, emotional, psychological, intellectual, social, and spiritual needs. The profession combines physical science, social science, nursing theory, and technology in caring for those individuals.

To work in the nursing profession, all nurses hold one or more credentials depending on their scope of practice and education. A licensed practical nurse (LPN) (also referred to as a licensed vocational nurse, registered practical nurse, enrolled nurse, and state enrolled nurse) works independently or with a registered nurse (RN). The most significant differentiation between an LPN and RN is found in the requirements for entry to practice, which determines entitlement for their scope of practice. For example, Canada requires a bachelor's degree for the RN and a two-year diploma for the LPN. A registered nurse provides scientific, psychological, and technological knowledge in the care of patients and families in many health care settings. Registered nurses may earn additional credentials or degrees.

In the United States, multiple educational paths will qualify a candidate to sit for the licensure examination as a registered nurse. The Associate Degree in Nursing (ADN) is awarded to the nurse who has completed a two-year undergraduate academic degree awarded by community colleges, junior colleges, technical colleges, and bachelor's degree-granting colleges and universities upon completion of a course of study usually lasting two years. It is also referred to as Associate in Nursing (AN), Associate of Applied Science in Nursing (AAS), or Associate of Science in Nursing (ASN). The Bachelor of Science in Nursing (BScN) is awarded to the nurse who has earned an American four-year academic degree in the science and principles of nursing, granted by a tertiary education university or similarly accredited school. After completing either the LPN or either RN education programs in the United States, graduates are eligible to sit for a licensing examination to become a nurse, the passing of which is required for the nursing license. The National Licensure Examination (NCLEX) test is a multiple choice exam nurses take to become licensed. It costs two-hundred dollars to take the NCLEX. It examines a nurses ability to properly care for a client. Study books and practice tests are available for purchase.

Nurses may follow their personal and professional interests by working with any group of people, in any setting, at any time. Some nurses follow the traditional role of working in a hospital setting. Other options include: Pediatrics, Neonatal, Maternity, OBGYN, Geriatrics, Ambulatory, or Nurse Anesthetists. There are many other options nurses can explore depending on the type of degree and education acquired. RNs may also pursue different roles as advanced practice registered nurses.

Nurses are not truly doctor's assistants. This is possible in certain situations, but nurses more often are independently caring for their patients or assisting other nurses. Registered Nurses treat patients, record their medical history, provide emotional support, and provide follow-up care. Nurses also help doctors perform diagnostic tests. Nurses are almost always working on their own or with other nurses. Nurses will assist doctors in the emergency room or in trauma care when help is needed.

How to know if Nursing is for you

Wondering about a career in adult, child or mental health nursing? How do you know if you could do it? Is nursing really for you? Nursing is a very emotionally, physically and spiritually demanding degree course and career path. And it's essential that have all the information to make this big step.

Steps

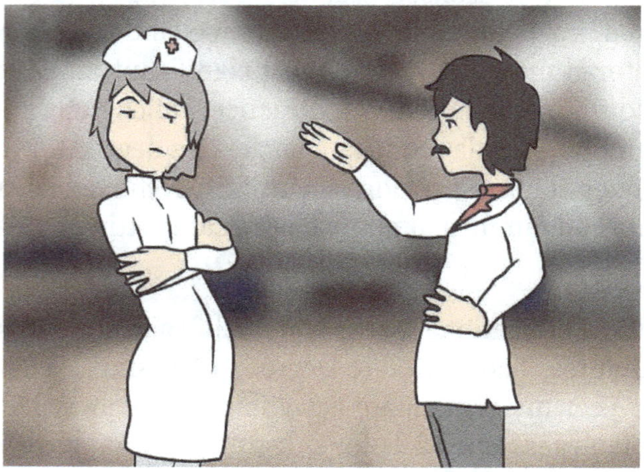

1. Consider how you deal with being told what to do. Do you have problems with authority? Are you okay with being told what to do and when to do it?

- When training to be a nurse and when qualified, you are told what to do all the time. Every day. This could be by patients, doctors, charge nurses, physio-therapists, occupational therapists, etc. If you have a problem with being told what to do, when to do it and how to do it, then you may need to rethink.

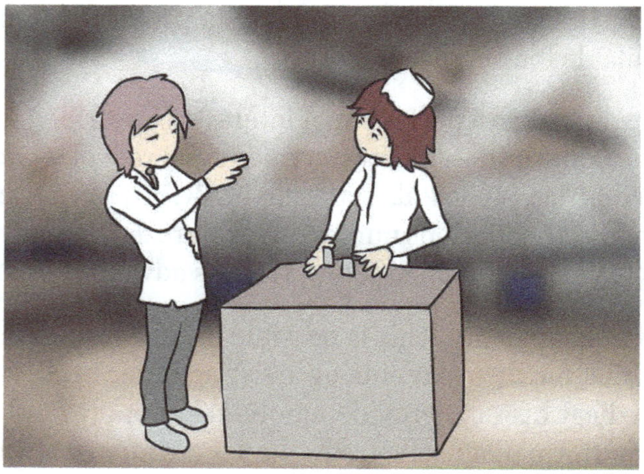

2. Think about whether you're all right with being second guessed. Are you okay with having your work scrutinized by other nurses, doctors, patients and patients families?

- When training to be a nurse you are scrutinized and assessed every second you are in placement. Staff report to the mentor on your progress, and you are assessed by your mentor in a book; where comments are made about every possible detail.
- When qualified, you are in charge of your patients. Staff, patients, doctors and patients families are quick to point out errors however tiny they may be.
- Can you handle this pressure? This ability to do everything to the best of your ability at all times (tired/hungry or not)? If you can, you could maybe handle it.

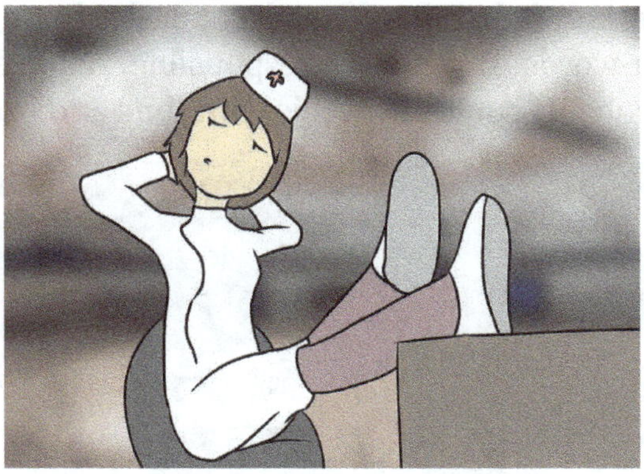

3. Examine your work ethic. Nursing is not a career that you can put your feet up for 5 minutes because you're "tired". A typical ward day is manic, and sometimes you are lucky to make it to your lunch breaks on time... if at all.

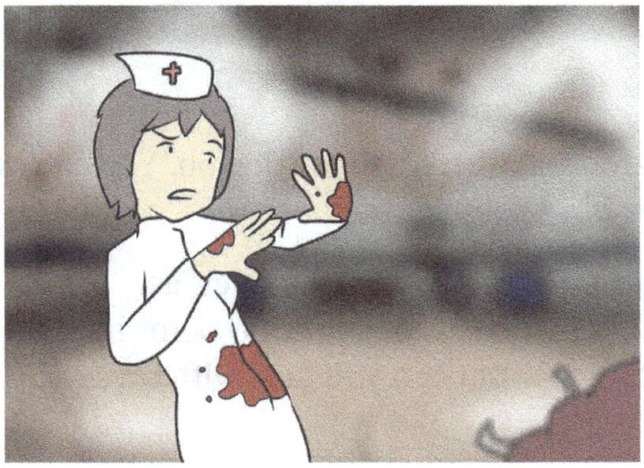

4. Be honest with yourself about how squeamish you are.

- You see puss, blood, mucus, urine, stool (Hard and watery), every possible substance that a human body can produce... Can you handle this without letting it show on your face?
- Can you smell these things without letting it show on your face?
- Can these things accidentally spill on you without gagging/fainting? ...Then maybe there's some hope for you!

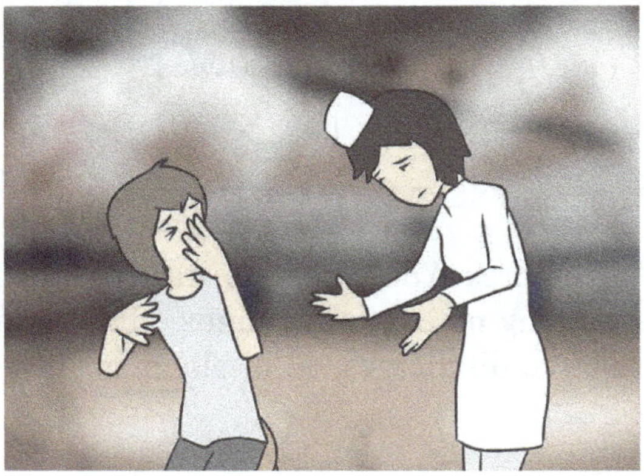

5. Consider your bedside manner. Can you build a rapport with strangers very fast? Can you be-

come a daughter, mother, brother, father, best friend, counselor but professional all at once and in about 5-10 minutes? In other words; If you are a responsible, reliable, likable, nice person with a good sense of humour you probably could learn this with time and practice.

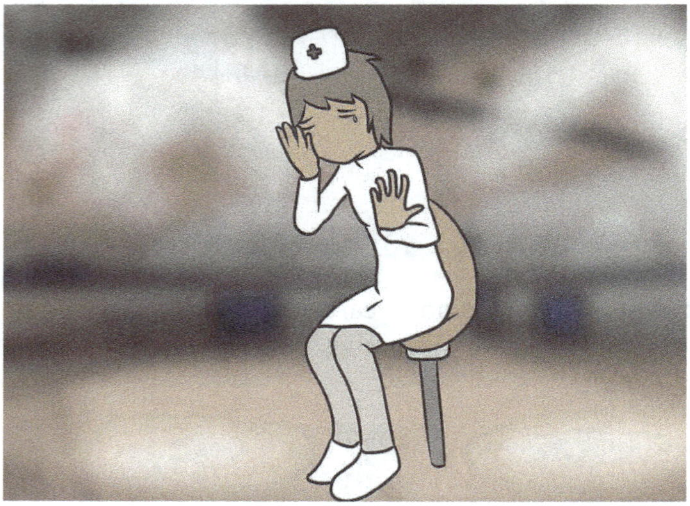

6. Remember that you need emotional strength for the job. You can be good friends with a patient one minute, and the next they have passed away.

- You have to be able to take any statements such as, "I don't want to die" or "I'm thinking about suicide" or "I'm worthless, there's no point in me living anymore"... You will be taught what to physically do. But can you deal with these questions emotionally when you go home?

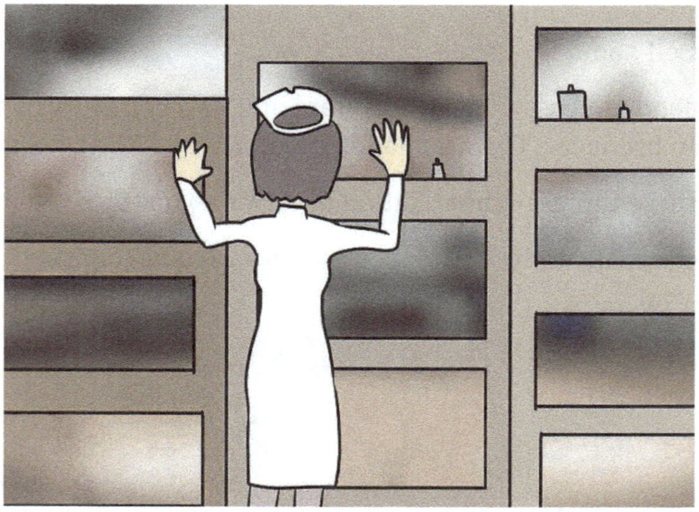

7. Think about how organized you area. You'll need to stay "on top of" social work referrals, dietitian referrals, food charts, nursing notes, ward rounds, observations, toileting, personal care, turning charts, fluid balance charts, discharges, admissions, medications, appointments and the list goes on and on and on.

- Are you responsible and pro-active enough to remember to do all of these things? And not just hand them over to the next nurse.

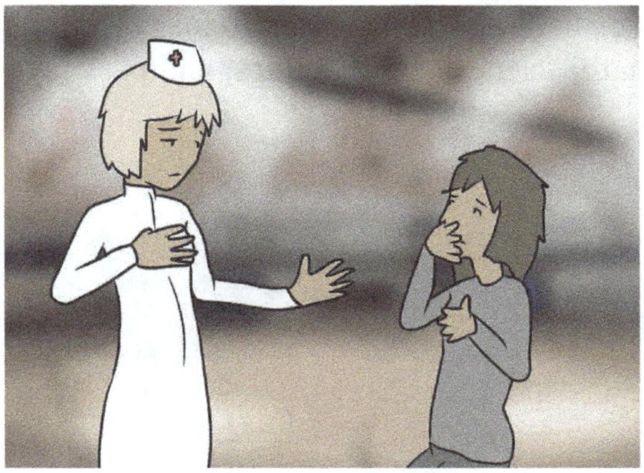

8. Think about how much you *care*. Can you care enough about a strangers well-being (no matter how nice/horrible they are) to give them the best care that you can possibly give?

- It's a tough balance between caring enough that you give amazing care, and not letting yourself get too emotionally attached and damaged.

How to be a Nurse

Nursing shortages are common. Nurses are needed in hospitals, clinics, doctors' offices, nursing homes, and home health care. Learning how to be a nurse is a great way to enter the healthcare profession.

Part 1

Starting Out

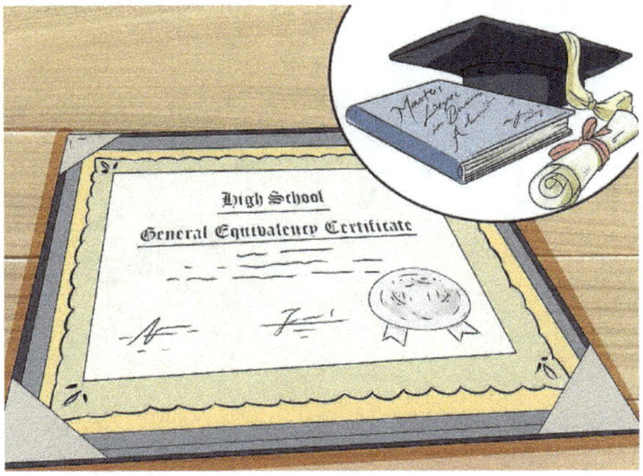

1. Get your high school diploma or GED. In order to complete the path to becoming any type of nurse (be it an LPN, an RN, or anything else), you need to complete high school. To get into a good nursing school, you need decent grades as well.

- Many nursing schools require a pre-entrance exam to be accepted into the nursing program as well. Many schools offer different programs, but know that all require prerequisite courses. Typical prerequisite courses have up to four years required from high school and college of English, math, science, social studies, and possibly even a couple years of a foreign language.

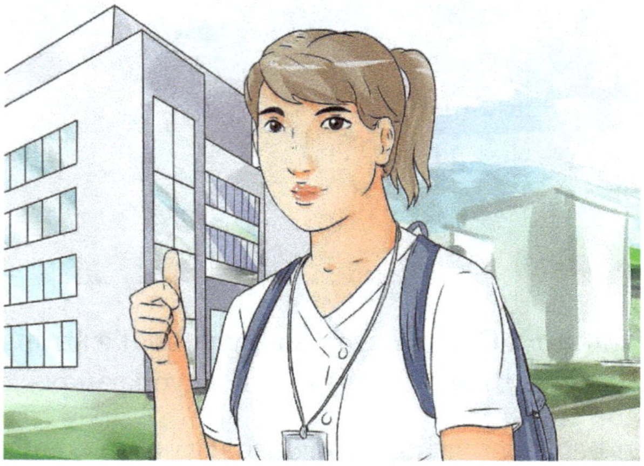

2. Get an entry-level job in the healthcare arena. While not always mandatory, some schools do require previous healthcare experience in order to be accepted to their program. If you have the time and desire to become a CNA (a Certified Nursing Assistant), that's a great first step. Not only will you start getting experience, but it proves you're serious.

- When you are CNA before a nurse, it gives you a good stepping stone into the healthcare world, and your future nursing coworkers will appreciate that you were an aide before a nurse.
- Even volunteering at a local hospital or doing admin work at a clinic looks great on your resume and exposes you to the environment. If you like the hospital environment, you'll have a better idea of the realities of nursing as a career. The more experience you have in this setting, the better—regardless of what kind of experience it is.
- Some may find that performing the aide work makes them realize nursing isn't for them as well.

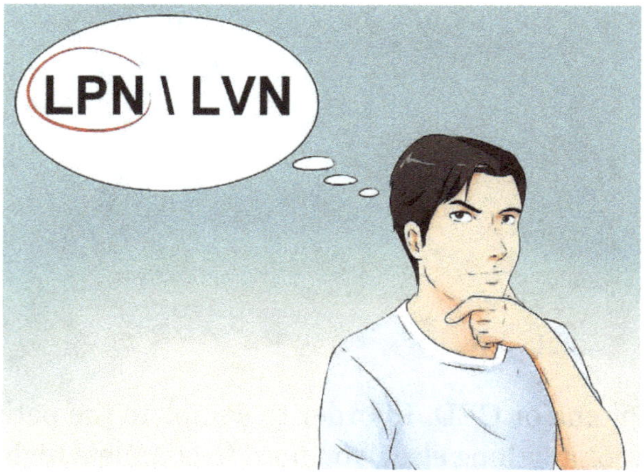

3. Decide if becoming an LPN/LVN is right for you. In a hospital, you'll likely run into CNAs, LPNs, and RNs. LPNs are Licensed Practical (Vocational) Nurses. A Licensed Practical Nurse (LPN) or Licensed Vocational Nurse (LVN) can do the basic essential care of the patient, pass medications,

and report the status of the patient directly to the Registered Nurse (RN) or the doctor, usually under the supervision of an RN. They're still nurses, just with less autonomy. Most nurses can become LPNs in around 18 months.

- LPN/LVNs take the NCLEX-PN examination, as opposed to the NCLEX-RN examination.
- Recent trends in the profession have shown LPNs fading out of the hospital setting and into long-term care facilities and offices.

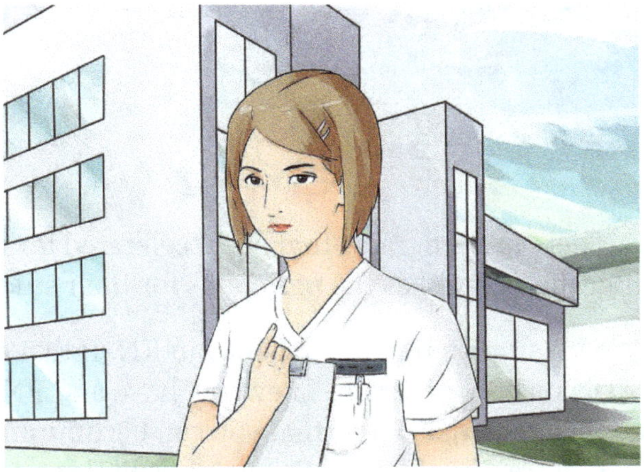

4. Decide if becoming an RN is right for you. RNs focus on the pathophysiology behind it all. Normally, there is an RN in "charge" of the LPNS, but along with that, the RN is responsible for the LPN's patients. Therefore, the LPN and RN need to understand and communicate with each other often for the safety of the patient.

- The RN must think critically on the job rather than simply performing tasks. Analyzing lab results, passing medications, educating patients why they take medications, performing plans of care, and supervisory roles are often part of the RN's job.

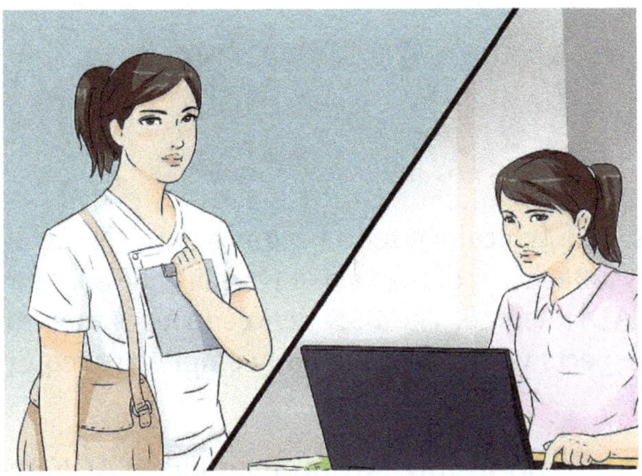

5. Decide which program best suits your needs. Becoming a nurse is easier than ever with online school and weekend options. The work is still difficult, but the flexibility is now available. Some programs are exclusively online. This may be ideal for those with families. Some students need a classroom setting to learn and benefit from that environment. Different options are available for each type of nurse.

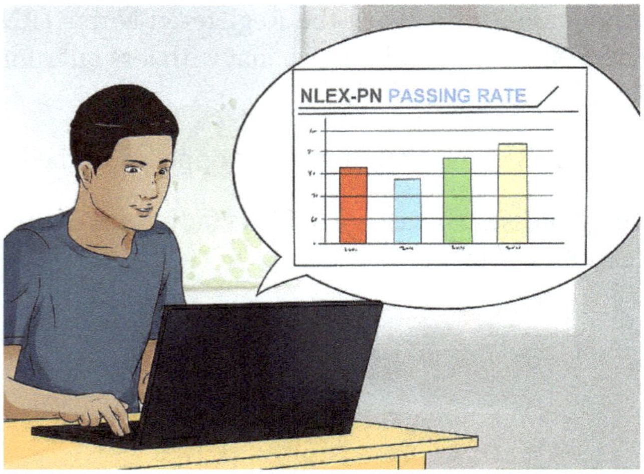

6. Look into LPN programs. There are programs that are accelerated for LPNs. Look into your specific state for accredited programs, as well as the pass rates for their students on the NCLEX-PN.

- For most, this is just a pit stop on the way to being an RN. If that speaks to you, talk to your school about their ADN or BSN program. They may have an LPN designation built in once you're halfway through. Otherwise, know that you can become an LPN after approximately eighteen months or so of training (mostly through hospitals or community colleges).

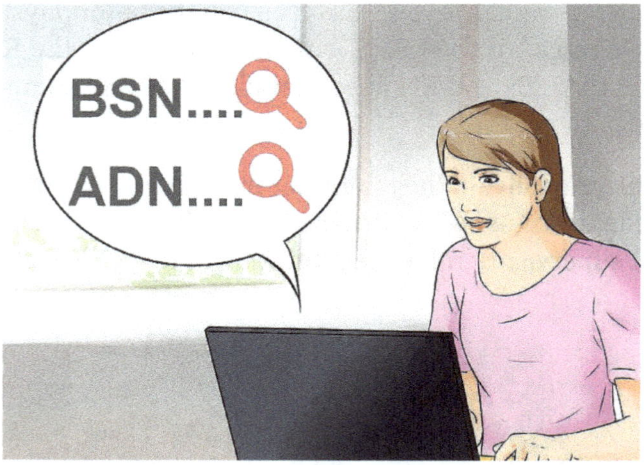

7. Look into RN programs. The typical route to becoming an RN includes an associate degree in Nursing (ADN) followed by a Bachelor of Science in Nursing (BSN). There is a recent push for RNs to have their BSN over an ADN degree. The BSN degree focuses more on the research in nursing. Nurses also have more prospects with a BSN as many employers require new nurse applicants to have it.

- You can expect to spend two-to-three years obtaining an ADN and a BSN is a full, four-year degree for a full-time student, which means the BSN is a much more expensive option.
- Both degrees allow recipients to sit for the NCLEX exam upon graduation.
- The leap in RN-to-BSN programs offered has grown more popular in recent years, a 22.2% leap between 2011 and 2012.

- Getting your BSN allows you to eventually pursue leadership positions, teach nursing students, lead the administrative side, etc. Having a four-year degree at all in today's society is invaluable as well.

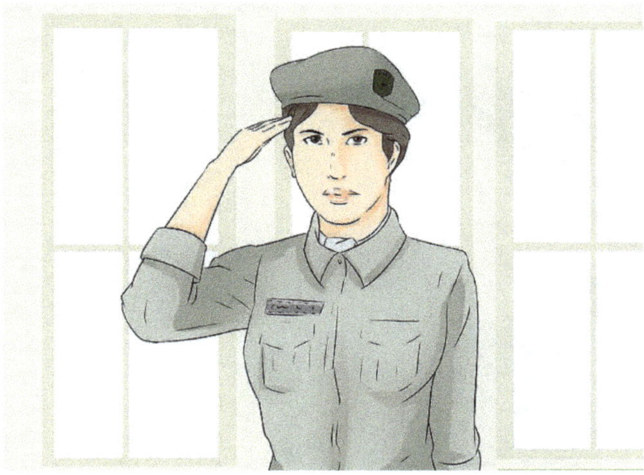

8. Consider alternate routes. A couple of other routes exist for becoming a nurse as well.

- Nursing diploma programs have dramatically decreased since the 1970s. Though these are becoming less and less common, it is still a viable option.
- Go through the military. You can train for two-to-four years through an ROTC Nursing program at a college or university.
- If you already have a four-year degree but it's not in nursing, you should be able to devise an accelerated program. All you need to do is send your transcripts to your new school and start asking questions. It's a very, very common thing. Some states even have special designations for this.

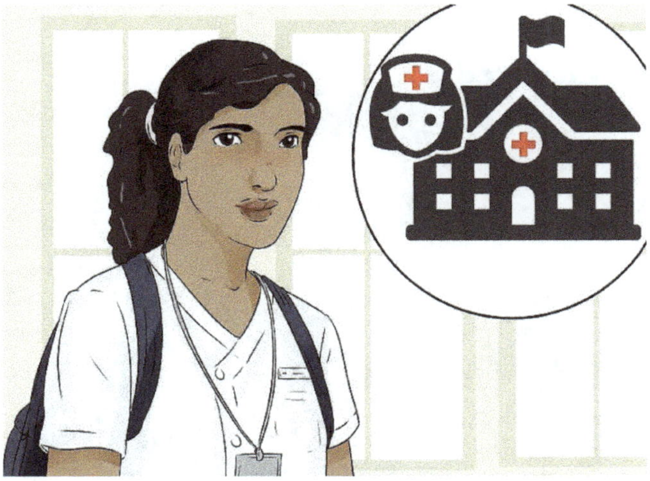

9. Apply to a nursing school. Once you've decided how you want to achieve this career goal, look at the schools and hospitals (some hospitals offer programs too) around you. You will have to decide if you want to take full- or part-time classes, how much you can spend, if you want to live in campus, and if you want to take any of the classes online.

- Be aware that the widely known nursing shortage has led to long waiting lists at some schools. It's best to inquire about this before you set your heart on one.
- If you already work for a hospital, see if any programs are affiliated with it. You may receive discounts if so.

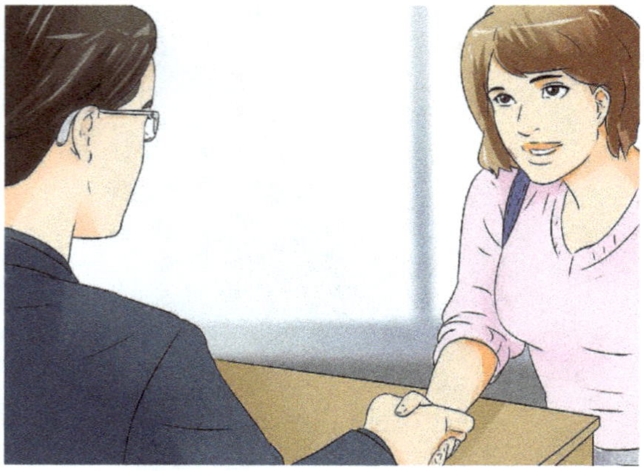

10. Get accepted. Once you've picked a school, you have to apply and get in. How do you do that? Most programs will require transcripts (high school or college), SAT/ACT scores, and essay and letters of recommendation. On-the-job experience is always a perk as well.

- If you can, get letters of recommendation from people who also work in healthcare. Ask the professional reference in person rather than by email. If you do not work in healthcare, request a recommendation letter from someone else who knows your work ethic and desire to become a nurse. Ask in advance. Don't rush the person.
- On the essay, don't write about what you think is a good answer; write what you believe. Using words from the heart will make you stick out from other applicants.

Part 2

Studying and Getting Licensed

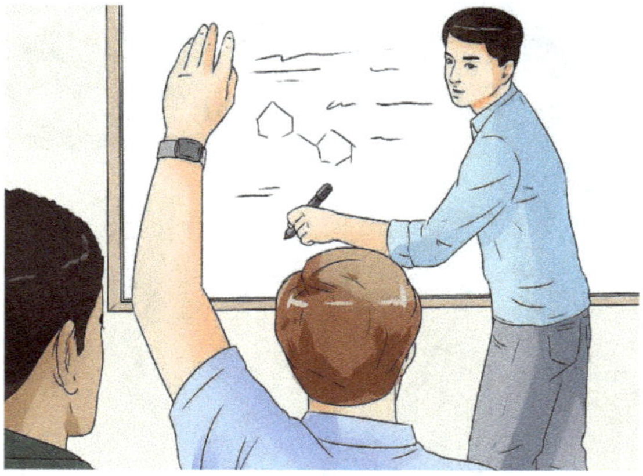

1. Be a top-notch student. You'll be studying anatomy, physiology, microbiology, chemistry, nutrition, psychology, and other social and behavioral sciences. Prepare to spend a lot of time studying hard to do well in such intensive courses.

- If you need inspiration to study, remember that people's lives will be in your hands once you're a nurse. If you need more motivation, remember that the graduation exam costs $200 to take each time. If you fail it, you can't take it for another 45-to-90 days.

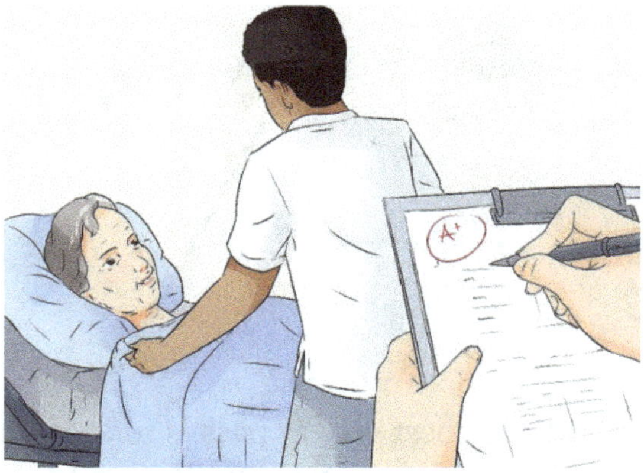

2. Ace your clinicals. Clinicals are part of your education, but they're out of the classroom and in the action. If you are a hands on learner, you'll really enjoy clinicals. Most clinicals are done in replacement of a school day and last throughout the entire nursing program. They focus on a specialization, such as medical-surgical, pediatrics, maternity, or psychiatric. You will learn many skills here, but you have to be willing and ready to learn.

- Clinicals are a normal working day, except not paid like residents in a medical-degree program.
- It's normal to be stressed during clinicals. After all, you're working with real people, and you're still a newbie. Everyone goes through this, and the feeling does go away. Continue to study and seek out opportunities.

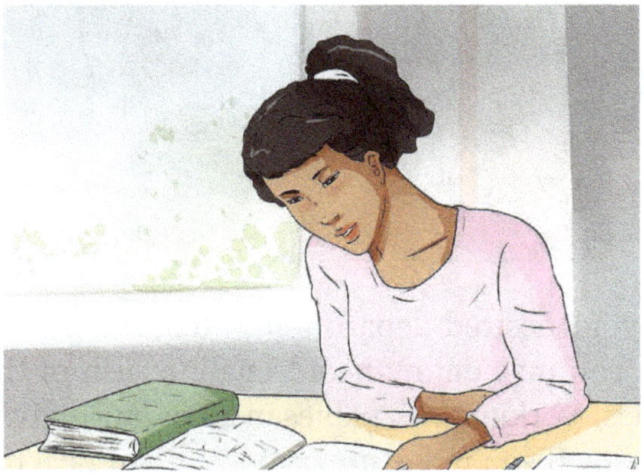

3. Prep for the NCLEX-RN. The exam is also known as "the boards." It's a series of questions (between 75 and 265) that will test your knowledge in a variety of different domains. You're given five hours to complete the test.

- The number of questions varies person to person. The test will continue until the computer feels it has accurately determined your knowledge level with 95% confidence. Finishing at 75 questions means you either did magnificently or very poorly, so don't worry about the number you get.

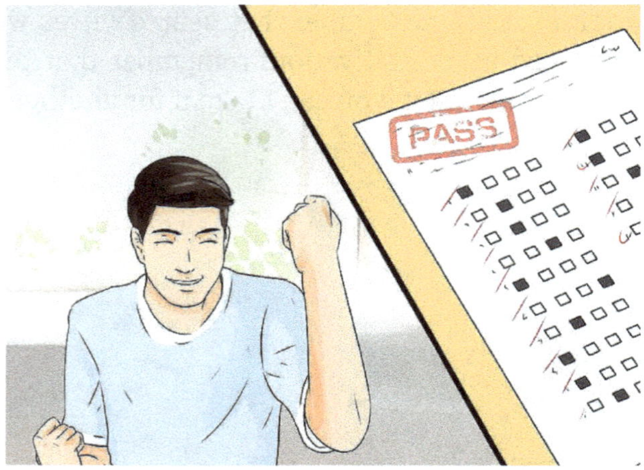

4. Pass the exam and get licensed. The best way to pass is to study hard and get plenty of sleep between studying. Know that 81% of candidates pass on the first try, so you have a great chance if you come prepared.

- Consider taking advantage of one of the prep courses available to help with studying the possibly overwhelming amount of information.
- The average number of questions is around 125, and the average test takes about 2.5 hours.

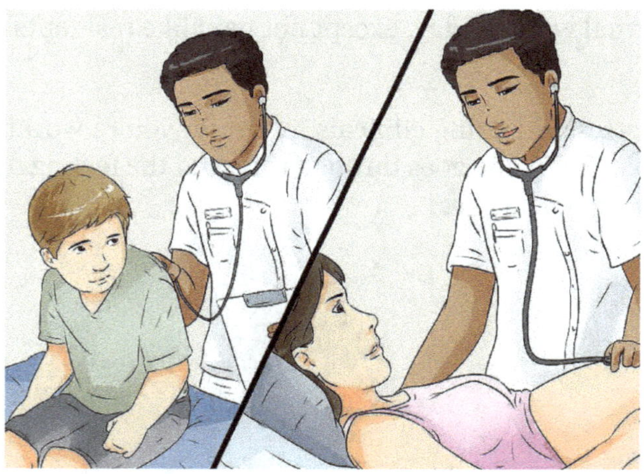

5. Look for employment in your desired department. Most nurses will have an idea where they want to work by this point. You may enjoy the adrenaline rush of the ER, the focus of the OR, working with kids in pediatrics, working with babies in labor and delivery, working with the elderly and long-term care patients, etc. If you're unsure, a medical-surgical unit will help with solidifying skills and prioritization.

- Consider the fact that baby boomers are pretty much taking over. Working with the 55+ demographic would ensure job stability.
- Working with children is great, but it can also be very sad. If you do choose to go into pediatrics, you'll be faced with a lot of situations that just aren't fair. There are a few options in the pediatric area, including general pediatrics, pediatric intensive care units, pediatric oncology units, and home care for pediatrics.

- Mother/baby units can be very difficult to get into. Everyone wants to work with patients who are happy, excited, and healthy. Remember, these areas are also very high stressed with two lives in your hands at one time. When it is sad in these units, it's very sad.
- If you do get into this unit, be ready to commit to a night shift job for many years because most nurses who work in OB do not leave.
- Most surgeries nowadays are scheduled. If you prefer working normal hours (plenty of nurses don't), being a surgical nurse may be down your alley. Otherwise prepare for the possibility of working night shifts.

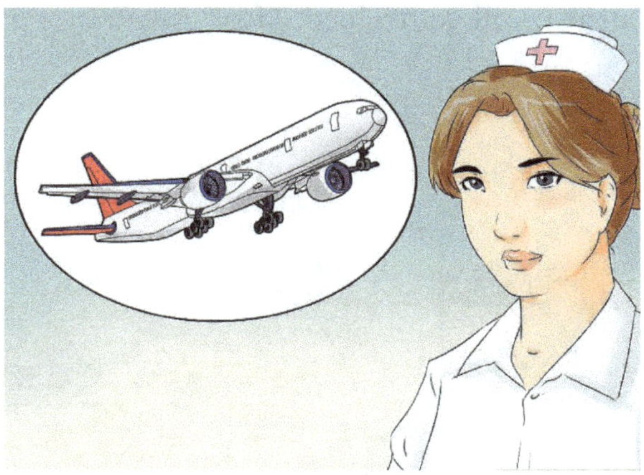

6. Consider your ideal work environment. Since nurses are needed everywhere and at all times, you can imagine the plethora of forms they take. They work in hospitals, of course, but they also work in private homes, in clinics, in doctor's offices, in nursing homes, etc.

- There's also the option of being a traveling nurse.
- Many places have nurses working third shift, on-call, or on standby. Your ideal environment may also allow you to choose between eight-, ten-, or twelve-hour shifts. Floating between different departments may also be an option.

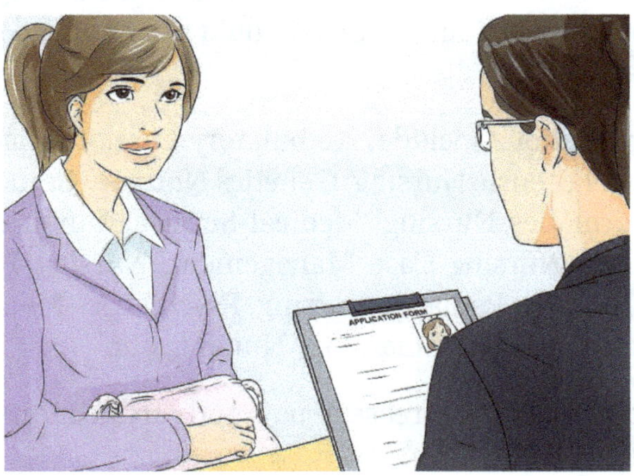

7. Apply for jobs. If you've been working at or through a hospital, that's your first go-to. If not, apply anywhere and everywhere you can. Unfortunately with the recent economic slump, it's getting harder and harder to find jobs, nursing jobs included.

- However, some places do prefer new grads (they cost less money), and the need for nurses is still booming.
- Practice interview questions often and be prepared for anything. Ask about your potential employer's turnover rate as well. If its 20% or higher, it may not be the place for you to start.
- Ask to shadow a day or two before you decide you want to work there. The attitudes of your fellow coworkers may have an impact on your decision.
- Ask about guidance. Expect that you will have training with a preceptor. It depends what unit you work on, but you will get trained. Most orientation programs last between 6-12 weeks.

Part 3

Advancing your Career

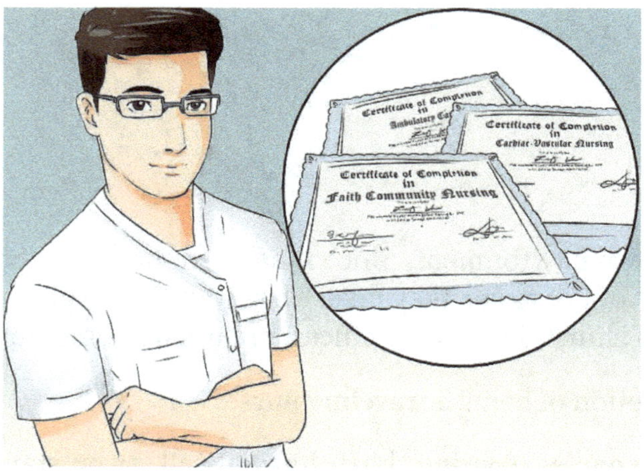

1. Get specialized. After X number of hours in your department, there's probably some certification you'll be able to get. Achieving a certificate makes you look like an expert in your field and may open doors for more opportunities. Your hospital should offer you a course, seminar, or training class to certify you in this area.

- Some available certifications include: Ambulatory Care, Cardiac-Vascular Nursing, Faith Community Nursing, Forensic Nursing, Genetics Nursing, Gerontological Nursing, Hemostasis Nursing, Informatics Nursing, Medical-Surgical Nursing, Nurse Executive, Nurse Executive - Advanced, Nursing Case Management, Nursing Professional Development, Pain Management Nursing, Pediatric Nursing, Psychiatric–Mental Health Nursing, Public Health Nursing - Advanced, Rheumatology Nursing, etc.
- With that should come a slight increase in pay, and certifications look great on a resume. If the opportunity comes, take it!
- You need so many hours on the floor of that department before you're even eligible for these certifications. Think of it more as a badge of honor instead of as a specialization or certification.

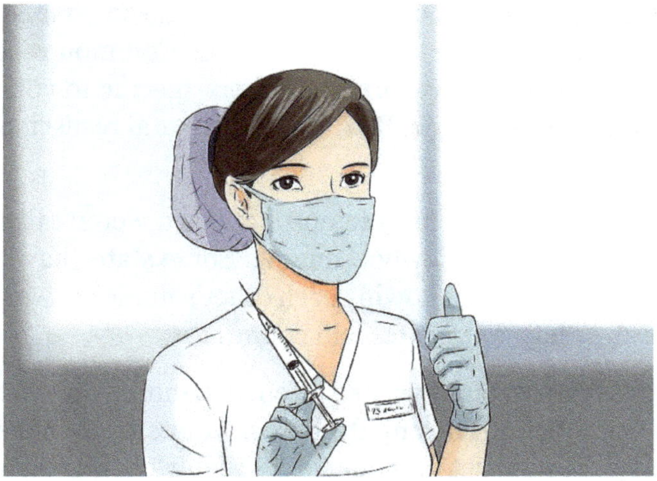

2. Be mentally ready. Nurses have to face many difficult situations. Whether it's a particularly nasty infection, vomit and excrement all over you, or a very sick baby, the job is hard. It is not for the mentally (nor physically) unfit.

- At one point or another, you may feel guilt for something that happened to someone, whether it was out of your control or not. This profession is not something that is always light on the spirit. If you have yet to pursue this as your career, think about this before you make the leap.
- Many institutions have groups for when incidents happen on units. These groups help debrief situations and are supportive emotionally to the staff.
- The schedule of a nurse can be pretty intense. You could work three twelve-hour shifts in a row before getting four days off. If you're working overtime, it could be more. It could also mean night shifts. You may even be on-call on your days off as well. Sleep may not be your constant companion. Stay aware of your schedule and avoid any states of fatigue.

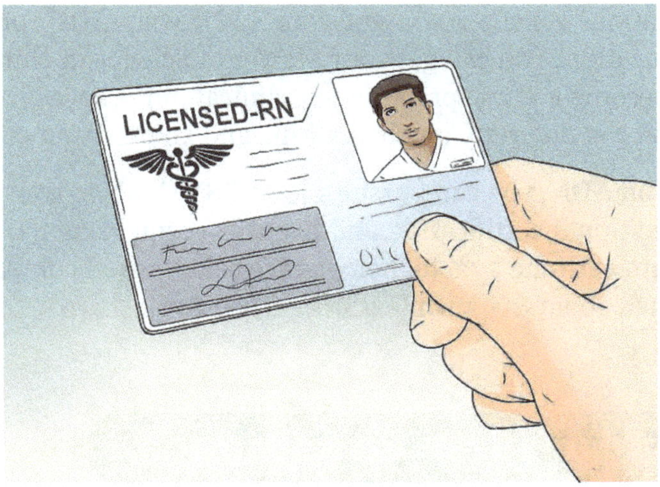

3. Maintain your licensure and credibility. Eligibility requirements for having a license vary by state or area, so maintaining yours depends on where you live. However, your employer will probably routinely have you in workshops, seminars, and certification classes to keep you up to date.

- It is still your professional responsibility to be up to date on your current certifications. Every department will have requirements for your job. Common requirements are basic life support, advanced cardiac life support, and others specific to your department of choice. For labor and delivery, for example, BLS, ACLS, neonatal resuscitation, and fetal monitoring are often required.
- It used to be that if you were licensed in one state, you weren't licensed in another. While that's still technically true, it's slowly changing. Some states have entered into the Nurse Licensure Compact Agreement, allowing each other's nurses to work within their boundaries. Currently it's at twenty-four states and counting.
- You'll need to retake your exams every so often, depending on where you live and whether or not you've been practicing. Look up the laws in your area to make sure your license stays active. By searching the internet for your state's requirement, you will find specific website for your state's board of nursing.
- Unless you lapse in renewal, you will never have to retake the NCLEX.

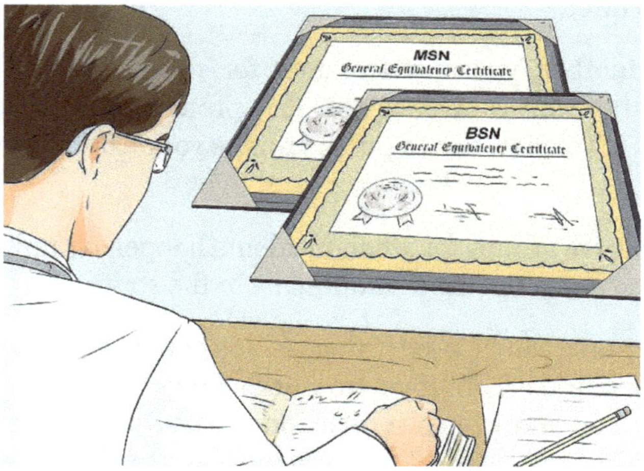

4. Pursue further education. Whether you got your LPN, your ADN, or your BSN, there's always room for more education. You can get your Master of Science in Nursing in only one or two years, allowing you to become a nurse practitioner, clinical nurse specialist, nurse anesthetist, or nurse-midwife. Then you can do pretty much anything and go pretty much anywhere.

- If you only have an ADN, you can pursue a joint BSN/MSN in two-to-three years. You will have to meet additional certification and licensure requirements. However, it's certainly worth looking into with the 27% higher average salary when compared to regular RNs. In 2011, ADNs earned about $64k while BSNs earned $76k.

How to become a Nurse Practitioner

Nurse Practitioners are one of several types of advanced practice nurses who are important partners in the healthcare industry. They blend their clinical expertise in diagnostics and treatment with an emphasis on disease prevention and health management. Often a Nurse Practitioner works alongside a general, family or specialized practice physician to set up and analyze health screenings, diagnose illnesses, and prescribe medications. The Nurse Practitioner also grants doctor referrals and arranges for preventative health as well as manages follow-up appointments. Becoming a Nurse Practitioner requires education and licensing as a Registered Nurse, graduate education and certification.

Part 1

Becoming a Registered Nurse

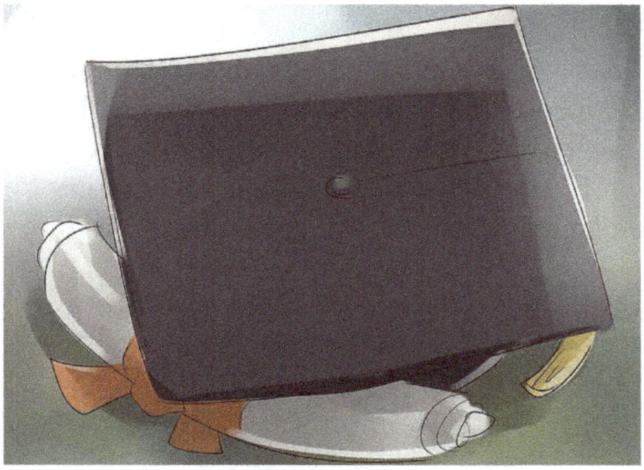

1. Get a high school diploma. Admission into a school of nursing requires a high school diploma or, alternately, passing the General Education Development (GED) test. If you want to be a nurse, pay attention courses like biology, physiology, and chemistry throughout high school. This knowledge will be very important in gaining qualification as a Registered Nurse (RN) and then a Nurse Practitioner (NP).

- The foundation of nursing is science. If you don't like science but find yourself interested in nursing throughout high school, speak with your school counselor about arranging a day or two to shadow a nurse.

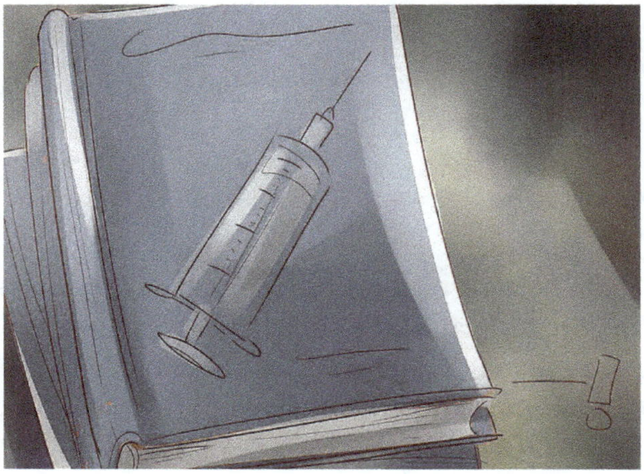

2. Undertake post-secondary education in nursing. There are three ways to become a registered nurse. In all cases, coursework includes physiology, biology, chemistry, nutrition, and anatomy.

- *Bachelor's degree in nursing (BSN).* This level of education is awarded by a college or university and usually takes four years to complete. Class offerings more diverse than other settings and include community health, pharmacology, health assessment, microbiology, human development and clinical practice. A BSN qualifies you for a higher pay grade and a wider variety of certifications and promotions on the job.
- *Associate's degree in nursing (ADN).* This is the most common way to obtain a registered nursing license and involves a two-year program at a community or junior college. Many students transition to BSN programs after having completed an ASN and holding an entry-level nursing position.
- *Diploma from an accredited nursing program.* You can also be eligible for licensure by completing a vocational nursing program. These accredited programs are often associated with a hospital and vary in length, though they are typically up to three years long. This education path is on the decline since the National Advisory Council on Nursing Education and Practice recommends that at least 66% of the workforce hold a BSN in nursing or higher.

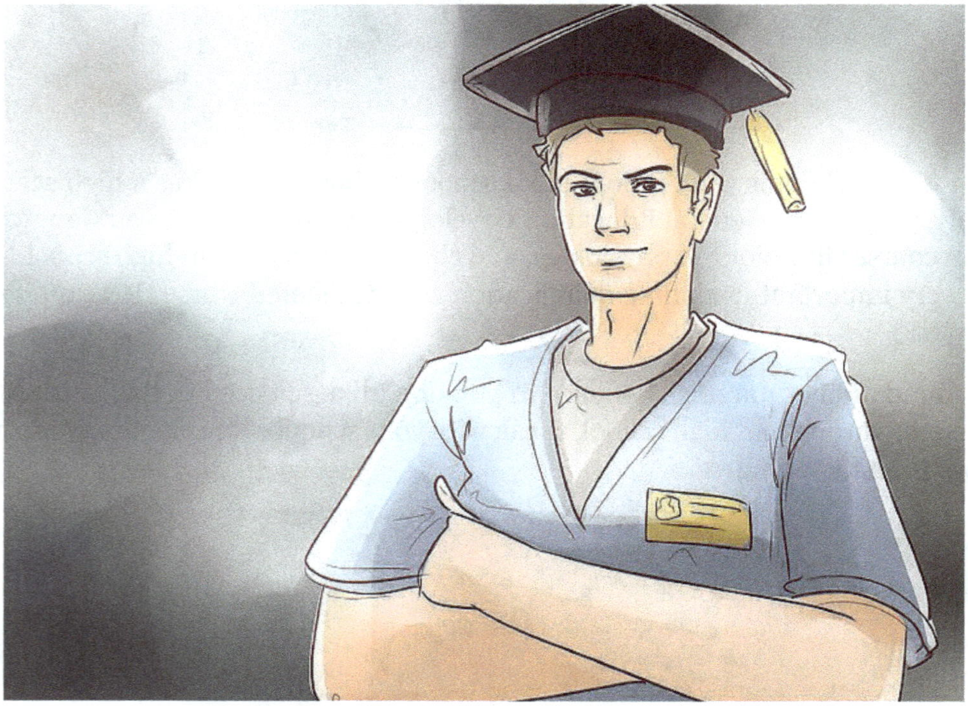

3. Note that you need a BSN to become a Nurse Practitioner. It is necessary to first become a Registered Nurse with a BSN before you can start a Master's of Science in Nursing (MSN) to become a nurse practitioner. With a diploma or ADN, nurses will be able to move on to their bachelor's degree through accelerated programs and potentially with the assistance of their employers via a tuition reimbursement program.

- You may also wish to earn a more advanced degree called Doctorate of Nursing Practice instead of the MSN.

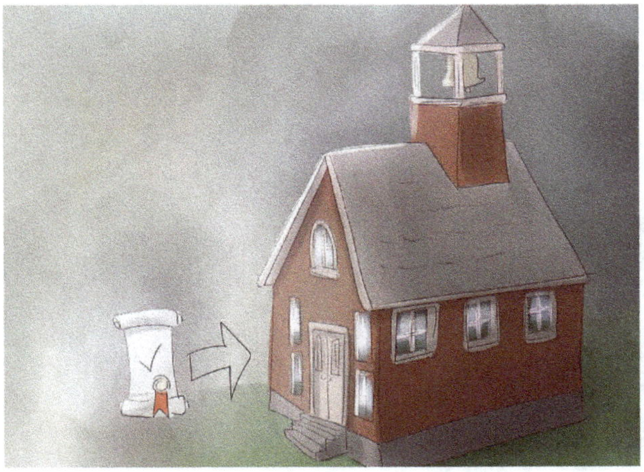

4. Make sure your school is accredited. The national accreditation agency for nursing schools is the Commission on Collegiate Nursing Education. This agency ensures the quality and integrity of bachelor, graduate, and residency programs in nursing. Accreditation is voluntary but ensures that colleges and schools providing nursing education are operating at the same professional level and educating future nurses in a manner which ensures that they can provide effective and standardized care.

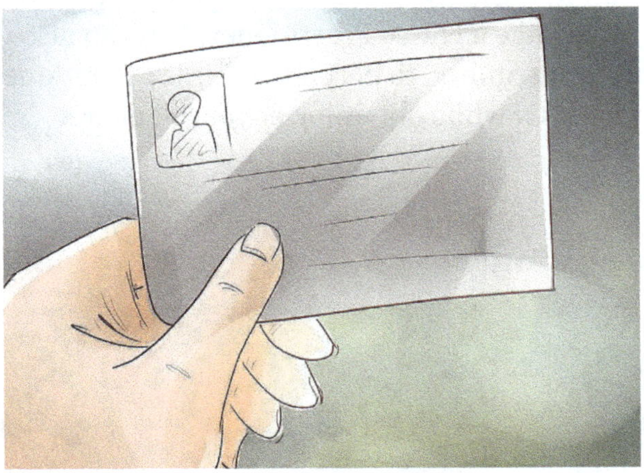

5. Get licensed. Registered Nurses in the United States must have a nursing license. Take the National Council Licensure Examination - Registered Nurse (NCLEX-RN) once you have graduated from your accredited program. This examination is the nationally recognized licensing exam for registered nurses. Prepare for the international equivalent, such as CGFNS International, if you plan to work overseas or if you are an international student planning to work in the United States.

- Prerequisites to and fees for the exam may differ between states. Check with the requirements for your state, or for the state you plan on practicing in.
- Be aware as well that each state has their own scope of practice for nursing. It is important to know scope of practice so you know what you can or can not do as a nurse in your state.
- Most states have reciprocal agreements, meaning that if you pass your exam in one state, you'll be able to apply for and receive a license in any other state without retaking the test as long as your license if free from any encumbrances (such as a felony conviction).

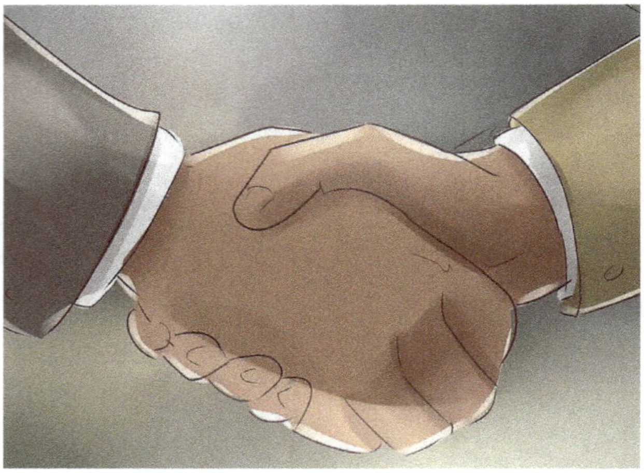

6. Find a job as an RN. Build some experience on the road to becoming a nurse practitioner by seeking entry-level work in a clinic or a hospital setting to get registered nursing experience. There are more than 2 million nurses in the United States, making the profession the largest in the healthcare field. There are a variety of settings in which a nurse can work, including hospitals, physician's offices, elderly care homes, prisons, college campuses and schools.

- Entry-level work as an RN usually serves as a stepping-stone to a higher-level career as an advanced practice nurse, like a Nurse Practitioner. You can also work as an RN as you pursue the further education required to become a Nurse Practitioner. There is great flexibility in being able to work as RN while obtaining advanced degree.

Part 2

Becoming a Nurse Practitioner

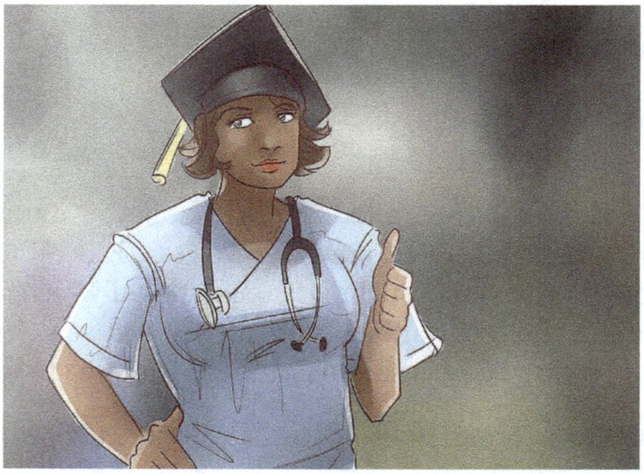

1. Get graduate education in nursing. Most Nurse Practitioners have obtained a Master's Degree of Science in Nursing (MSN). Master's programs are often designed around the needs of a working professional and frequently offer night and weekend classes. A MSN may take between two and seven years to complete, depending upon if the applicant is pursuing the degree full-time or part-time. Make sure to choose a graduate program that has been accredited by either the Commission on Collegiate Nursing Education (CCNE) or the National League for Nursing Accrediting Commission (NLNAC).

- To be admitted to this graduate program, you will be required to have a Registered Nurse's license, a bachelor's degree, and a minimum GPA in the bachelor's degree as determined by the prospective school. Applications often require a statement of purpose, personal history or professional history. Applications may also require an interview.
- A MSN degree, particularly one with a Nurse Practitioner concentration, prepares students for careers beyond entry-level and allows them to choose a specialty such as pediatrics, women's health, family care or geriatrics, among other fields.
- Be aware that there is a growing movement to require all Nurse Practitioners to have a Doctor of Nursing Practice (D.N.P.) degree, or basically a doctoral degree. This degree requires three to four years of further education after a bachelor's degree in nursing.

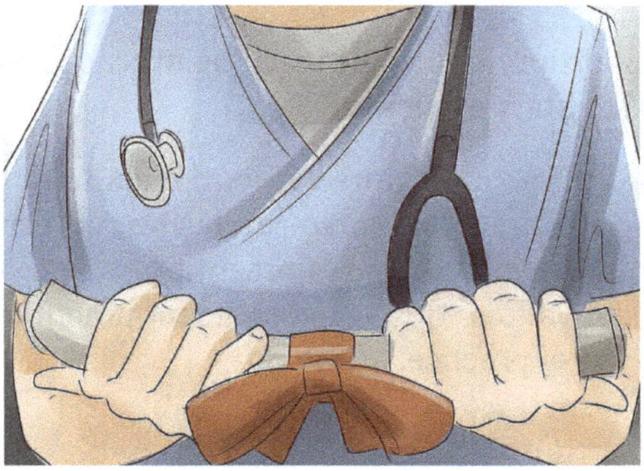

2. Get certified to work as a nurse practitioner. After earning a MSN, take the certification examination administered by the American Nurses Credentialing Center (ANCC) or the American Academy of Nurse Practitioners (AANP).

- Specialties that require certification in addition to licensing include pediatrics, family health, mental health, acute care, diabetes management and school nursing.
- Once certified, Nurse Practitioners can also choose to take a specialty examination that certifies they have additional knowledge and ability to practice. These specialty certifications include pain management, rehabilitation, cardiac rehabilitation, college health nursing, forensic nursing, diabetes management, nurse executive, pediatrics, and school nursing.

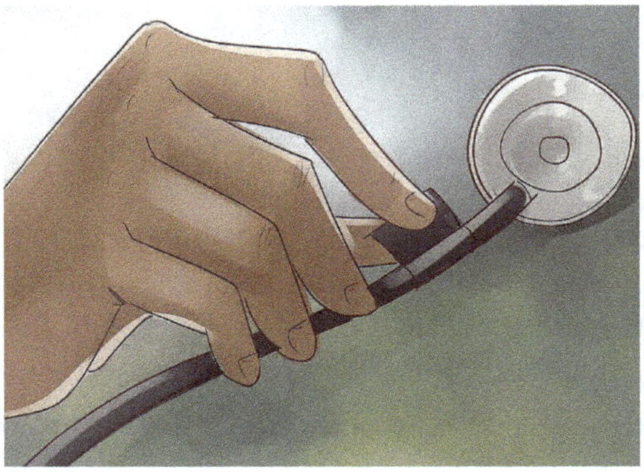

3. Get a job as a Nurse Practitioner. Nurse practitioners are valued members of the healthcare

team, providing cost effective care in the diagnosis, treatment and management of many acute and chronic illnesses. This variety in practice and ability to specialize offers practitioners many options in the work place. Jobs are available in hospitals, private practices, nursing homes, clinics, health departments, urgent care settings, healthcare technology companies, and Health Maintenance Organizations (HMOs), among many other institutions. Different ways of getting a job include consulting online job websites, contacting headhunters in nursing, consulting local hospital job postings, and networking with physicians, nursing managers and community clinics, among other methods.

- The average salary of a NP is is $90,583 and the job outlook for NPs is considered excellent at present. This is because the numbers of primary care physicians is decreasing as the demand for healthcare services is rising thanks to the aging baby boomer generation.
- Other professional opportunities include teaching in schools and universities and working for governmental and military agencies.
- Note as well that about 15% of all Nurse Practitioners have their own private practices. There are also a growing number of nurse-run healthcare centers in the United States in which all healthcare is provided by nurse practitioners and other professionals. Keep in mind that not every state allows this — independent practitioners can only do this if it is within their state's scope of practice.

Part 3

Understanding Nursing

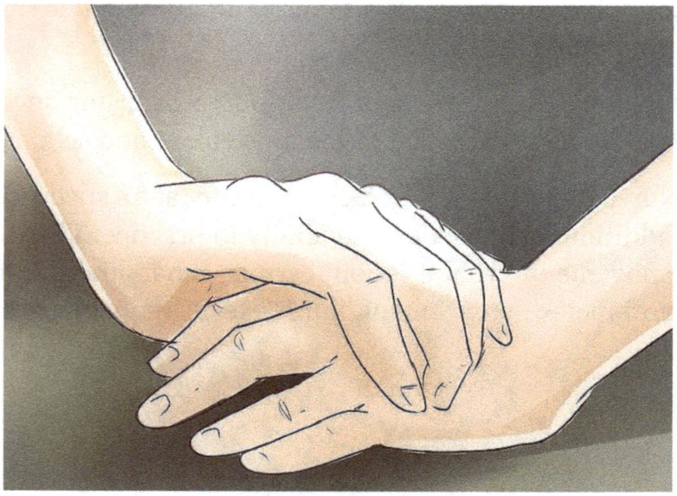

1. Understand the nursing profession in general. According to the American Nurses Association, nursing today is designed for the protection, promotion and optimization of health and the prevention of illness and injury. Nurses are advocates in the care of individuals, families and communities. The standardized education of today's nurses, in contrast to the past, reflects the high expectations communities and physicians have on the men and women who fill these roles.

- The nursing profession is not just for women; there are over a hundred thousand registered male nurses working in the US.

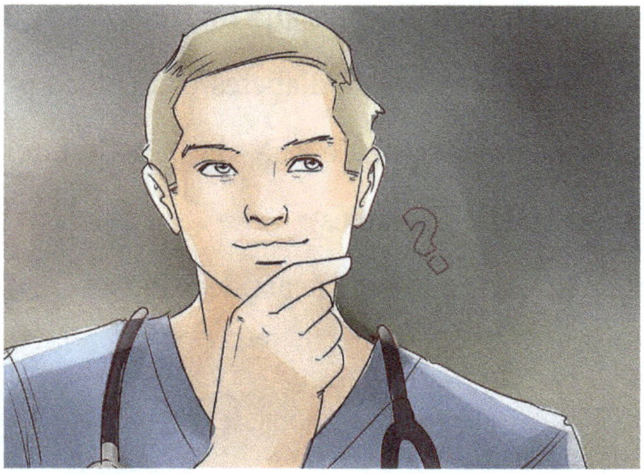

2. Determine if the general responsibilities of nursing interest you. The foundation of all nursing practice is based in human anatomy and physiology. The chief mission of the nursing field is to protect, promote and optimize health. Key responsibilities for nurses include:

- Performing physical examinations and taking medical and family histories.
- Providing counseling and education about health promotion and injury protection.
- Administering medication and providing wound care.
- Coordinating care and collaborating with other professionals including doctors, therapists and dietitians.
- Directing and supervising care and providing education to patients and family, which enable patients to be discharged sooner.

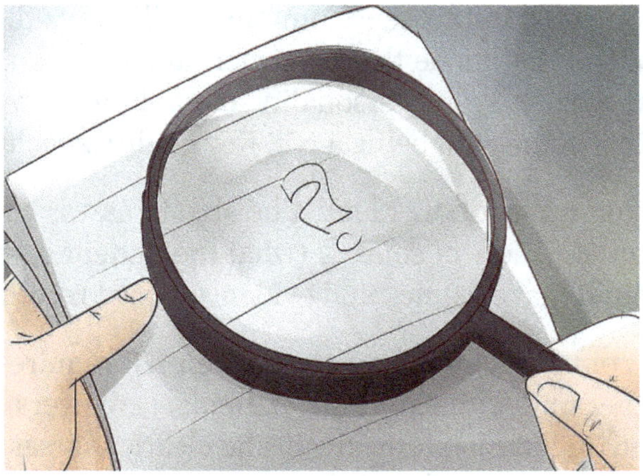

3. Consider the specific job of a Nurse Practitioner. Nurse Practitioners are advanced practice nurses who have obtained graduate education which in turn increases their professional responsibilities. Nurse practitioners can serve in multiple roles, including providing direct care to patients, research in healthcare, consulting and education. Some of their duties can include:

- Undertaking physical examinations of patients
- Providing immunizations

- Diagnosing and treating common illnesses and injuries
- Managing chronic health problems (e.g., diabetes, high blood pressure, etc.)
- Ordering and interpret diagnostic tests (e.g., X-rays, EKGs, etc.)
- Prescribing medications and/or therapies
- Counseling patients on lifestyle and healthcare decisions

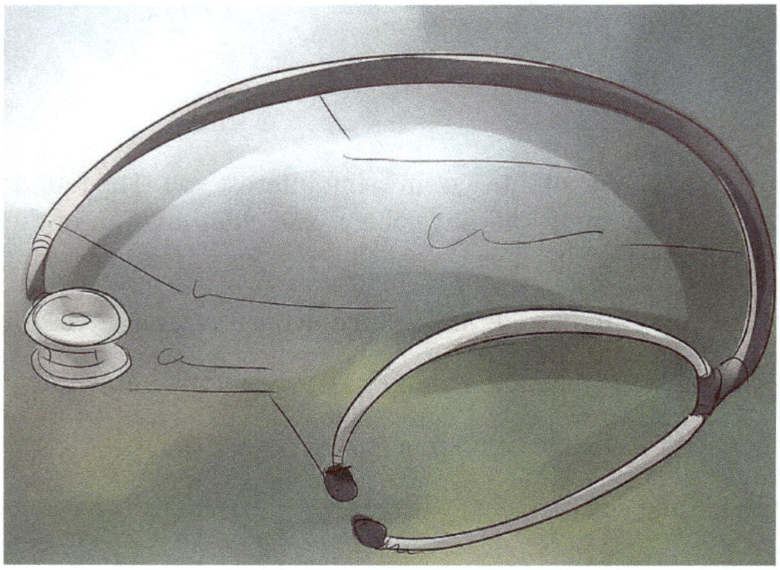

4. Know the skills and qualities required of Nurse Practitioners. Beyond having a breadth of knowledge in medicine (and being someone who does not get squeamish easily!), a Nurse Practitioner must also be skilled in other areas. In this sense, nursing is like any other profession in that there are specific individual qualities that make the job easier and a more natural fit for some people. It's important to determine whether your personality and abilities can accommodate the various responsibilities and tasks that come with being a NP. Key qualities include:

- *Critical thinking*: Nurse Practitioners must be able to assess changes in the health status of their patients from a variety of sources (what the patient says, diagnostic tests, clinical examinations, etc.) and make a quick and evidence-based recommendations.
- *Interpersonal and communication skills*: Being an NP requires working with people everyday—doctors, other nurses, technicians, patients, caregivers, and others. To communicate information and do their jobs effectively and clearly, nurses need strong interpersonal skills, patience, and the ability to break down complex information into something that is accessible for ordinary people (i.e., non-specialists).
- *Compassion*: Caring and empathy are valuable when taking care of individuals who are in sick or injured. Remember that patients may be scared or in pain and need to be comforted, reassured, and motivated to fight through their illnesses.
- *Detail-oriented and organized*: NPs often work with multiple patients and healthcare professional at a time and so they need to be able to keep track of what has been done and what

needs to be done. In addition, attention to detail is key; one small mistake can have a big impact on a patient's condition and life.

- *Effective coping with stress*: Nurse Practitioners should be able to cope with stress in effective and healthy ways because they often work in urgent, emergency and/or other sensitive situations and face continual workplace pressures and stressors.

How to become a Registered Nurse

Registered nurses provide medical care, education, and emotional support to patients. Employment for nurses is expected to increase by 19% from 2010 to 2022, which is a faster growth rate than most other occupations. This is a rewarding field that will make a real difference in your community and has a wide array of options for advancement.

Part 1

Understanding Nursing

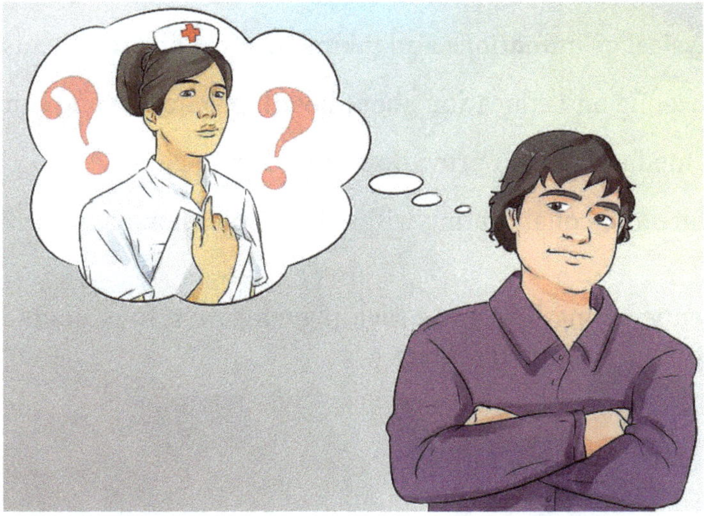

1. Understand the profession. According to the American Nurses Association, nursing today is designed for the protection, promotion and optimization of health and the prevention of illness and injury. Nurses are advocates in the care of individuals, families and communities. The standardized education of today's registered nurses, in contrast to the past, reflects the high expectations communities and physicians have on the men and women who fill these roles. In recent years, the employment of nurses has grown and will continue to grow in part because of the aging of the baby boomer population and the associated growing rate of chronic conditions like diabetes.

- The nursing profession is not just for women; there are over a hundred thousand registered male nurses working in the US.
- People with chronic diseases, such as heart and lung disease, are living longer than ever, which equates to sicker patients living longer and requiring skilled medical services.

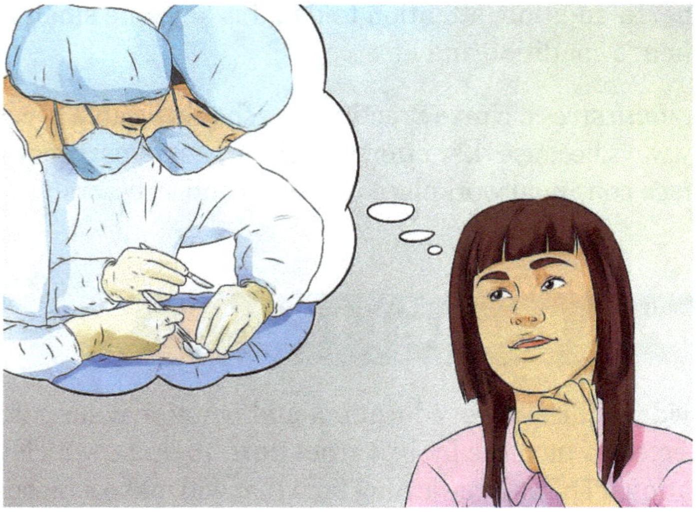

2. Determine if the roles and responsibilities of nursing interest you. The foundation of all nursing practice is based in human anatomy and physiology. The chief mission of the nursing field is to protect, promote and optimize health. Key responsibilities for nurses include (but are not limited to):

- Triaging and assessing injury levels in emergency situations.
- Performing physical examinations and taking medical and family histories.
- Providing counseling and education about health promotion and injury protection.
- Administering medication and providing wound care.
- Coordinating care and collaborating with other professionals including doctors, therapists and dietitians.
- Directing and supervising care and providing education to patients and family, which enables patients to be discharged sooner.

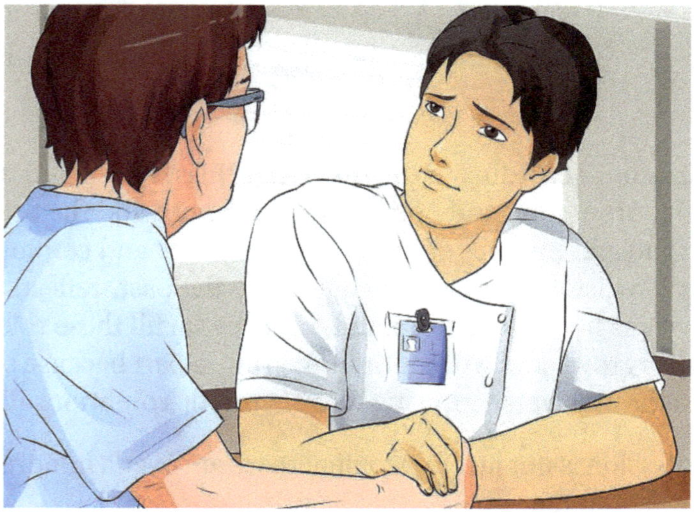

3. Know the skills and qualities involved in nursing. Beyond having a breadth of knowledge in medicine (and being someone who does not get squeamish easily!), a nurse must also be skilled in

other areas. In this sense, nursing is like any other profession in that there are specific individual qualities that make the job easier and a more natural fit for some people. It's important to determine whether your personality and abilities can accommodate the various responsibilities and tasks that come with being a nurse. Key qualities include:

- *Interpersonal and communication skills*: Being a nurse requires working with people every day—doctors, other nurses, technicians, patients, caregivers, and others. To communicate information clearly and do their jobs effectively, nurses need strong interpersonal skills, patience, and the ability to break down complex information into something that is accessible for ordinary people (i.e., non-specialists).
- *Compassion*: Caring and empathy are valuable when taking care of individuals who are sick or injured. Remember that patients may be scared or in pain and need to be comforted, reassured, and motivated to fight through their illnesses.
- *Critical thinking*: Registered nurses must be able to assess changes in the health status of their patients and make a quick referrals.
- *Detail-oriented and organized*: Nurses often work with multiple patients and healthcare professional at a time and so they need to be able to keep track of what has been done and what needs to be done. In addition, attention to detail is key; medication needs to be given on time and emergency protocols must be followed to the letter.
- *Stamina*: Nurses are often required to perform physical tasks, such as lifting patients, and also work long shifts of between eight and 12 hours, which may include night shifts.

Part 2

Obtaining the Correct Education and Credentials

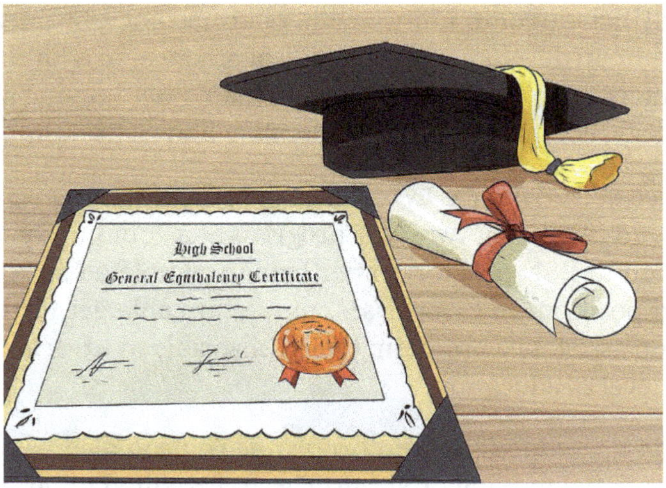

1. Get a high school diploma. Admission into a school of nursing requires a high school diploma or, alternately, passing the General Education Development (GED) test. If you want to be a nurse, pay attention to your performance, skill, and interest in courses like biology, physiology, and chemistry throughout high school. The knowledge from these courses will be important in your post-secondary education.

- A good foundational knowledge and understanding of how the human body works is necessary in the field of nursing and begins already in high school.
- Don't get discouraged if these subjects don't come easily to you. Consider hiring a private tutor to help you in your math and science courses in order to improve and develop effective study and learning strategies.

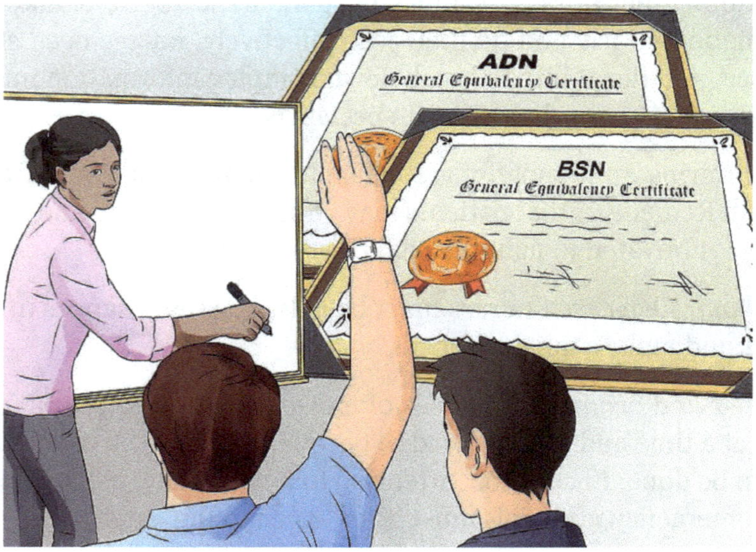

2. Undertake post-secondary education in nursing. There are three ways to become a registered nurse. Whatever path you choose, the coursework involved will include physiology, biology, chemistry, nutrition, and anatomy.

- *Bachelor's degree in nursing (BSN).* This level of education is like a bachelor's program in all other fields. It is awarded by a college or university and usually takes four years to complete. Classes will include community health, pharmacology, health assessment, microbiology, chemistry, human development and clinical practice. In addition, bachelor's programs usually include more training in social sciences than other nursing programs. You may take courses in sociology, communications, leadership, and critical thinking.
- *Associate's degree in nursing (ADN).* This is the most common way to obtain a registered nursing license and involves a two-year program at a community or junior college. Many students transition to BSN programs after having completed an ADN and holding an entry-level nursing position. In these cases, nurses are able get further education using an employer's tuition assistance program; they're also able to work and earn an income while getting the next level of education.
- *Diploma from an accredited nursing program.* You can also be eligible for licensure by completing a vocational nursing program. These accredited programs are often associated with a hospital and vary in length, though they are typically up to three years long. In this program, classroom learning, clinical practice, and on-the-job training are combined. This education path is on the decline since hospitals have placed a limit on the number of diploma graduates they can hire due to recommendations by the National Advisory Council on Nursing Education.

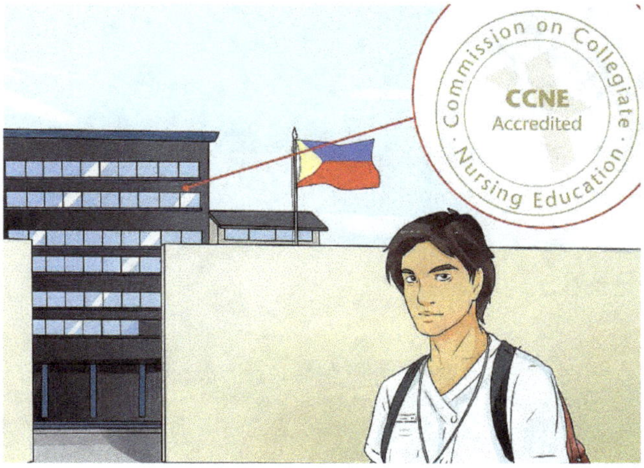

3. Make sure your school is accredited. The national accreditation agency for nursing schools is the Commission on Collegiate Nursing Education. This agency ensures the quality and integrity of bachelor, graduate, and residency programs in nursing. Accreditation is voluntary but ensures that colleges and schools providing nursing education are operating at the same professional level and educating future nurses in a manner which ensures that they can provide effective and standardized care.

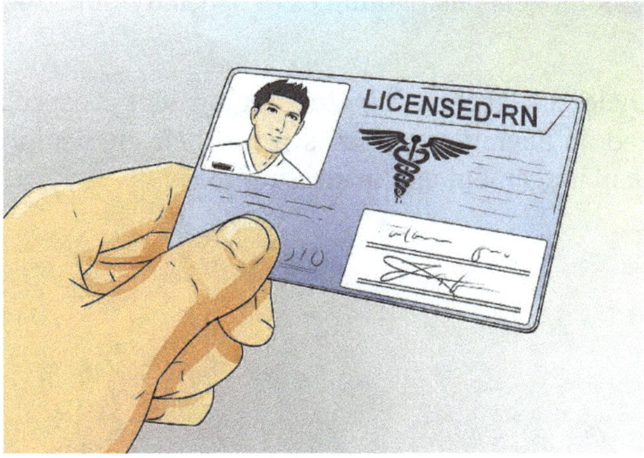

4. Get licensed. Registered nurses must have a nursing license. Take the National Council Licensure Examination — Registered Nurse (NCLEX-RN) once you have graduated from your accredited program and thus have completed the appropriate education requirements. This test is the nationally recognized licensing exam for registered nurses.

- Prerequisites to and fees for the exam may differ between states. Check with the requirements for your state, or for the state you plan on practicing in.
- Note the following requirements in order to sit the licensure examination:
  - Application for the examination must include a U.S. social security number.
  - Individuals must be accompanied by a recent passport-style photograph.
  - Application must identify the school from which the applicant graduated. Transcripts must be forwarded to prove that the individual met all educational requirements.

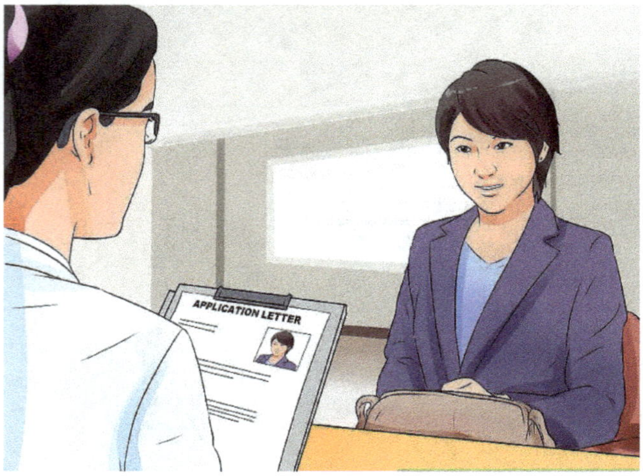

5. Find a job as a nurse. There are more than two million nurses in the United States, making the position the largest in the healthcare field. There are a variety of settings in which a nurse can work, including hospitals, physician's offices, elderly care homes, prisons, college campuses and schools.

- Newly certified nurses should consider working in a specialty unit, as the patients in these facilities are more homogeneous. Examples of specialty units include orthopedic and pediatrics units.
- Nurses with a bachelor's degree have better employment prospects than those who do not; they are recognized as having capabilities from their curriculum that prepare them for management, case management and leadership roles.

Part 3

Growing in the Field

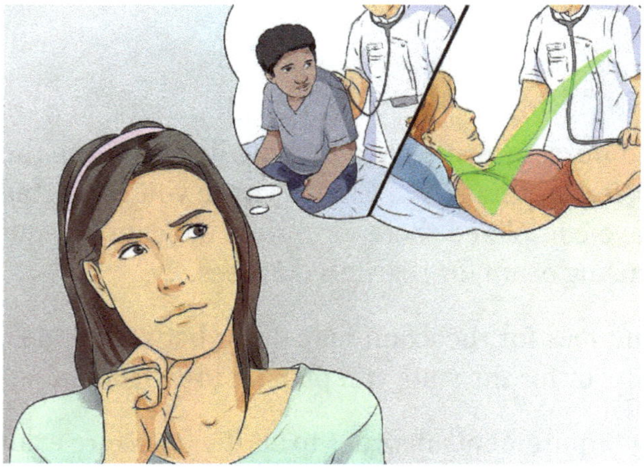

1. Decide what specialty interests you. There are a variety of fields for nurses to practice, including pediatrics, adults, OB/GYN, geriatrics, community health, occupational health, rehabilitation, surgery, neonatal, intensive care, and emergency. You will likely have already started thinking about this during your RN educational training. Each RN program gives their nursing students clinical rotations through which they gain experience in these various areas of the hospital and community.

- Nursing students may have a full semester in a particular clinical rotation, such as pediatrics, adult or community health. They will also experience several hours in an intensive care unit, emergency room and neonatal unit. Not all schools will give nurses rotations through a physical rehabilitation unit for patients following strokes or spinal cord injuries. Most schools will expect that nurses get experience with geriatric care while caring for adults.
- Once you know what field of nursing you'd like to work in, you can apply for jobs in that field.

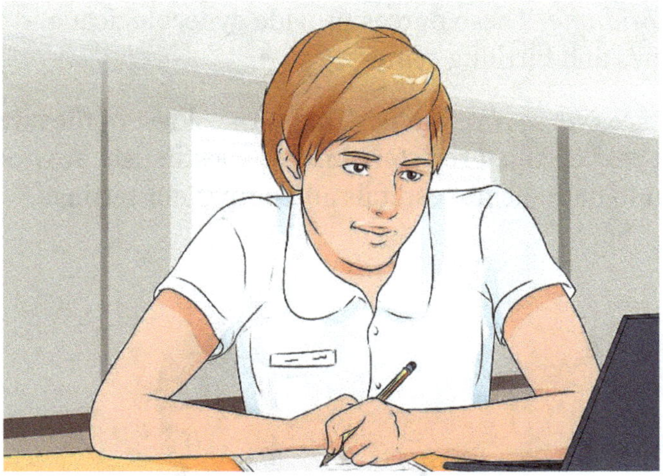

2. Stay up-to-date with your practice. Even after completing the required education and certification, nurses should continue to read medical journals, be aware of the policies of the healthcare organization they work for, and take additional courses in medicine. Scientific and medical knowledge and technologies are constantly changing and evolving and so staying up-to-date is key to providing effective healthcare.

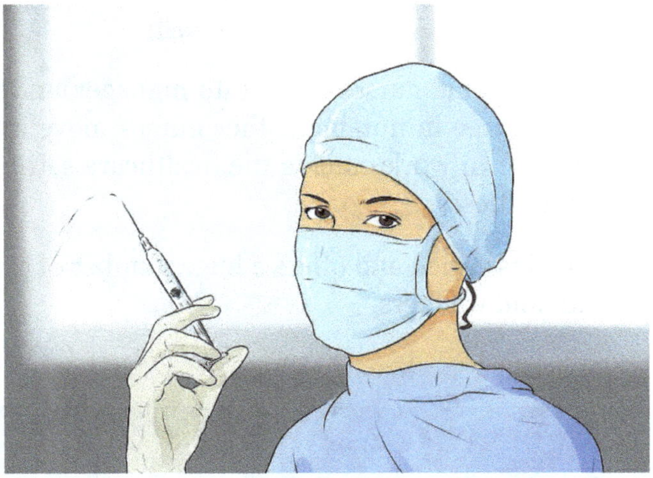

3. Consider becoming an advanced practice registered nurse (APRN). The term advanced practice registered nurse is an umbrella term used for nurses who have achieved at least a master's degree in nursing (MSN). The academic program to become an advanced practice nurse is one to two academic years, depending upon the specialty, school, and your previous work experience. There are four main advanced practice settings in which nurses can practice under this APRN umbrella:

- *Clinical Nurse Specialist.* These nurses typically work in hospitals, clinics and nursing homes. They handle a wide variety of physical and mental health problems and may work within the fields of research, education and administration.
- *Nurse Practitioner.* These advanced practice nurses may work in clinics, and nursing homes, hospitals or private offices. They see a wide range of primary and preventative health patients. In most states, nurse practitioners can prescribe medication, diagnose illness, and treat minor injuries.
- *Certified Nurse Midwife.* These nurses provide gynecological and low risk obstetrics care in hospitals, homes and birthing centers.
- *Certified Registered Nurse Anesthetist.* This is the oldest of the advanced practice nursing specialists. Each year certified registered nurse anesthetists provide more than 65% of the anesthetics given to patients in hospitals and outpatient settings.

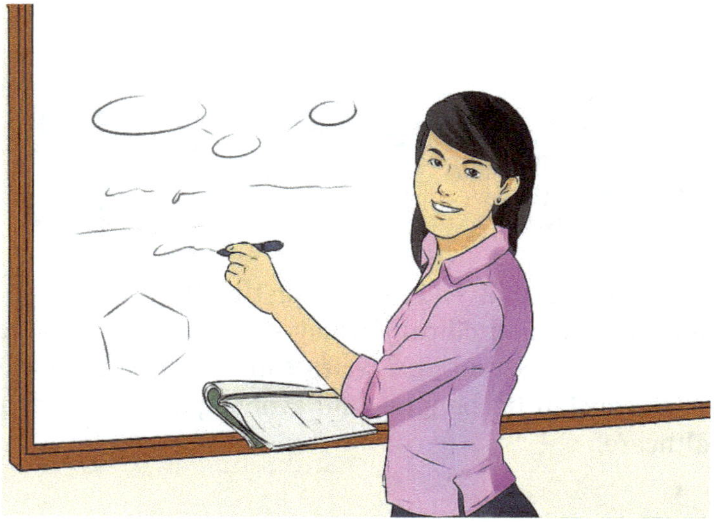

4. Be aware of other career paths. Some nurses move into management positions, which are increasingly requiring a graduate degree in nursing. Other nurses move into the business aspects of healthcare, while still others opt to work outside the healthcare setting directly by becoming instructors in colleges and universities.

- All in all, the nursing field is varied and offers a huge number of opportunities for individuals interested in health and wellness.

How to become a CNA (Certified Nursing Assistant)

CNAs (Certified Nursing Assistants) are professionals who help nurses by performing routine duties at hospitals and other care facilities. CNAs help bathe and clothe patients, check vital signs and other statistics like weight and height, and reposition patients who are unable to move themselves, among other responsibilities. Read the steps below to learn how to become a CNA, and how to be a good CNA when you get a job in the field.

Method 1

Getting the Job

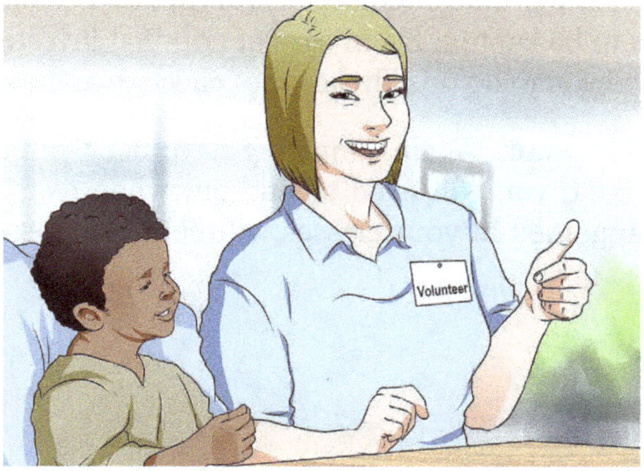

1. Enter a training program. Becoming a CNA requires a high school diploma plus some additional college-level courses, in almost all cases. You can typically sign up for a CNA program through your local community college.

- Prepare for a time commitment. CNA programs vary in length, but average between six weeks and five months of extra school. The special CNA classes you have to take are set up so that you can take them in a specific order.
    - CNA classes are divided between study sessions and hands-on practice sessions.
    - Because CNA programs usually end with a special certificate rather than a degree, electives are not required.
- CNA programs can be competitive. Consider volunteering at a hospital or nursing home to boost your chances of acceptance.
    - Volunteering is also a good way to gauge whether or not you will enjoy being a CNA, as some of the duties you're likely to perform are similar to those a CNA performs.

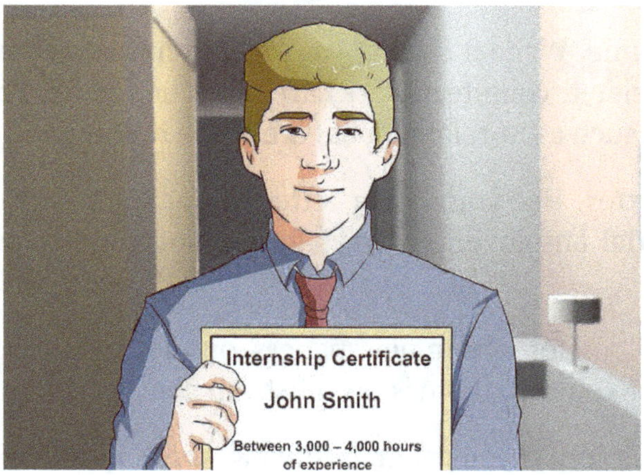

2. Get certified. Usually, an accredited training program will take care of some of the legal details

for you, but because CNAs are health professionals, additional certification and verification is required before you'll be able to work as a CNA.

- File your fingerprints. Most states require health care and education system employees to submit fingerprints to be kept on file in case of criminal investigations. Chances are your CNA program helped you to do this already, but check to make sure.
- Take the certification exam. Again, this may have been integrated into your training program, but if it isn't, you will need to find out when tests are and sign up for one. The knowledge you gained in your classes will help you pass the exam and earn your certificate.

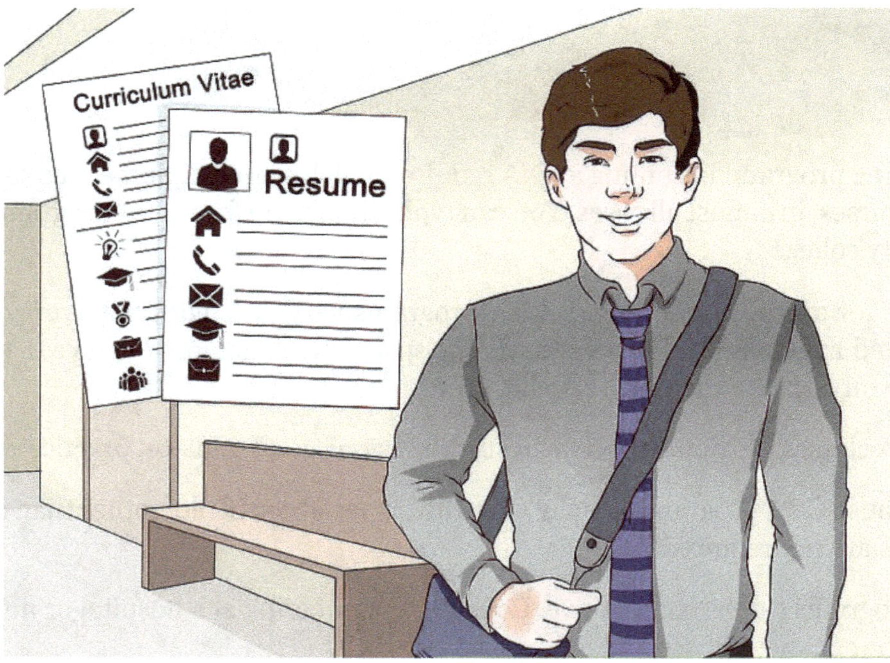

3. Apply for work. Now that you're a fully-certified nursing assistant, it's time to get a job in the field. Prepare a resume and a cover letter, and begin looking for work.

- Organize your resume. Write it so that your most impressive qualifications (such as your certification and related volunteer work) are near the top, and items that have less to do with being a CNA (such as unrelated jobs) are at the bottom.
- Prepare a cover letter. Use your cover letter to put the information on your resume in context for potential employers. Always have a cover letter on hand in case you need one.
- Look everywhere. Look for jobs in newspapers, online, and through word of mouth. Apply in person whenever you can; there is no substitute for a personal appearance.
- Make a good impression. If you get an interview, show up well dressed and on time, speak clearly, make plenty of eye contact, and smile.

Method 2

Being a Great CNA

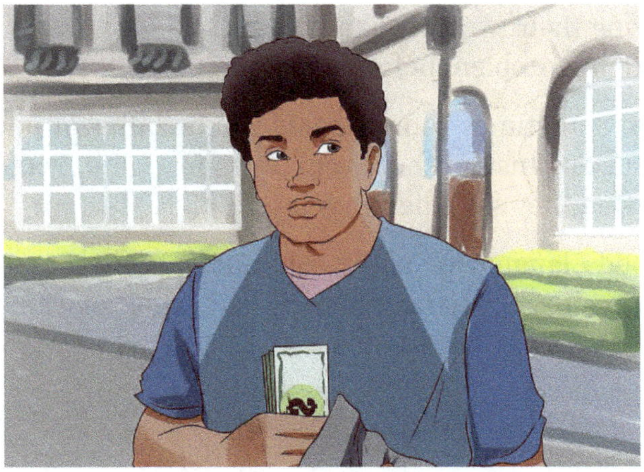

1. Follow the rules. This might sound absurdly simple, but more than one CNA has been let go for not doing things according to code. This includes technical problems, such as forgetting to do something repeatedly, as well as more serious violations like drug theft.

- Don't steal from your workplace. Being a CNA is stressful and can seem thankless at times, but stealing prescription medications for recreational use or illicit sale isn't the right way to ease the pressure. Find other ways to relax and focus yourself instead.
- Do whatever the nurse says. Do it with a smile and without complaint. You'll make a strong good impression on the nurse, who is probably also feeling harried and overworked. If something sounds unsafe, feel free to ask why you have been told to do it; otherwise, just do it.
- Take pride in your work. Even though you're probably a ways down on the healthcare totem pole, you're doing an important and vital job that helps save lives. Treat your job like it matters, because it does. Do everything as well as you possibly can.

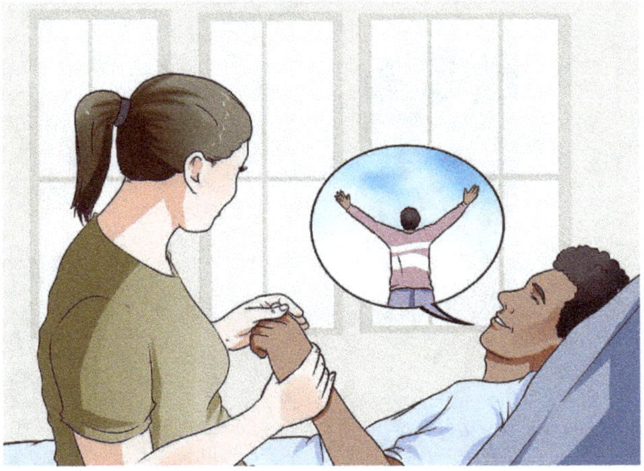

2. Be a good listener. Take the time to talk to patients when you are able. Be gracious and respectful. Remember, the people you're serving don't usually want to be where they are. Having a kind and polite person around who will listen to them makes a powerful positive impact.

- If you have any free time, swing back by your patients and make small talk with them. They'll love you for it.
- Always take patient concerns and questions seriously. If you can answer them, do so; if you're not sure, bring their worries to the nurse. In a busy ward, your attentiveness might help catch a developing problem before it gets serious.
- Develop thick skin. Sometimes your patients will be bitter or miserable and looking for a person to take it out on. Just let them vent and stay polite. People who are scared and in pain rarely mean what they say when they lash out.
- Pay attention to body language. People communicate their emotions through body language. If you stay sensitive to changes in body language, you can better guess how to speak with your patients each time you see them.

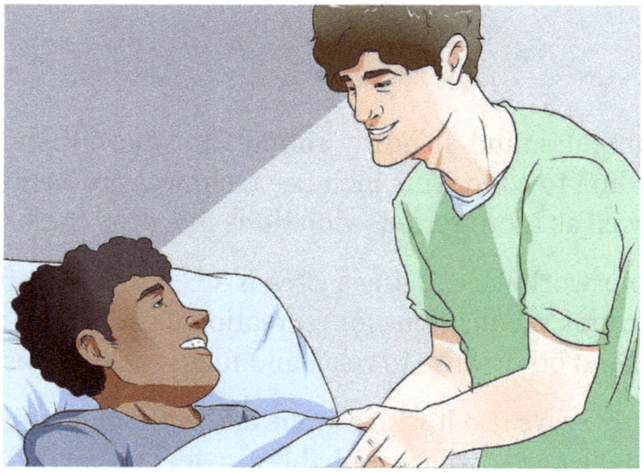

3. Be gentle. Speak clearly but softly, and approach your patients at a calm, measured pace. In nursing homes, where the people you take care of may be suffering from Alzheimer's disease, sudden movements and loud noises can cause severe agitation. Adopt a soft touch and keep things as pleasant as possible for your patients.

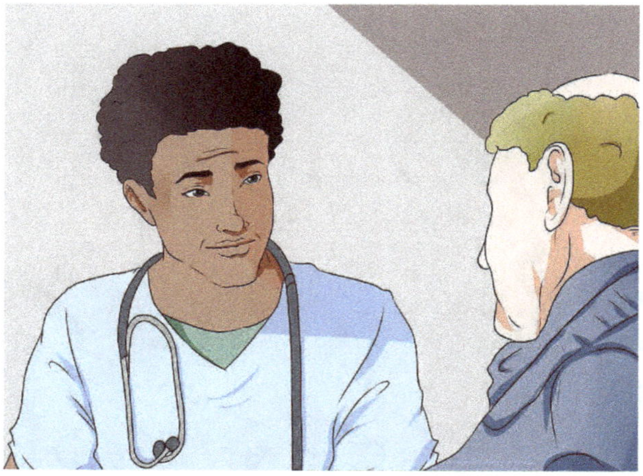

4. Be patient. Having patience is imperative. There may be times when you will have to repeat yourself multiple times when communicating with residents or patients due to an impairment. It is important to allow the resident to communicate at their own speed.

- Be patient with your higher-ups as well. They may snap at you or forget to give you important information. If you remain patient, steady, and calm, they will usually catch themselves and stop treating you poorly.
- Try creative communication methods. When trying to speak with a person suffering from Alzheimer's or another disease or condition that impairs communication, unusual approaches are sometimes required.
  - Try communicating using objects and body language instead of words, or by pointing and nodding at things.
  - Don't simply raise your voice as though the patient can't hear you. It's disrespectful and generally ineffective.

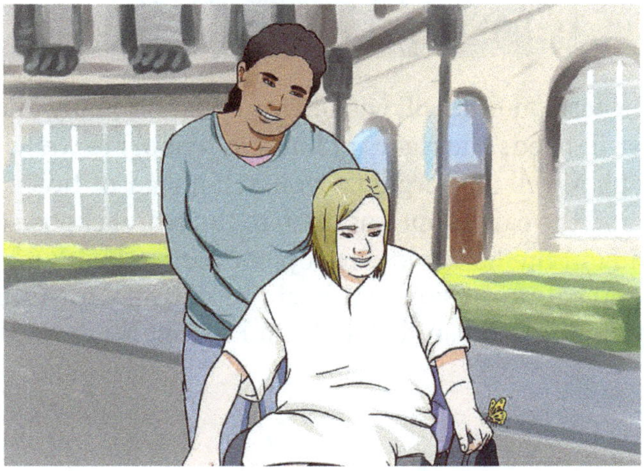

5. Learn to prioritize. There may be moments when several things need to be done at the same time. As in emergency medical treatment, it is important that you learn to triage them by immediate importance. Use your head and learn from experience which tasks are best done before the rest.

- Don't rush your patients. Your time crunch isn't their fault; it's the schedule's. You can politely explain your situation, but don't put pressure on them to do anything faster than usual. It is unacceptable to cause them unnecessary stress or worry.
- Never hesitate to ask for help. You may not always get it, but if you're feeling overwhelmed, it won't hurt to ask. You may find that there is another employee nearby who has a bit of free time and will be glad to split some of your workload with you for a little while.
- Use your time wisely and productively. Downtime is precious, but unless you're on a lunch break, try offering to help out other CNAs instead or perform extra duties. Not only will this ease everyone else's load and make work go more smoothly, it will pay itself back later when you get swamped and other workers remember how you helped them out.

Chapter 2 Preparing for Nursing School

Nursing is a significances expounding professional. To become a professional nurse, an individual needs training in order to acquire a license. Professional nursing is best understood in confluence with the major topics listed in the following chapter.

How to Prepare for Nursing School

Nursing is a wonderful profession that will challenge you emotionally and mentally and help you comfort and care for those in need. The rigors of nursing school are well documented, but you can succeed in school if you plan well and organize yourself ahead of time. Understand the various types of nursing degrees and the career options open to them and choose the one that's the best fit for you. Meet those already in the field and develop connections with fellow students to increase your knowledge of the medical profession and begin to network for future jobs. Once you're in school, key steps like developing good study habits and finding ways to relieve stress will contribute to your success.

Method 1

Deciding on a Degree

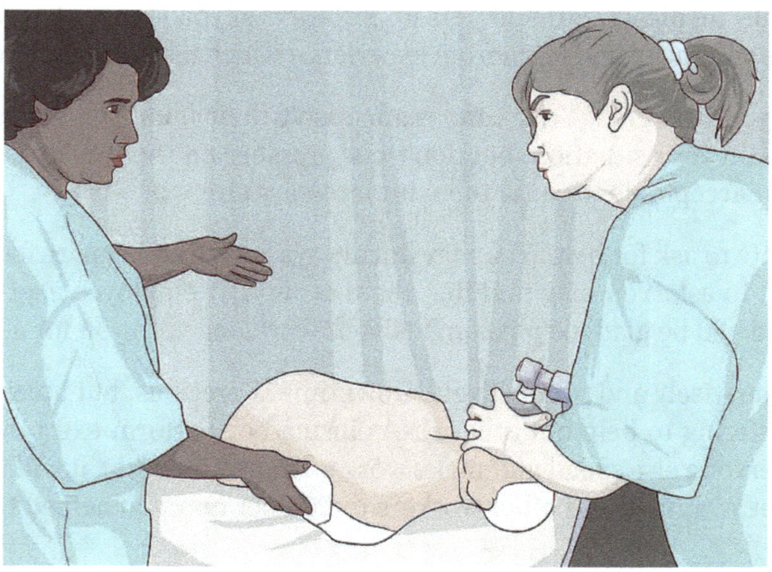

1. Complete a certified nursing assistant (CNA) training program. CNAs work as aides to nurses, completing tasks such as cleaning, filing, or scheduling. You can receive your CNA certificate after approximately 72 hours of training.

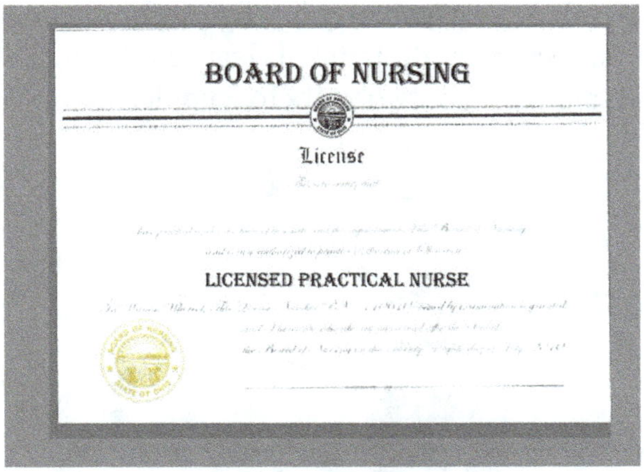

2. Become a licensed practical nurse (LPN). Earning an LPN degree typically takes one year of full-time study or two years if the courses are taken part time. LPNs are considered dependent practitioners, meaning they are always under the direction and supervision of another professional, such as a registered nurse. With this degree, you can administer medications, collect vital signs, and collect specimens from patients.

- In Texas and California, LPNs are referred to as LVNs (licensed vocational nurses).
- Classes in an LPN program are heavily focused on anatomy and physiology, and the majority of the curriculum is clinical practice.
- LPN degrees are offered at a range of settings, such as technical schools, hospitals, community colleges, and privately owned nursing schools.

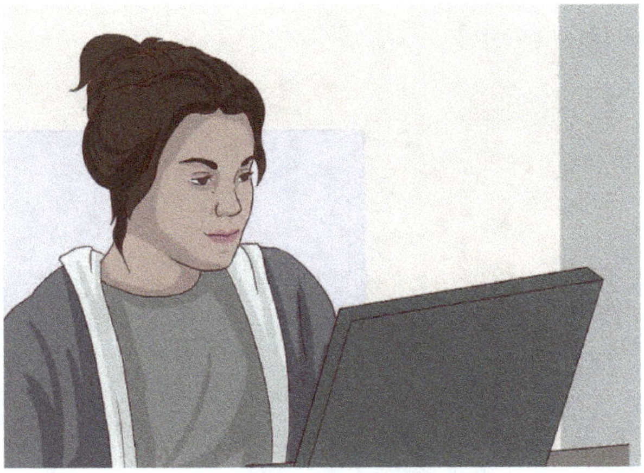

3. Explore how to become a Registered Nurse (RN). RNs can perform a variety of jobs within the healthcare world, including trauma nurses, occupational health nurses, psychiatric nurses, or intensive care nurses. To achieve this certification, you will need to either complete an associate of science in nursing (ASN) or an associate's degree in nursing, which typically takes two years at a community college. Another option is to pursue a bachelor of science in nursing (BSN), which is a four-year degree.

- Attaining an associate's degree in nursing is the quickest way to become a nurse, but BSNs typically hold supervisory positions, so the extra schooling may be of interest to you.

- If you have an associate's degree, you may be eligible for an accelerated RN-to-BSN degree program, in which you receive credit for skills learned through work experience and previous schooling. This typically takes two years to complete.

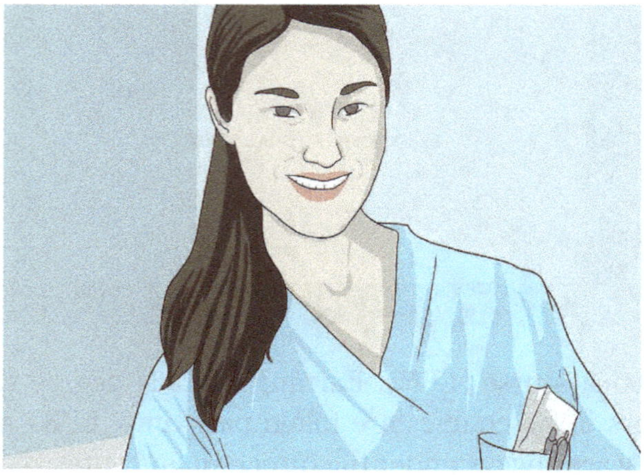

4. Consider pursuing a master of science degree in nursing (MSN). To further specialize in the nursing field, you can complete an MSN program in fields such as nurse-midwifery, nursing education, or geriatrics. You will also be able to teach at the college level if you hold an MSN degree, which usually takes about two years to complete.

- Nursing professions collectively known as advanced practice nurses, like nurse anesthetists, nursing administrator, or clinical nurse specialist, require a MSN.

Method 2

Learning More About the Field

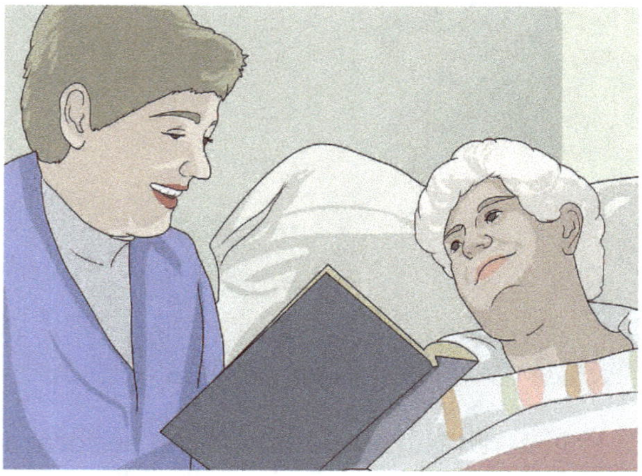

1. Volunteer at a local clinic or hospital. Healthcare settings are almost always in need of volunteers, and you will be able to learn more about nursing, and healthcare in general, by immersing yourself in a medical setting. Contact local nursing homes, VA hospitals, or children's hospitals and ask about volunteer opportunities.

- Volunteering will help you confirm that a career in nursing is what you want, and you will be helping others in the process.

- You will be able to make some valuable contacts while volunteering.
- You may also be able to shadow a nurse while volunteering if you sign a confidentiality form. This can give you a glimpse into what an average day on the job is like.

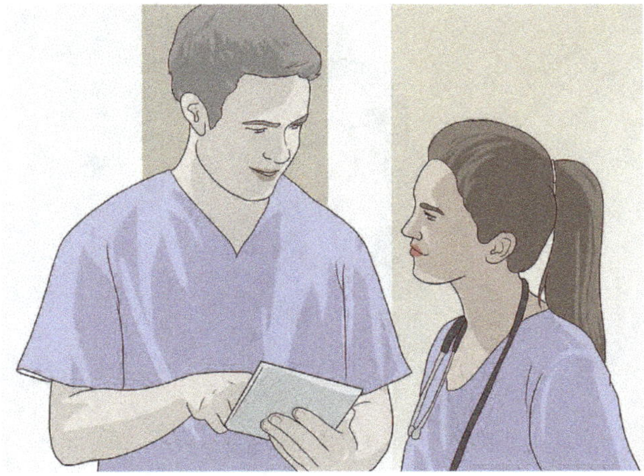

2. Network with local nurses. Call the human resources or outreach departments at local hospitals and ask to set up interviews with nurses. Tell them you are a prospective student and want to learn more about the field and what to expect in school.

- Nurses will be able to give you advice about how to handle your studies and maintain a school-life balance. They will also be able to offer their expertise on how to study for and pass the licensure exams.
- Some of the nurses you connect with may agree to mentor you throughout nursing school.
- Your nursing connections may also be able to help you find a placement when it is time to complete the clinical portion of your studies.

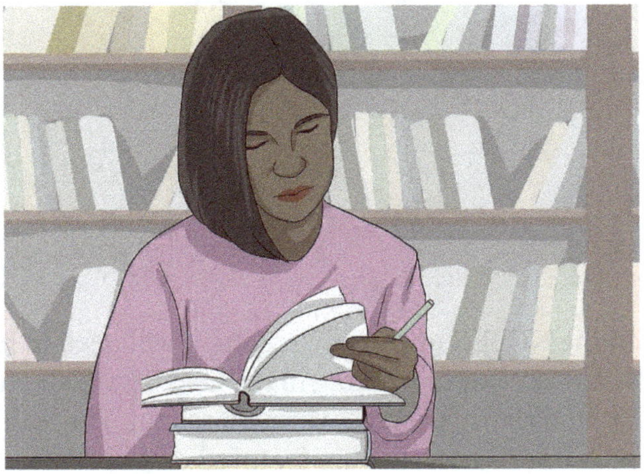

3. Educate yourself about current happenings in nursing. Read as much as you can about the nursing profession and medical field so that you are aware of current trends or issues. Subscribe to newsfeeds from healthcare news sites. This will help you bring a real-life focus to your studies.

- Online nursing forums are a good resource for current issues in the medical community.

Method 3

Setting yourself up for Success

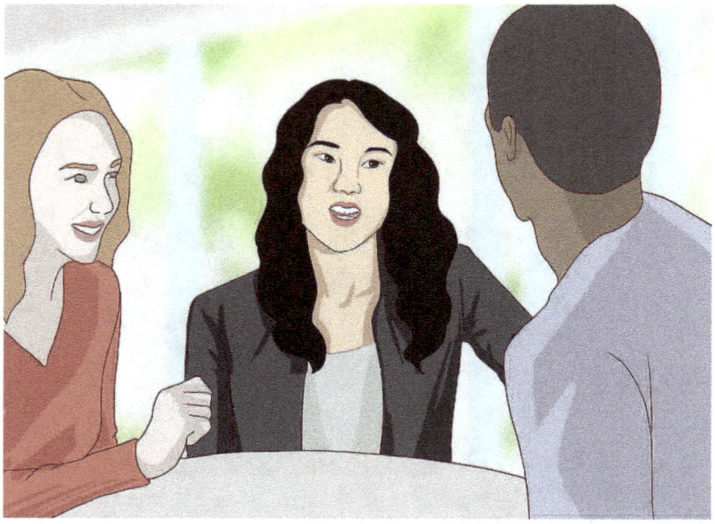

1. Meet some future classmates. If your school hosts social events or get-togethers before classes start, plan to attend them. Nursing school can be stressful, and it will be helpful to have a set of peers who understand and can help you through the challenges you'll face as a nursing student.

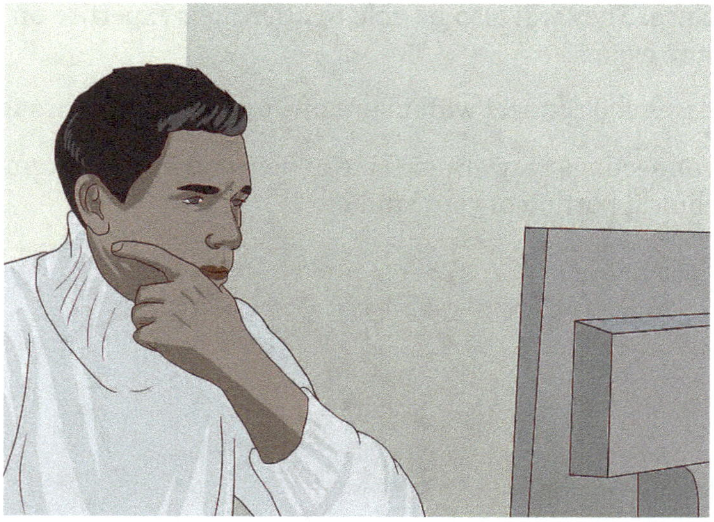

2. Familiarize yourself with the NCLEX exams. Every nurse will need to pass the National Council Licensure Examination (NCLEX) prior to working in the field. Review a study guide for the NCLEX before you start your studies and as you progress through school. This will help you understand the types of questions asked and the subjects that are featured on the exams.

- There are different versions for registered nurses (NCLEX-RN) and licensed practical nurses (NCLEX-PN).
- You will not have to worry about the NCLEX if you plan to become a CNA. CNAs do not take the NCLEX. They take a separate exam for CNAs.

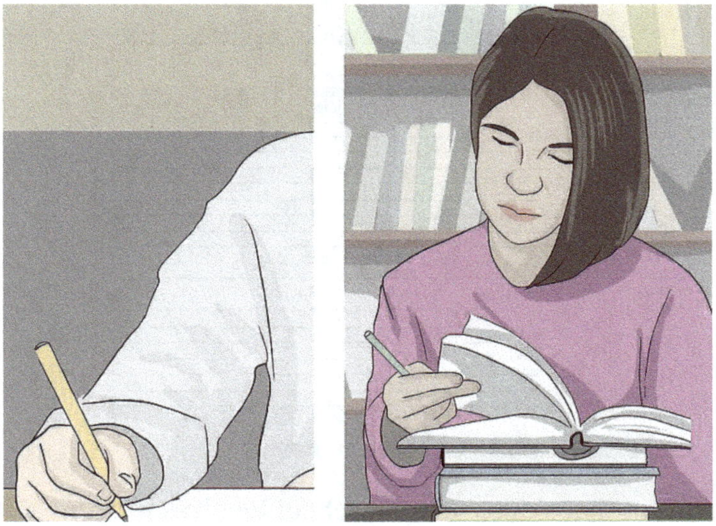

3. Set good study habits. It is easy to become overwhelmed with the sheer volume of work involved in nursing school, as well as the wealth of knowledge you need to master. Schedule study time in your planner and develop good habits, like studying a little each day and reviewing your notes during your down time.

- Your professors will undoubtedly assign numerous chapters to read each week. Instead of trying to memorize all of them, focus more attention on the material covered in class.
- Keep in mind that you will using what you learn when treating patients. You may understand and master the material better if you think, "How will this information help me treat patients?"

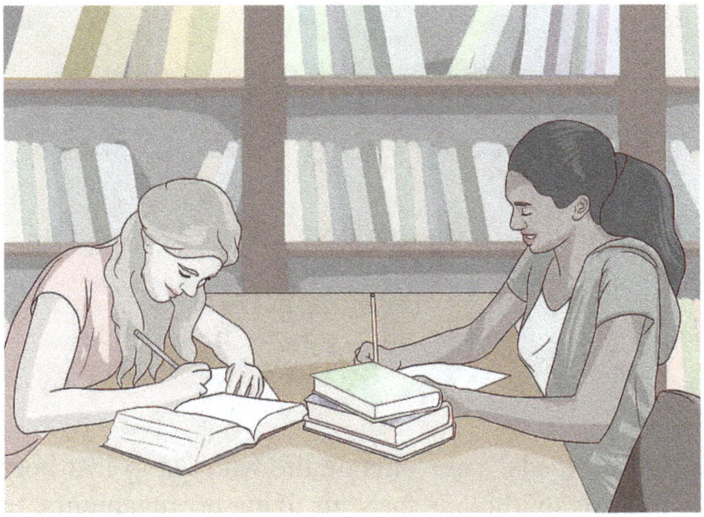

4. Join or start a study group. Your school may already have study groups set up, or you could form one with some friends. With a study group, you can compare notes, study for tests, and practice demonstrating skills.

- You will retain more knowledge and be less stressed if you study, either with a group or alone, on a regular basis rather than cram the night before exams.

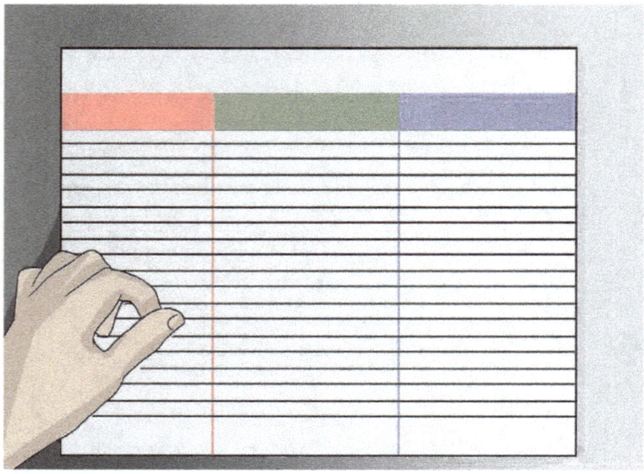

5. Develop strong organizational skills. Nursing school involves learning a lot of material, sometimes in a short period of time. Since you will also be busy with other aspects of your life, you will need to figure out a way to remain organized and on top of things. Use either a daily planner, a wall calendar, or an online scheduling program to block out time for studying, projects, and all of the reading you will need to do.

- Use the alerts on your smart phone to keep track of upcoming exams and paper deadlines.
- Keep all of your nursing gear in one place at home, so you always know where it is.
- Organize other aspects of your life as well, like scheduling time for errands and household chores.

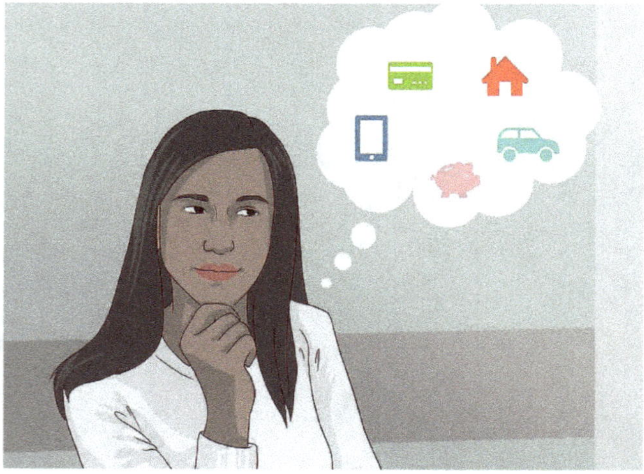

6. Take care of your logistical needs. Your outside life won't stop just because you're busy with nursing school. Be sure to have solid plans for your living arrangements, transportation, and income stream before starting your program.

- If you can, live at home with your parents or find a roommate to share expenses with. This type of living situation can also be helpful because household chores won't fall only on you.
- If you plan to work during school, be upfront with your supervisor about your schedule. It will typically change every 8 weeks, so flexibility is a must for your job.

Method 4

Preparing yourself Emotionally and Physically

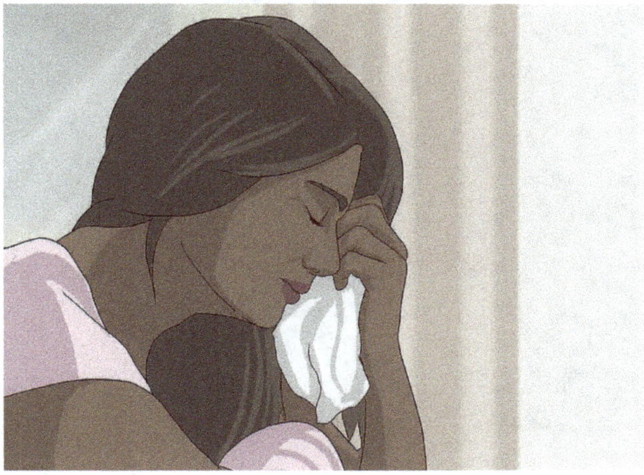

1. Be aware of the emotional issues you may face. Nursing school can be grueling and emotionally taxing, and these feelings can be amplified when you begin to deal with patients in your clinical rotations. Essential coping skills can include confiding in fellow students or a therapist if you become overwhelmed emotionally. Taking the time to find joy and humor each day, even if you're surrounded by very sick patients, can help as well.

- Remind yourself that your patients are depending on you, and that you are impacting their lives in profound ways. This can be helpful on days that you feel sad or upset by your job.
- Remember that even the best nursing care cannot solve every issue.

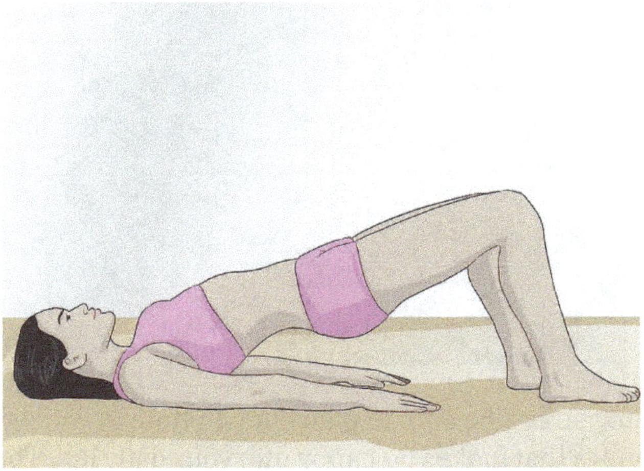

2. Start or continue your exercise program. Not only can exercise help relieve stress and anxiety, but it will also keep you in shape physically. Nursing school can involve physically taxing work, like lifting or moving patients. To keep in shape for these demands, you should aim for at least 30 minutes of exercise five times a week to reap the most benefits.

- Incorporate strength training, particularly for your core, and flexibility exercises into your routine to prepare you for the physical demands of lifting and moving patients.

- Some students find it useful to combine study sessions with exercise, like comparing notes with a classmate while taking a walk or a job.

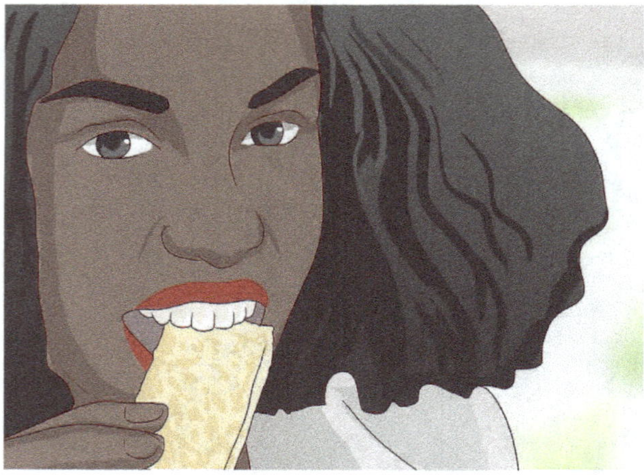

3. Remember to eat well, even when busy. On days when you're rushing from class to clinicals, sitting down for a meal may be the last thing on your mind. But you won't study effectively or treat patients well if you're not properly nourished. Plan your meals on the weekend and then shop accordingly to help you have healthy food throughout the week.

- Keep healthy snacks on you at all times. Good options include granola bars, nuts, fresh or dehydrated fruits, and beef jerky.
- You can turn some study sessions into healthy potluck gatherings.

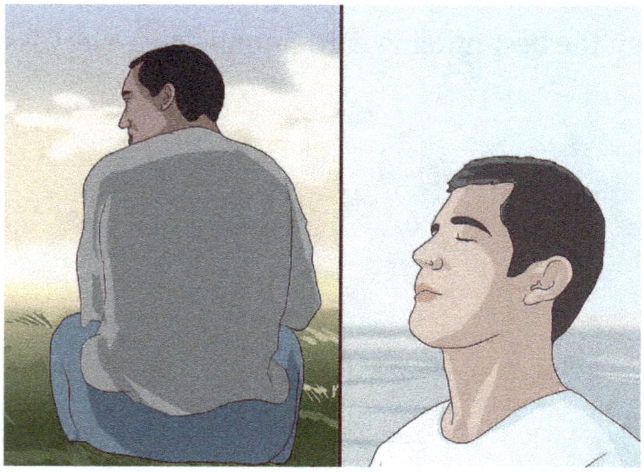

4. Make a plan for managing stress. Be sure to plan enough time in your schedule for life outside of school, and incorporate things that make you happy into your daily life. The rigors of nursing school can be stressful, so you want to have outlets so you can bring your best self to school each day.

- Think about things that boost your mood, like taking time for a relaxing cup of coffee or tea or chatting with a friend. Remember to incorporate those into your days as often as possible to keep yourself emotionally healthy.
- If possible, take advantage of a school break by getting away, even if it's just a day trip. A change of scenery can be beneficial in clearing your mind and lifting your spirits.

How to Prepare for the Nursing School Entrance Exams

Getting into nursing school can be a competitive process. In addition to high grades, work experience, volunteer experience, and a successful interview, applicants must take a nursing school entrance exam when applying to any accredited nursing program. If you are interested in attending nursing school, you must learn how to prepare for the nursing school entrance exams since these tests are a crucial part of the application.

Part 1

Preparing for the Exam

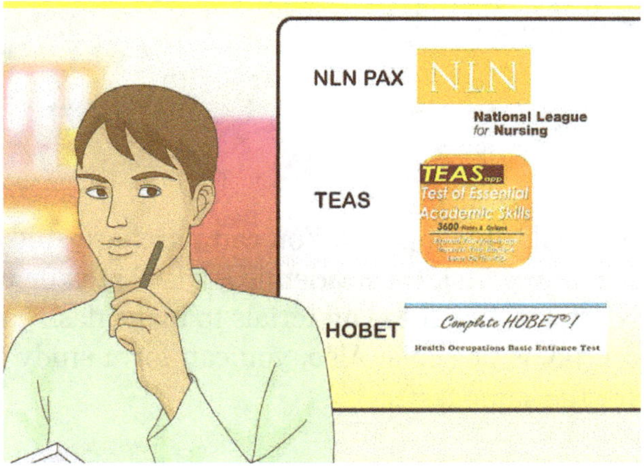

1. Identify which exam you need to take. In order to study for a nursing school entrance exam, you need to know which test you will be taking. The most common nursing school entrance exams are:

- National League for Nursing Pre-Admission Exam (NLN PAX)
- Test of Essential Academic Skills (TEAS)
- Health Occupations Basic Entrance Test (HOBET)

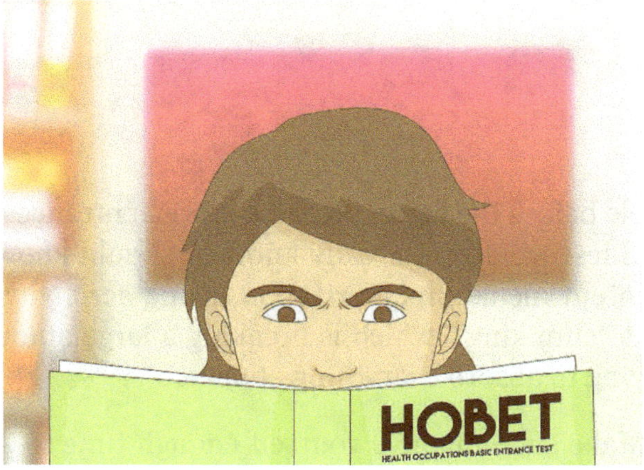

2. Know the nuances of that exam. Nursing school entrance exams are different. Knowing the

parameters of each test will allow you to focus on specific areas while studying. For example, the HOBET exam gauges your social skills and ability to cope with stress while the TEAS test is simply gauging your basic math, reading and science skills.

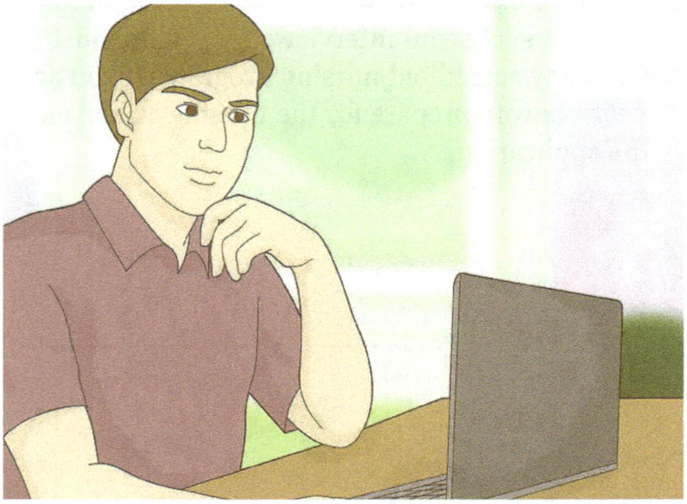

3. Acquire the necessary materials and support. You can purchase study materials from any reputable bookstore or online resource. Ask the academic advisor at your prospective school for any recommendations for study guides. Use these materials to make flash cards and notes and absorb as much about the test material as possible. Also, you can form study groups if you know other people who are preparing for the same test.

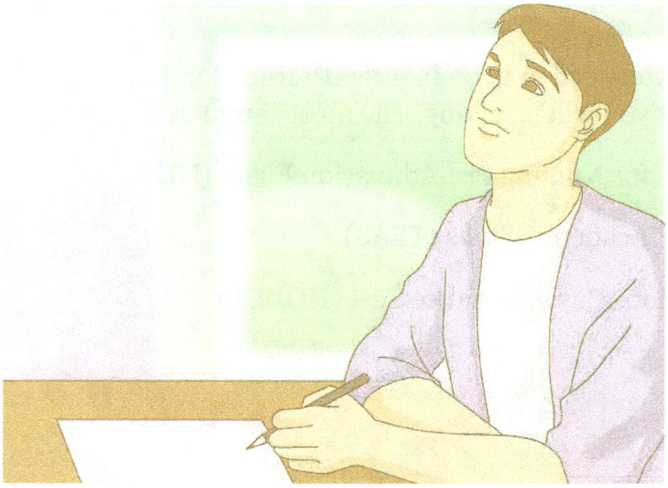

4. Study as much as possible before the exam. Nursing school entrance exams are content driven, which means that they will test what you already know or should know. Techniques that can be successful for studying content include memorization, using acronyms, and using associations. Another type of studying is "chunking," which is breaking a large amount of material down into smaller units instead of trying to absorb everything at once.

- Avoid cramming. Make sure you give yourself enough time to study. If you have already worked and volunteered in the field, you will likely already know a lot of the information, but don't use that as an excuse to wait to the last minute to study.

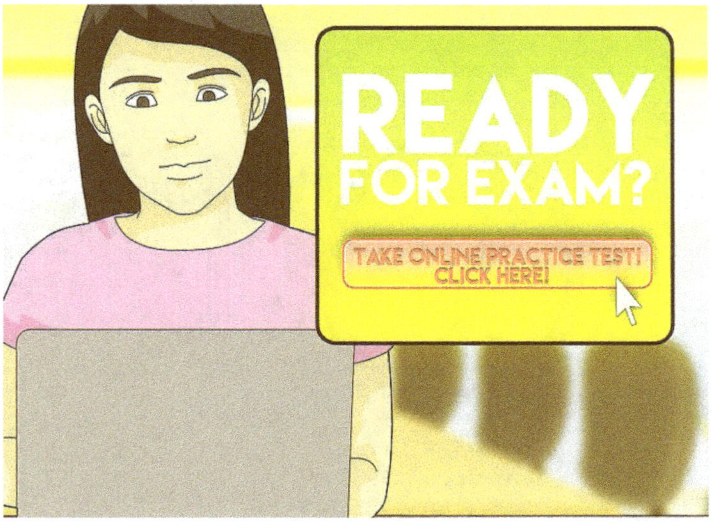
READY
FOR EXAM?
TAKE ONLINE PRACTICE TEST!
CLICK HERE!

5. Take practice exams. We've all heard the phrase "practice makes perfect." Find a practice test for the type of nursing school entrance exam you will be taking online, in your study guide or at a local community center or college. Taking this practice test can help you identify areas in which your performance was weak and fix it before taking the actual exam.

- Take as many different practice tests as you can, as they will cover different material.
- If you identify areas of weakness, spend additional time studying this material and seek out the help of a tutor.

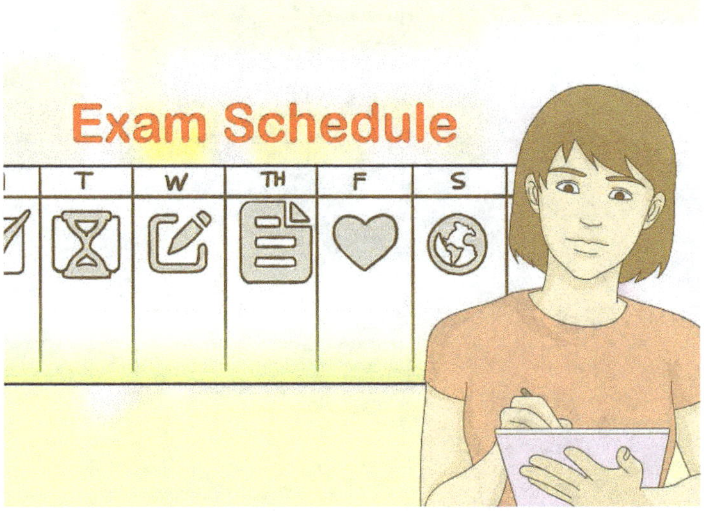
Exam Schedule
T
W
TH
F
S

6. Schedule the exam. Arrange an exam date that will give you plenty of time to study, but will also allow you to submit your application materials, along with the test score, to your prospective school before the submission deadline.

- It is wise to check your calendar and make sure you do not have any scheduling conflicts on the day of your exam or in the days that immediately precede it. Preparation is a huge part of success on standardized tests and your will want to be sure you have the days leading up to exam free for study and preparation.

Part 2

Taking the Exam

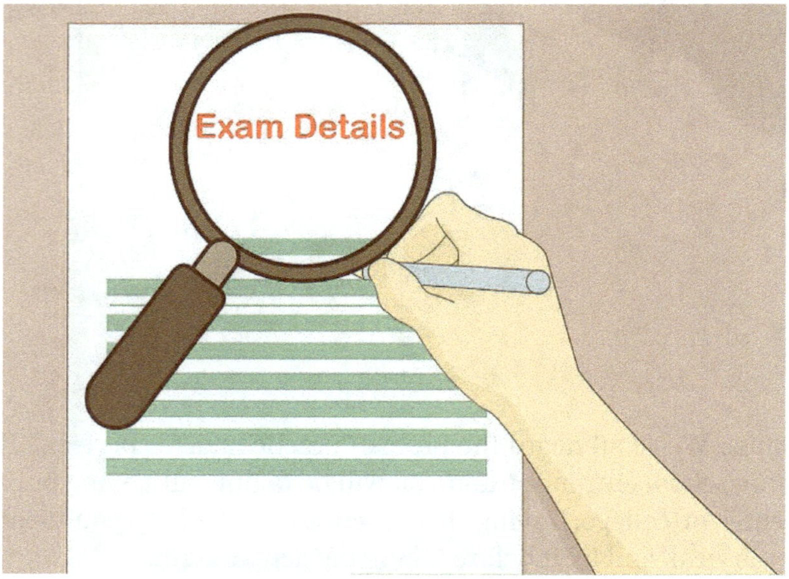

1. Know the details of your examination. Identify when, where, and in what format your nursing school entrance exam will be administered well before the exam date. Make sure you get a good night's rest before the exam and leave yourself time for a final review of the materials.

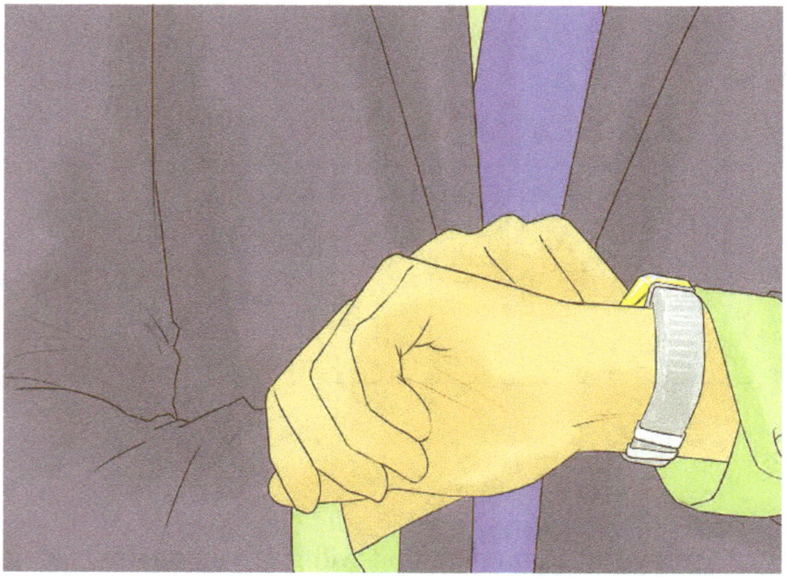

2. Arrive early. Arrive at the testing site at least 30 minutes early on the day of your exam. Bring your picture ID and pencils, if necessary. Do not bring your cell phone, calculator, food, drinks, or any study materials into the exam room.

- Noise-canceling headphones may be issued at formalized testing centers, as there are often many people taking exams at the same time.

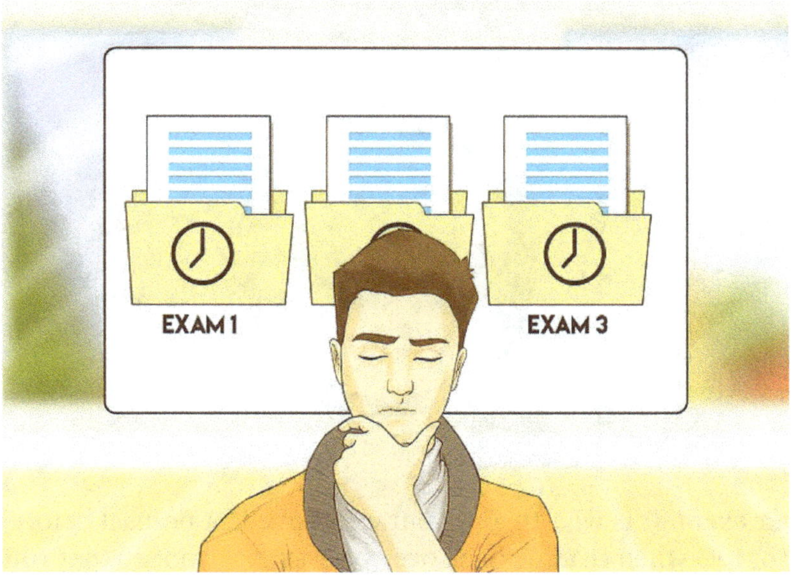

3. Have a section plan. As is the case with most standardized tests, nursing school entrance exams break down into various sections and the overall exam has a set time limit. Knowing this, plan to spend a pre-determined amount of time on each section and stick to it. Also, don't forget to allow yourself some time to review your answers in each section before moving on.

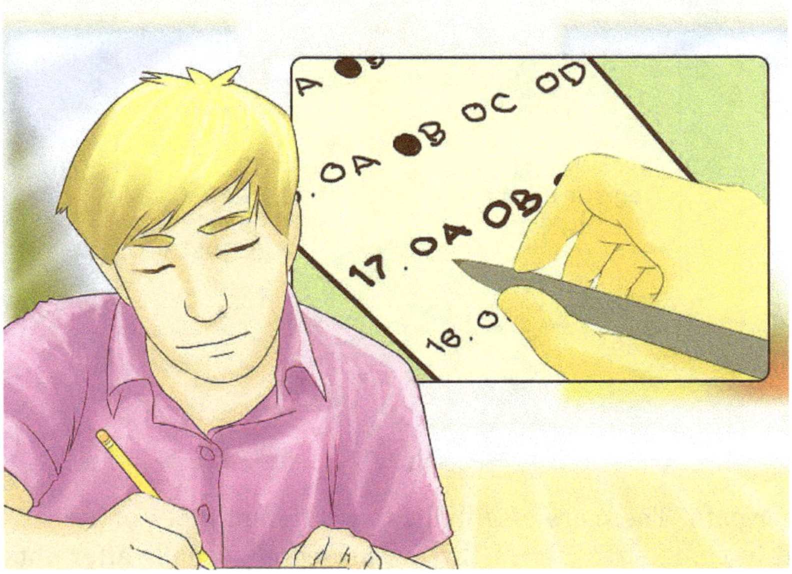

4. Take the exam. The majority of these exams are comprised of multiple choice questions. Read and answer each question carefully. If you get caught up on a question, skip it and come back to it during the review period you allotted for yourself. Never leave questions unanswered. If you don't know the answer, guess. You may get lucky and get some extra points.

- You may want to look into strategies for quickly answering multiple choice questions. For instance, first cross off any obviously wrong answers. Answers with absolute qualifiers like "always" or "never" are typically not the correct answer; however, relative qualifiers such as "generally" or "sometimes" are usually found in the correct answer.

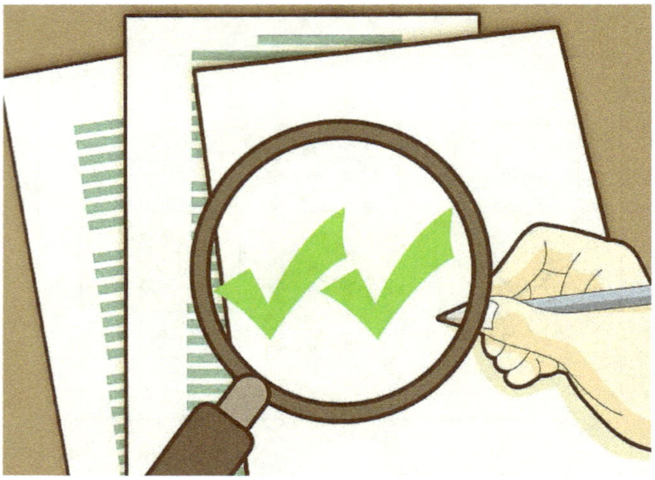

5. Double check your exam. It is wise to give your exam one last perusal before handing it in. You may catch an error or two when reading back over your exam or notice that you failed to answer a question here or there.

Part 3

Deciding which Test to Take

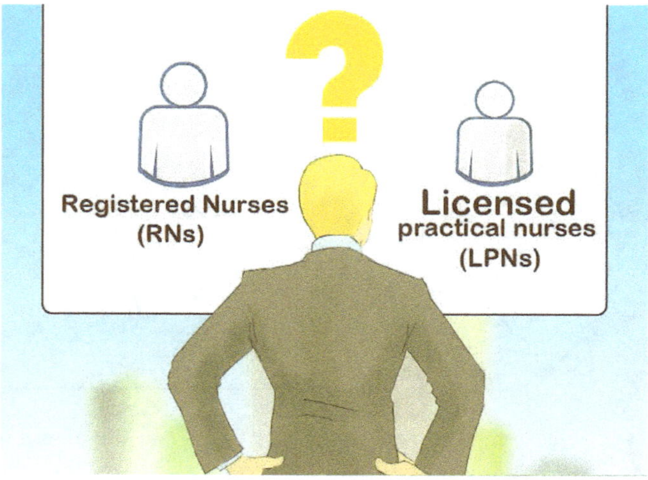

1. Decide on a career path. There are essentially two different types of nurses. Registered nurses (RNs) are expected to complete a two or three year degree, usually after obtaining a bachelor's degree, are more often employed in hospitals and are expected to take on more important tasks that involve a greater degree of critical thinking and decision making. Licensed practical nurses (LPNs) usually obtain a nursing certificate after about a year of nursing education. LPNs are more often employed in long term care facilities, filling administrative roles and overseeing the basics of patient care (changing bedpans, linens, IVs, etc.).

- In settings where LPNs and RNs work together, RNs outrank LPNs and undertake more intensive and critical duties.
- Most nursing school entrance exams offer separate tests for LPN and RN programs.

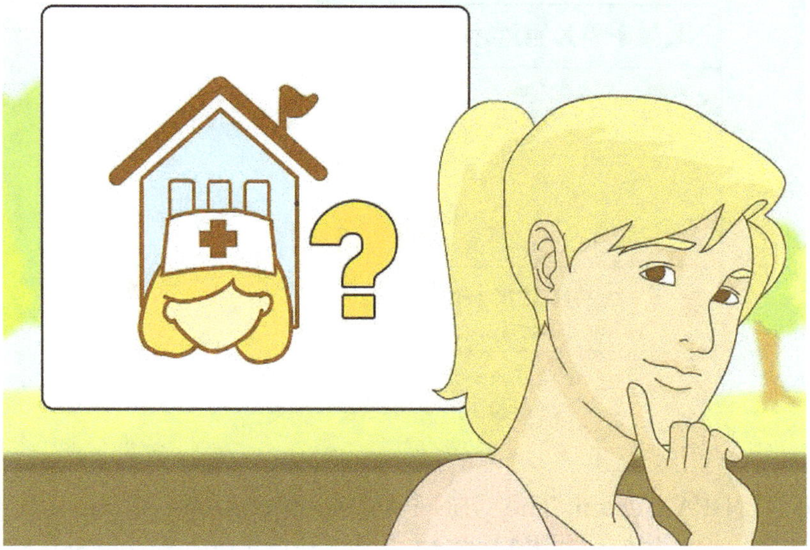

2. Select nursing schools. Once you have chosen between becoming a RN or LPN, choose one or more nursing schools that can provide you with your desired degree or certificate through the completion of their program.

- Make sure that the school you choose is an accredited school.
- The school will specify which entrance exam is necessary to apply to the nursing program you want.

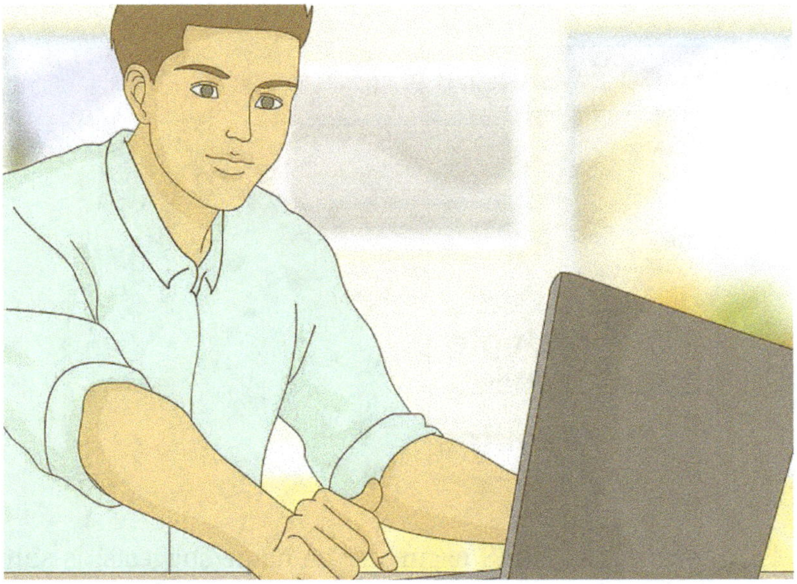

3. Learn the specifics of the test. Find out the specifics of the test you will take so that you know how to study for it and what material to focus on. The exams typically take between 2 and 3.5 hours to complete. The exams may be administered on a computer or using pencil and paper. You will find out your scores immediately after completing the computerized version of the test.

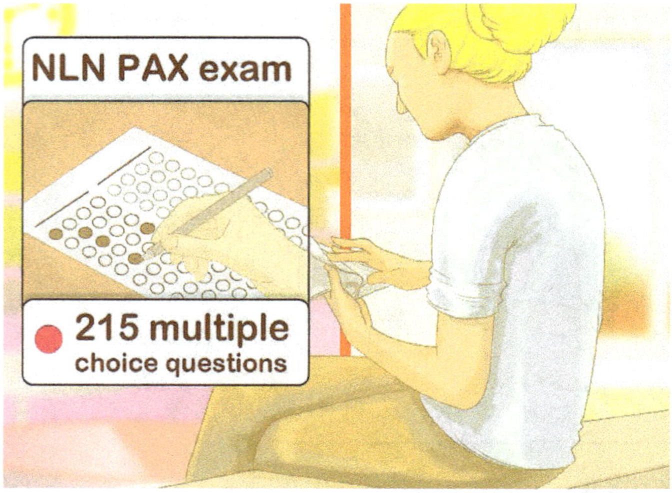

4. Prepare for the NLN PAX exam. The NLN PAX exam consists of about 215 multiple choice questions. The questions on the NLN PAX exam break down into verbal skills, math and science sections. Some of the questions on this exam will not be graded, as they are simply used to gauge responses for future testing. However, you won't know which questions will or will not be graded at the time of the exam, so answer each one to the best of your ability.

- You can't use a calculator for this exam.
- The exam takes about 3 hours to complete and costs about $60 to $100.
- You will not be allowed to retake this exam for six months after the initial testing date.

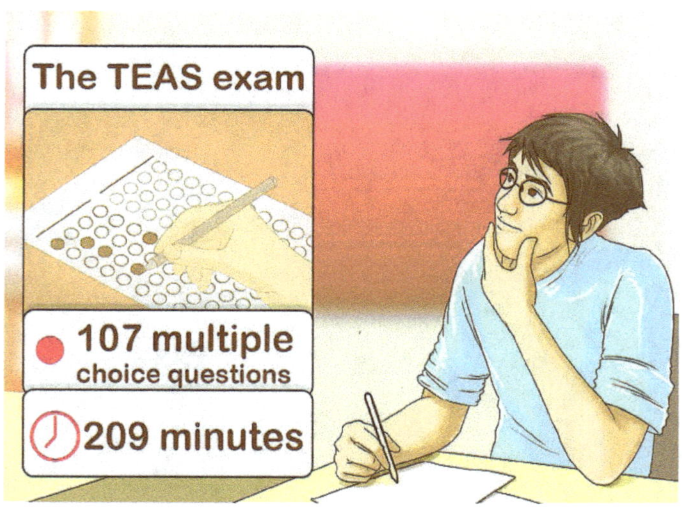

5. Prepare for the TEAS exam. The TEAS exam, as the name suggests, is simply a test of basic knowledge that you should have learned in high school. This exam breaks down to English, reading skills, science and math sections. The TEAS exam contains 107 multiple choice questions that must be answered in 209 minutes.

- You will not be allowed to use a calculator.
- Fees for this exam can range between $20 and $60.

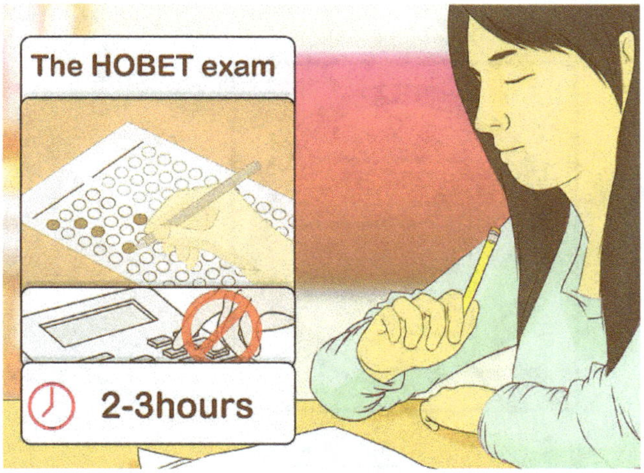

6. Prepare for the HOBET exam. The HOBET exam is administered by the same company that operates the TEAS exam and tests candidates for the same generalized knowledge, but also gauges an individual's potential to work in healthcare. The HOBET exam gauges basic math skills, reading comprehension skills, test taking skills, critical thinking skills, social interactions, your ability to cope with stressful situations and your learning style. The math section requires knowledge of algebra, fractions, percentages, statistics and other math functions. The reading comprehension section tests to ensure you have attained a tenth-grade reading level.

- The test takes between two to three hours to complete and you will not be allowed to use a calculator.
- While you can take the HOBET exam multiple times, many schools limit the number of tests for its candidates, citing the belief that if you fail to achieve success in your first few tries, you are probably not an ideal candidate for healthcare work.
- The fee for this exam varies by school.

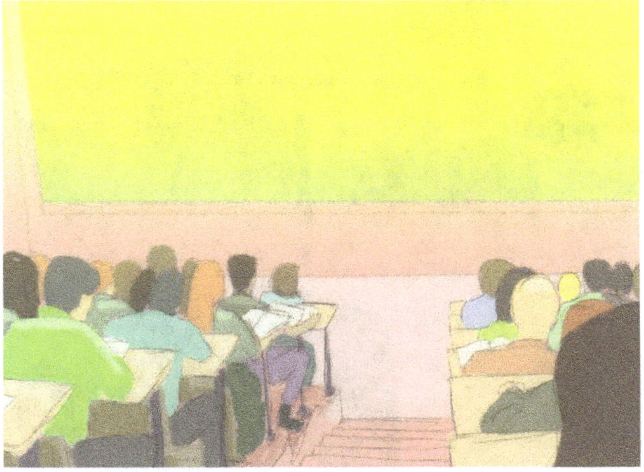

7. Know where the exam is offered. Find out where you can take your nursing school entrance exam in your area and how to register. Be aware that there is a fee for a nursing school entrance exam. This is all information that you can get from your prospective school or from websites maintained by the exams' administrators. Give yourself enough time to study before your registered test date.

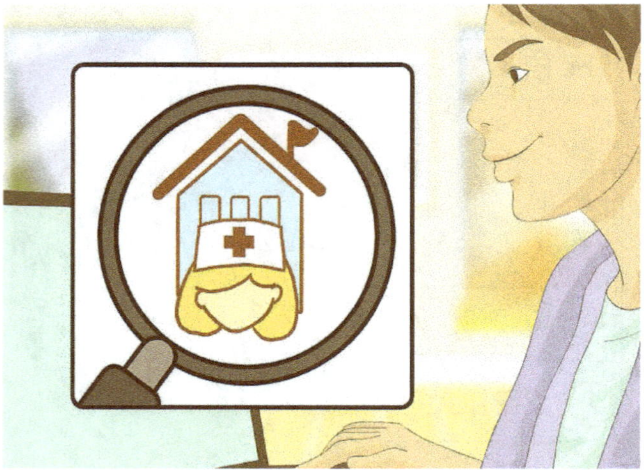

8. Know how your test will be weighted. Do some research about the nursing program you intend to apply to. Some schools weigh your grade history and personal history more heavily than your entrance exam, while others consider your exam scores to be more important.

How to get into Nursing School

Getting into nursing school can be a tough and detailed process. The application materials can be extensive, taking several months to complete. Dedication and motivation are required to complete the process. Nursing programs are very competitive, but you can increase your chances of acceptance with proper preparation and planning.

Part 1

Preparing for Nursing School

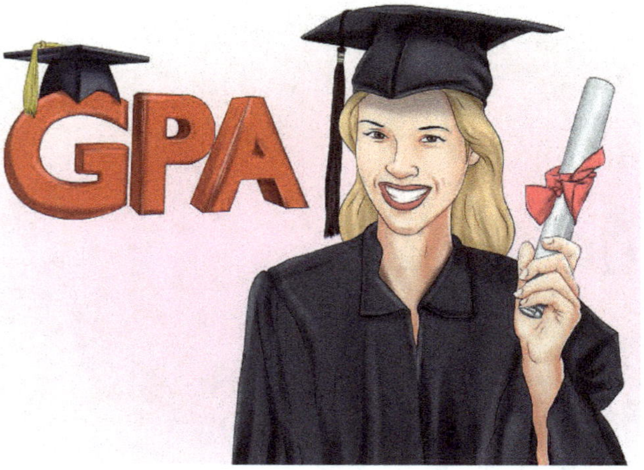

1. Graduate from high school. Graduating from high school or the equivalent is required to get into any nursing program. You should try to make very good grades and have a high GPA. You should also do well in your science coursework.

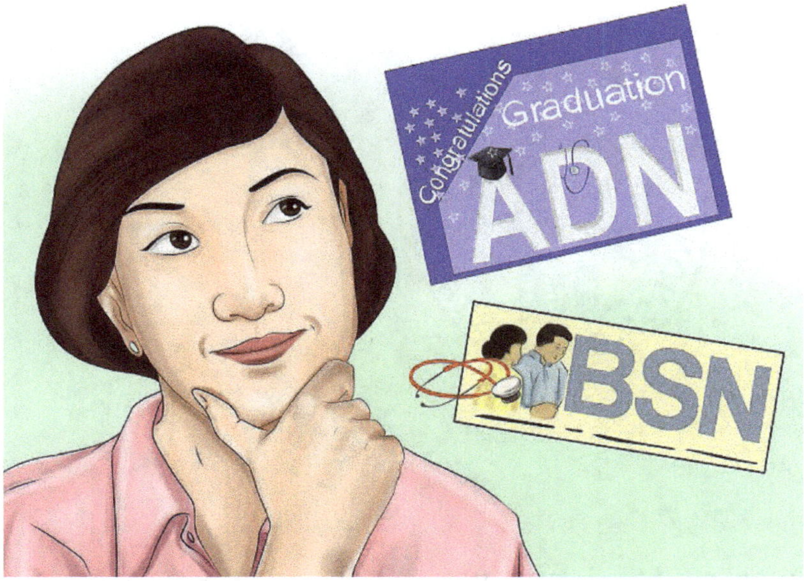

2. Decide which nursing degree you will pursue. You can go to school for an associate degree (ADN) or a baccalaureate (BSN) degree. BSN programs are more competitive and have tougher admission standards. ADN programs take only two years to complete and are less expensive. BSN programs require additional coursework and take four years to complete. Having a BSN degree will provide you with more job opportunities, a higher salary, and more career advancement opportunities.

- There is also a licensed practical nursing degree, which is the lowest level nursing degree. It is usually an 11 month program for licensed practical nursing.

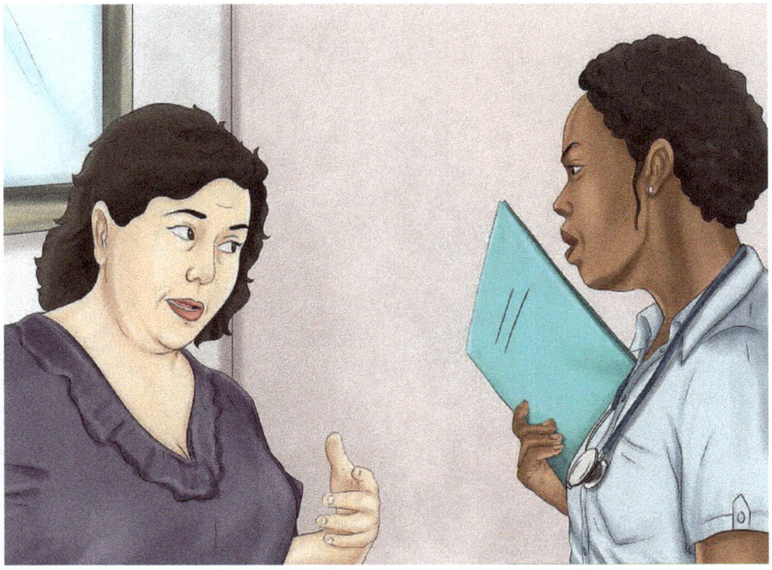

3. Talk with current nurses. Speaking with someone who is already working in the profession will give you a better idea of life as a nurse. If you do not know any nurses personally, you can contact a doctor's office or hospital and let them know you are a prospective nursing student. Most likely, they will happy to speak with you.

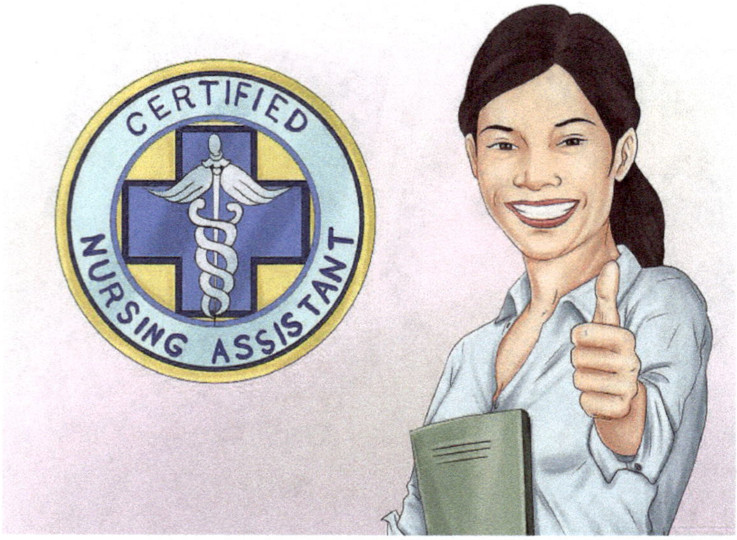

4. Get experience in the healthcare field. You can volunteer or work part-time in the healthcare field. This will help you decide if nursing is the right career for you. You can also put this experience on your resume when you apply to school. Many hospitals have volunteer programs.

- It is imperative that new incoming nurses have a realistic and accurate degree of their job responsibilities as well as know the responsibilities of their allied professional help. A great way to do this is by beginning as a certified nursing assistant.

Part 2

Choosing a School

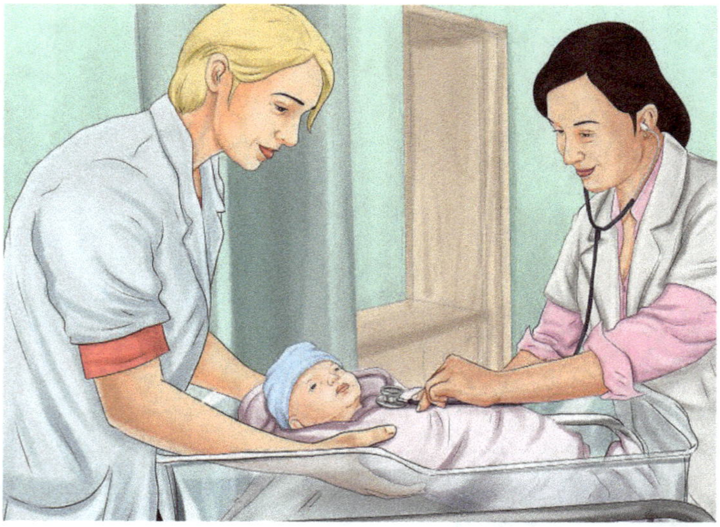

1. Develop your criteria. You should create a checklist by which you evaluate each school. Your checklist should include personal factors that are important to you, such as the location, tuition prices, and your career goals. Other important considerations are the pass rate on the National Council Licensure Examination (NCLEX), graduation rate, career placement services, and the faculty.

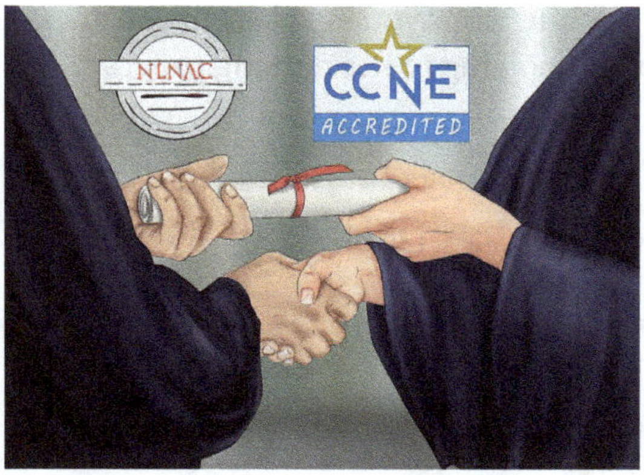

2. Determine the school's accreditation status. The school you choose should be accredited by the National League for Nursing Accrediting Commission (NLNAC) or the Commission on Collegiate Nursing Education (CCNE). The school should also be approved by a state board of nursing.

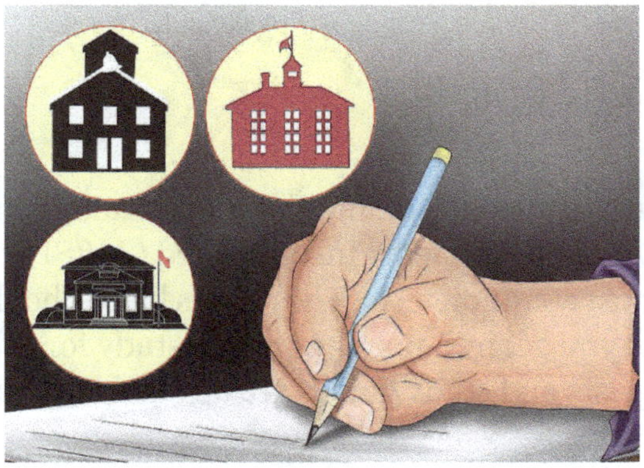

3. Make a list of schools that you will apply to. This list will help you stay organized throughout the application process. Your list should include the application deadlines and the application requirements. Also pay attention to any prerequisites you may need.

- Some nursing schools will admit students on the basis that all general education coursework is complete before the start of the program. These courses may include anatomy and physiology, microbiology, general psychology, and human development.

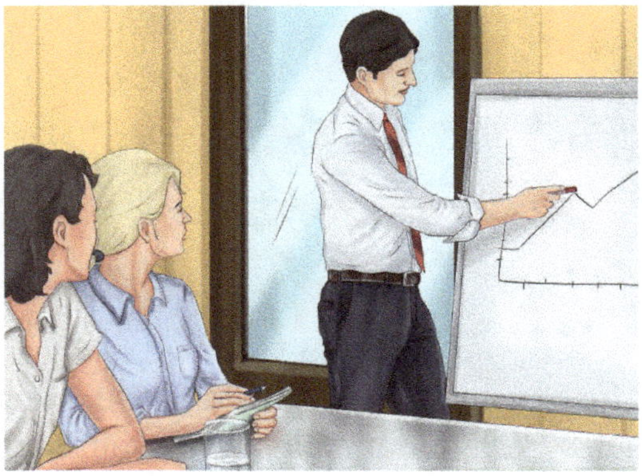

4. Attend an information session or open house. Many schools invite students who are interested in applying to an information session. These sessions discuss the application process, program

curriculum, and tuition. Ask any questions you may have if you are attending one of these sessions. Note that this is not the same as applying to the nursing program.

Part 3

Preparing your Application Materials

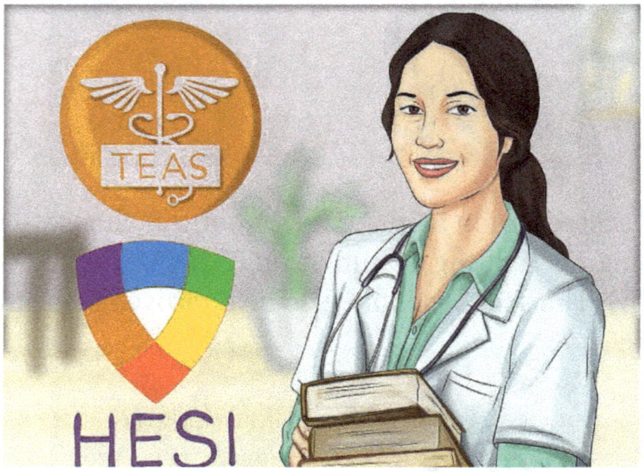

1. Take necessary admission assessments. Nursing classes demand that you have math, reading, and language skills. The Health Education Systems Incorporated (HESI) and the Test of Essential Academic Skills (TEAS) are the most common tests. These tests help schools decide if you will do well in nursing school. To ensure that you get into nursing school, study for this test beforehand so you can do your best. Online practice tests and study guides are available for both the TEAS and the HESI.

- Do not forget to sign up for any other testing the school may ask for. One example is the College Placement Test, or CPT. This is to determine if you are ready for college in general. You might need to study for this exam to make sure you get the highest scores possible.

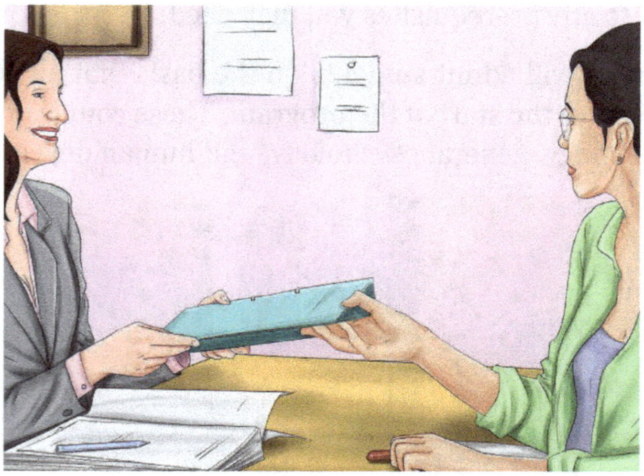

2. Request official transcripts for any and all colleges you have attended. Some schools also want high school transcripts; if you are fresh out of high school, your high school transcript alone will suffice. Many schools have an online transcript request form you can fill out and they will send it electronically, cutting out some of the footwork you have to do. There may be a fee to send transcripts, no matter if they're paper or electronic.

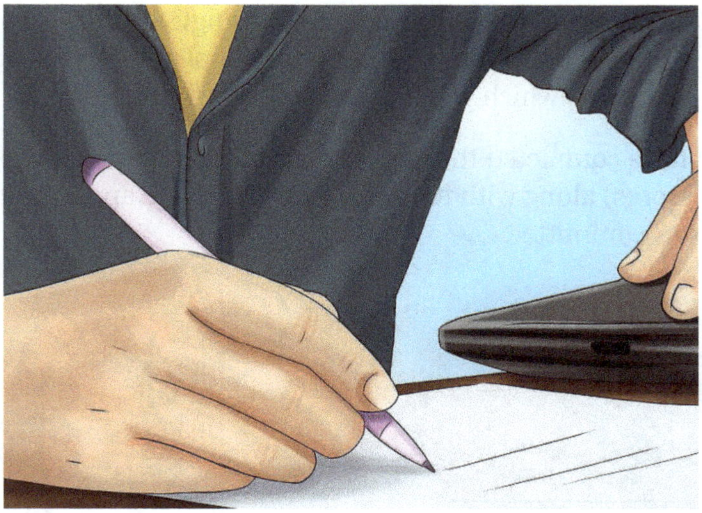

3. Write your admissions essay, if required. Many nursing schools require potential students to write an essay on why they want to be a nurse or on the roles of a nurse. The essay will allow the administration to see who you are as a person. Follow the instructions they give you and make sure your essay has no spelling or grammatical errors. If you know someone who has successfully gotten into nursing school, ask to see their essay for inspiration. You should also let someone else give you feedback on your essay.

- Schools will be checking to see that you have a good understanding of the reality of nursing. It is a tough job and one that is physically, emotionally, and intellectually demanding.

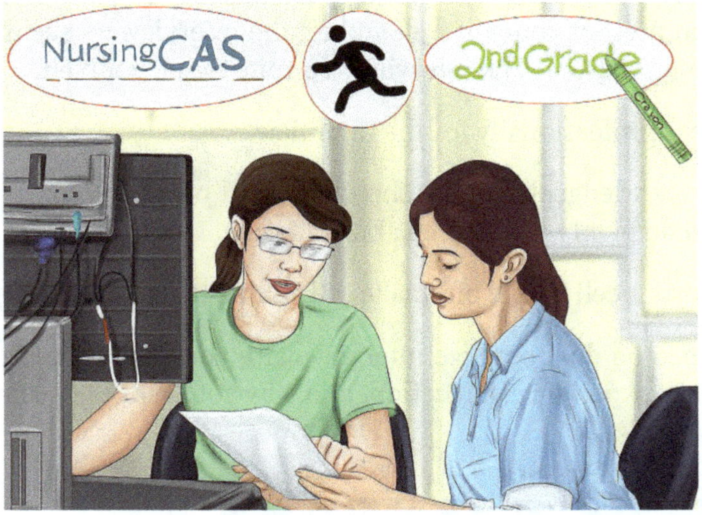

4. Complete the application. It is important that you pay attention to application deadlines and submit your application as soon as possible. Turn your application packet in as early as possible, as some schools review them on a first-come, first-served basis, and nursing is extremely competitive.

- Nursing schools look at many factors when choosing applicants. Your grades, extracurricular activities, and references are important as well. Schools are looking for well-rounded people.

- The Nursing Centralized Application Service (NursingCAS) allows you to apply to multiple schools using a single application. All nursing schools do not participate in this service. Make sure the schools to which you are applying use this system.
- Make sure you have completed the application fully and submit any supplemental materials (essay, test scores) along with it. An incomplete or late application will not be reviewed by the admissions committee.

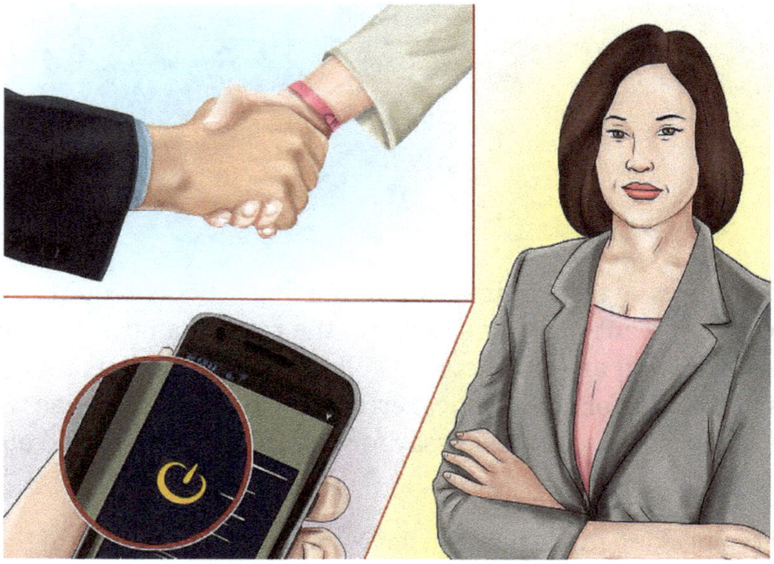

5. Prepare for your interview. Some schools require an interview as part of the application process. It is important that you present yourself well and let the interviewers see that you will be a great addition to their nursing program. The interview is a time to sell yourself.

- You should dress professionally for the interview.
- You should be knowledgeable about the school and program for which you are interviewing. You should do plenty of research ahead of time.
- Be sure to turn your cell phone off, make eye contact, and have a firm handshake.
- Have another person do a practice interview with you. You should practice talking about your career goals, experience, education, and why you want to become a nurse.

How to Pay for Nursing School

If you've decided on a career in nursing, then your next step is probably figuring out how to pay for nursing school. In addition to paying for tuition and book fees, student nurses are also responsible for lab fees, uniform fees, personal health insurance and required immunizations, and other costs that don't apply to most students. If you need assistance, there are a variety of loan programs, grants, scholarships and work repayment programs that can help you pay for nursing school, whether pursuing an RN designation or a degree.

Method 1

Applying for Grants and Scholarships

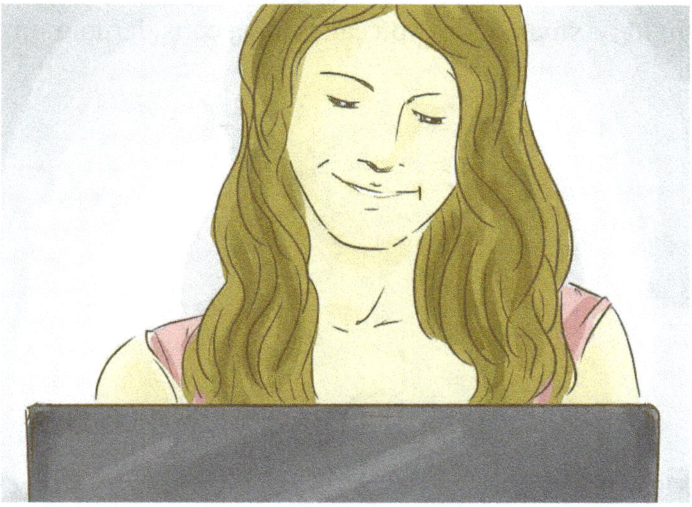

1. Research scholarship and grant opportunities. Search the internet for reputable scholarship and grant opportunities. If you've already applied and been accepted to a nursing program, start with its website. Your college program's site will likely offer helpful links that compile opportunities and offer helpful information about applying.

- Check the financial aid resources listed on the website of the American Association of Colleges of Nursing (AACN).
- Remember, the more scholarship and grant money you can accumulate, the less you have to pay out of pocket and the less debt you have to pay back in the future.

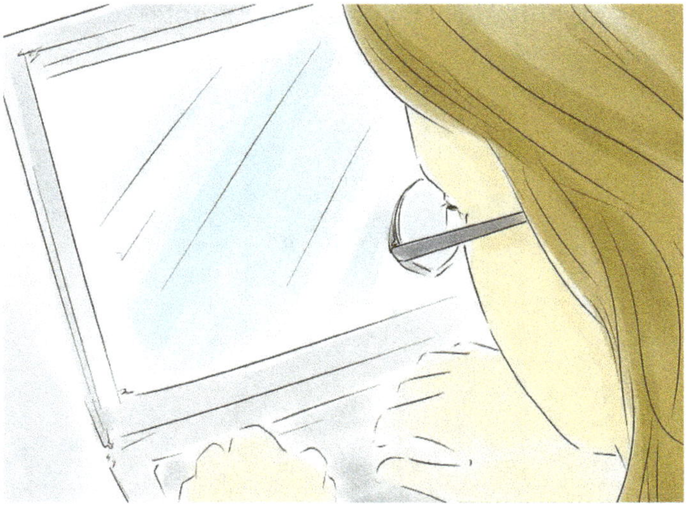

2. Apply for nursing scholarships. With a shortage of nurses in certain sectors of the medical field, there are a number of public and private organizations that provide scholarships for nursing students. Some scholarships are designated for students looking to earn a bachelor's or master's degree in nursing, so read descriptions carefully and only save links to relevant opportunities.

- Keep in mind that hundreds or thousands of students apply for major national scholarships.
- Try applying for local scholarships as well, as they will have smaller applicant pools. Individually, they might be smaller, but you can build a considerable sum of money by winning several of them.

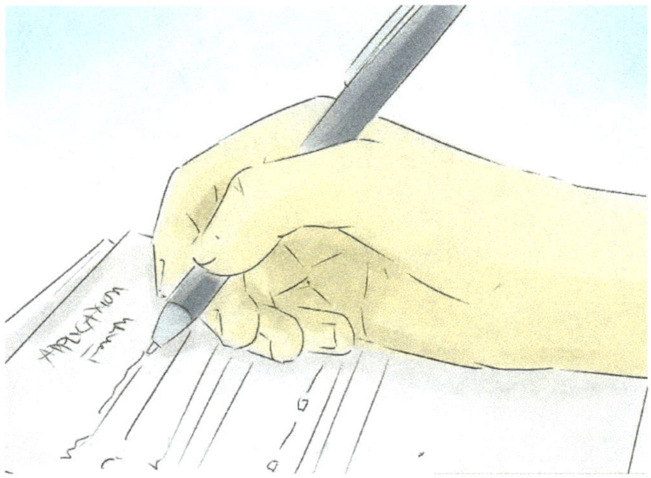

3. Apply for nursing school grants. Look into state government-funded grants for nursing students. The U.S. Department of Health and Human Services sponsors a number of grants to help in-need students pay for nursing school. Other, private grants may require you to have reached a certain level in your education (such as completing one semester of your program), or may require that you agree to work for a specified time in a particular area of nursing. However, you don't have to repay any of the money you're awarded out of pocket. That'll help you graduate from a nursing program as debt-free as possible.

- Professional nursing organizations may also offer grants.

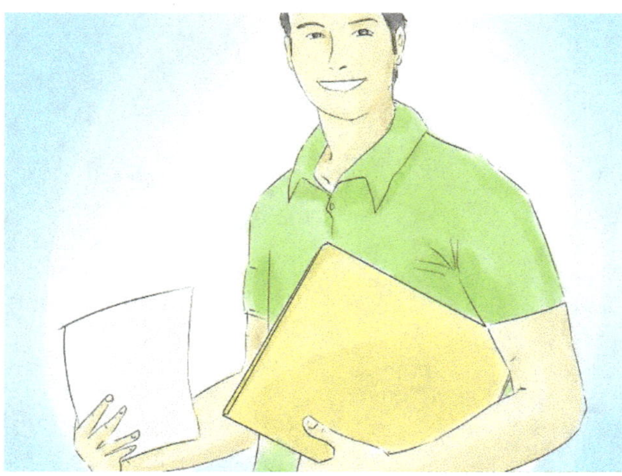

4. Stay organized and keep application responses handy. Once you've researched scholarship and grant opportunities, make a calendar or use a calendar app that specifically lists application deadlines and other important related dates. Once you've applied to a few, keep any digital files saved on your computer, or make copies of applications that had to be submitted in writing.

- List dates in your calendar in advance of application deadlines, or set reminders to work on an application. Give yourself reminders to begin and complete applications several days before they're due.
- Keeping application info, from basic info to essay responses, will help streamline the process so you can maximize the number of applications you send.

Method 2

Consulting with your Program and Financial Aid Office

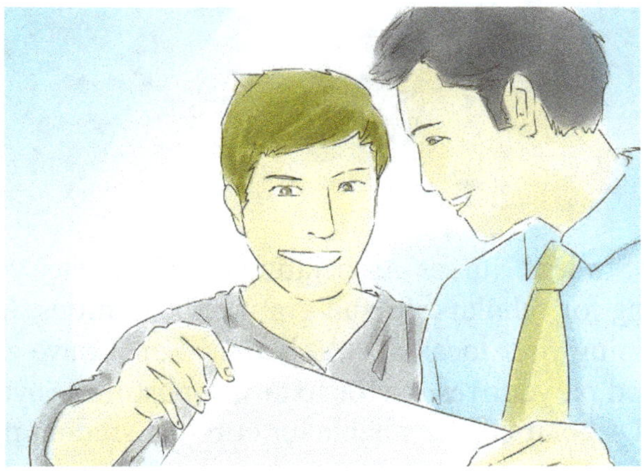

1. Discuss financial aid options with your nursing program. As you apply to and are accepted into a nursing program, talk to anyone you come into contact with about financial aid. Look at your program's website for financial aid info that's specific to the program. Look for the contact info of relevant people, such as the program director or the department's student advisors.

- Ask them about local scholarship opportunities, work-study programs, and how other students commonly pay for that particular program.

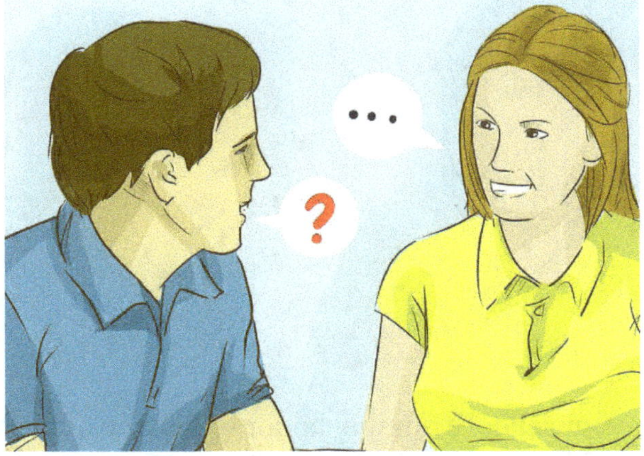

2. Inquire with the college financial aid office. Talk to your college's financial aid counselors about securing aid and about the process of paying for nursing school. If there is federal financing available, the office will instruct you on how to apply. Federal aid is usually a loan, so you will need to repay the borrowed amount.

- If you're applying for a program in the United States, fill out a FAFSA, or Free Application for Federal Student Aid. Your school will provide you with information about deadlines.

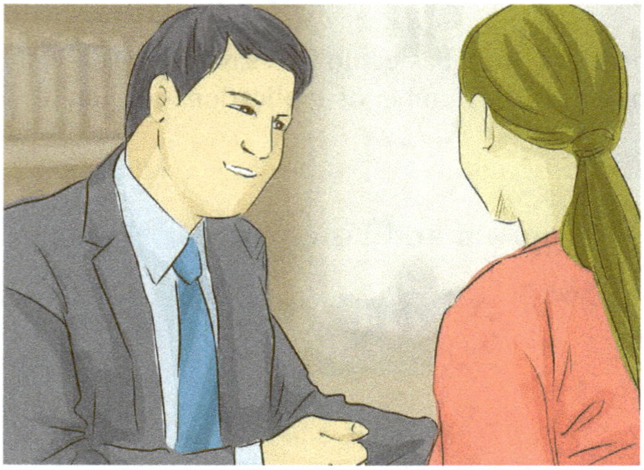

3. Join your local National Student Nurses' Association (NSNA). Once you're enrolled in a nursing program, don't stop looking for scholarship and grant opportunities. Continue to make yourself a winning applicant by joining your local NSNA chapter. You'll have access to great networking opportunities, it'll look good on your resumé or to any opportunities you apply for, and you'll be informed about grants and scholarships available for enrolled student nurses.

- Take a leadership position in your local chapter for even more networking opportunities, to learn more, and for a resumé booster.
- Your nursing professors will provide you with information about how your program participates in the NSNA and other relevant organizations.

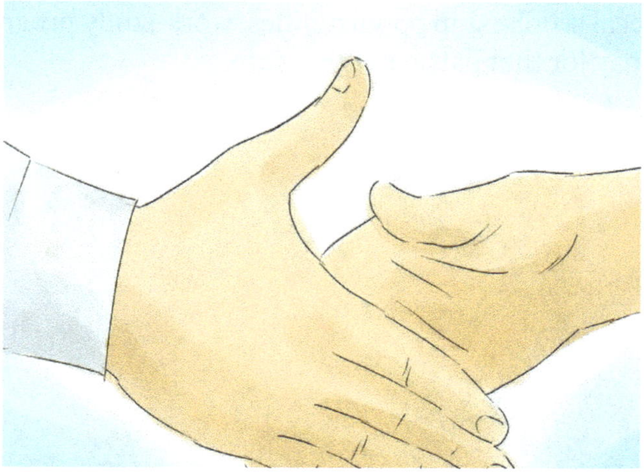

4. Join Sigma Theta Tau or your school's nursing honor society. In addition to joining your school's NSNA, find out if your school has a local chapter of Sigma Theta Tau, which is the international honor society for student nurses. If not, find out if your college participates in another nursing student honor society, and how to get accepted into it. Keep your GPA up, and once again, take a leadership position if any are available to make yourself a more appealing enrolled applicant for scholarships and grants.

Method 3

Graduating with as Little Debt as Possible

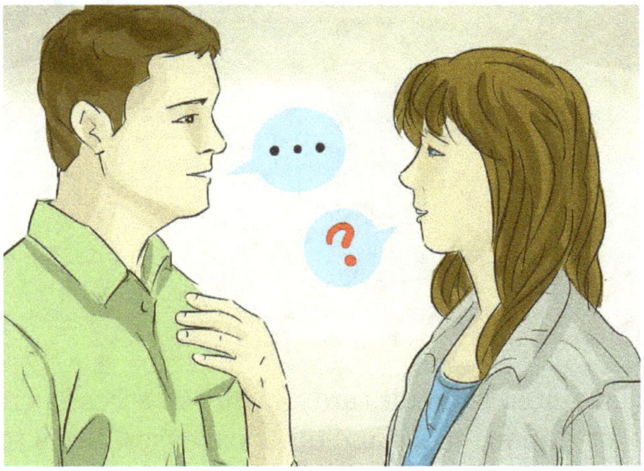

1. Ask a family member to borrow money. Being indebted to a family member at a very low or zero rate of interest is definitely preferable to being indebted to a federal loan servicer. You can avoid a lengthy application process and years of outside debt if you have a family member who's in a position to loan or give you the money needed for school.

- Any loan agreement, even those between family members, should be put into writing.

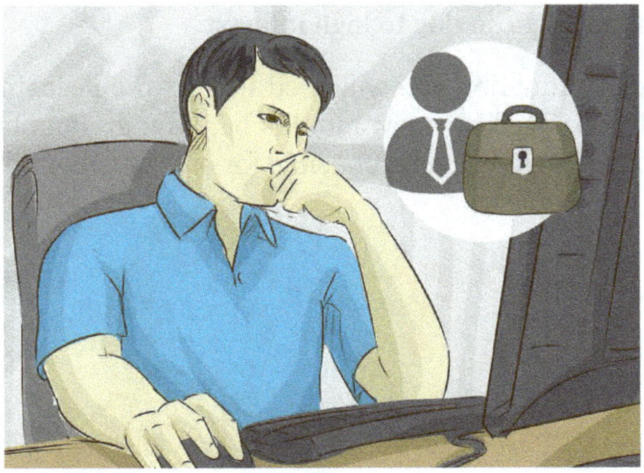

2. Seek part-time work that can help you pay for some of the costs. Most nursing programs are very demanding, and you'll need to devote your focus to completing your coursework, externships, and clinical rotations. If you can manage it, consider obtaining a part-time job to cover part of your tuition, living costs, or other expenses, especially one that's relevant to your studies. Various private and public hospitals offer jobs for student nurses as Undergraduate A.I.N. (Assistant in Nursing), which is also helpful for the course itself.

- Speak with your program's advisors or look for on-campus part-time work.
- Look for doctors in need office help. Check listing online, in classified ads, or visit offices in person.

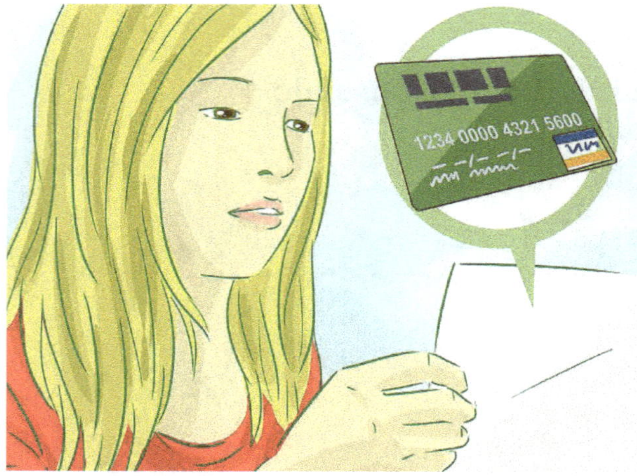

3. Use an interest-free or low-interest credit card. If you can access a credit card with a minimal interest rate, use it to pay for tuition, books and other expenses. Use a rewards or cash back card to earn rewards off the amount you charge to the card. If a grant and scholarship awards are only paying partial tuition, and if you have good enough credit, you can potentially access an interest rate lower than what you'd pay for federal student loans.

- If you've been awarded a total financial aid package that only covers part of your tuition, consider using a card to pay off the rest.
- Be careful of high interest rates when using a credit card. Don't end up paying more money than necessary in the long run due to high interest.
- Be aware that after graduation you will need to pass the licensing test and gain employment. There could very well be a few months between graduation and your first nursing job, so be aware of when you'd be responsible for any loan or credit card repayments.

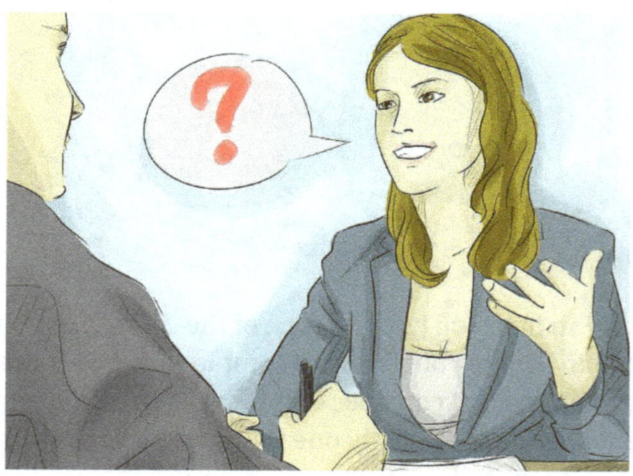

4. Find out about work repayment and student loan forgiveness options. When you're applying for nursing jobs, consider getting a job that offers loan repayment or forgiveness options. This type of financial aid requires that you work for a particular agency or within a particular field of nursing, such as end of life care, for a certain number of years. In return, your employer offers a repayment option once you begin employment.

- Look for federally funded programs, such as the Nursing Education Loan Repayment Program.
- Look for local programs that also offer work repayment and loan forgiveness, such as state health departments.

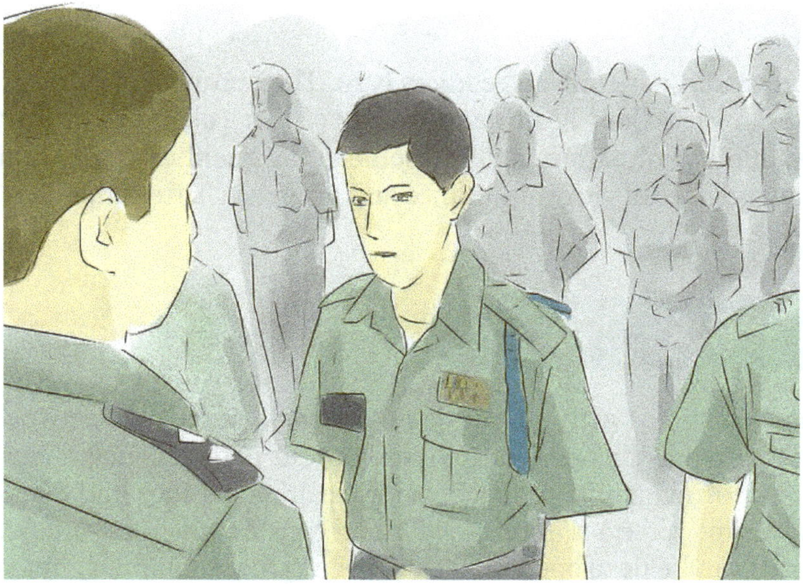

5. Join the military. In addition to public health service, military service can also offer full forgiveness of federal student loan debt. Debt forgiveness programs for public and military service often include consolidating loans to renegotiate a smaller monthly payment. After 120 on-time monthly payments, the remaining balance is forgiven.

Chapter 3 Developing Nursing Skills

Nurses nurture and treat a person who requires care. They provide physical and mental care to persons in order to improve their health and quality of life. Talking to patients, assessing their health, having the ability to empathize, etc. are some of the qualities of a good nurse. The aspects elucidated in this chapter are of vital importance and provide a better understanding of nursing.

How to be a Good Nurse

Being a nurse is more than just getting your degree. Being a nurse requires you to have very specific skills in order to provide the best possible care to your patients, including the core attributes of genuine caring, nurturing, ability to teach, being health conscious and a good communicator. Being a good nurse means you excel at these skills and consider them essential to the work you do everyday. These skills can be developed in advance of a career in nursing, but you may not know your success performing some of these skills until you're on the job.

Method 1

Preparing yourself to be a Good Nurse

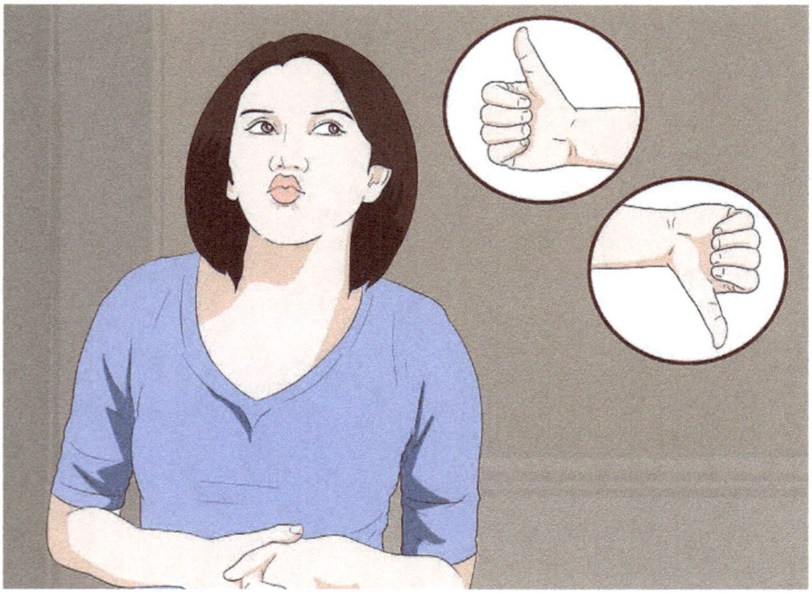

1. Think critically. Nursing is a lot like a game of chess. It's complex and you have to think several moves ahead. You need to be able to assess a patient critically to determine his medical needs, while taking multiple factors and potential outcomes into account.

- Critical thinking is a process by which you review the situation, analyze what's going on, and question what you don't know. You can break the process down into 5 steps:
    - Step 1: Identify the goal, the problem, or the issue.
    - Step 2: Review and diagnose the goal, problem, or issue. What information do you have available about the goal, problem, or issue? Based on the information you have, what's the best resolution?
    - Step 3: Explore your options. Think about what the resolutions may be, and how and who would actually achieve them.
    - Step 4: Actually carry out the resolution. Get it done.
    - Step 5: Reflect on your success or failure. What went well and what didn't go so well? What can you do better or differently next time? How do we learn from this experience?

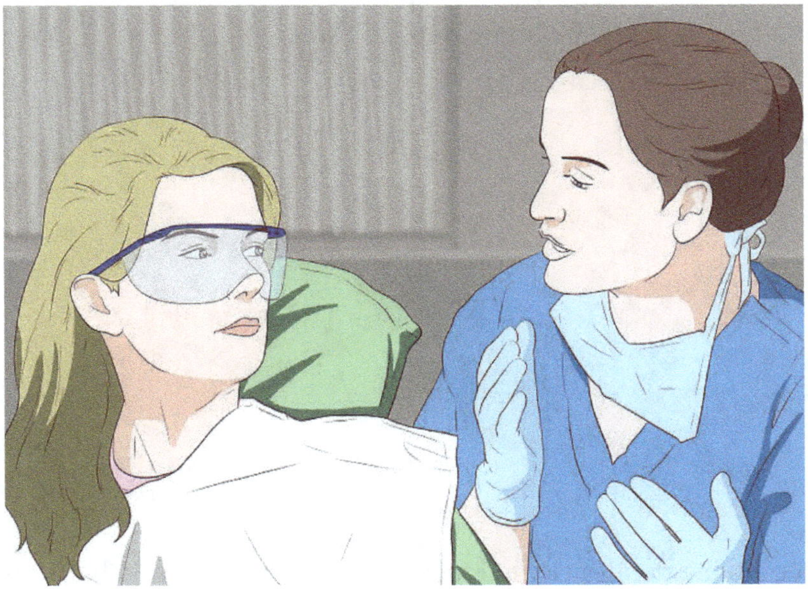

2. Communicate effectively. Nurses need to be able to communicate with their patients in order to understand how their patients are feeling and what they are concerned about. Communicating effectively means you can listen well when someone else is speaking to you, and that you can speak clearly and concisely to someone else (e.g. patient, doctor, other nurses, family members, etc.). As a nurse you're also likely to make a lot of notes whether in a physical chart or on the computer, therefore you must also be able to communicate effectively in writing as you may not be there in person to explain what you meant.

- Keep in mind that you will be dealing with many different nationalities, including people who may not speak the same language as you or the doctor. Find out what services are available to the patient to help them communicate effectively – are there interpreters on staff? Are you aware of any cultural beliefs or practices that might interfere with their health?

- As a good nurse you need to be able to listen to a doctor's instructions and carry out those instructions quickly without needing to clarify every detail. In order to do this you need to be able to listen to the doctor in what is likely a fast-paced and hectic environment while you're doing something else. At the same time, don't hesitate to ask questions to clarify what is needed. Doctors, just as nurses, need to communicate effectively. If it is not clear what the physician/provider is trying to relay, keep asking questions.
- An exceptional nurse not only listens and carries out instruction, they advocate for their patients. Because of your excellent listening skills, you've developed an understanding of your patients, how they feel, and what they want. You should also understand that your patients may be a little intimidated speaking up and asking their doctor specific questions, or making requests. As their nurse, you may need to do the speaking up for your patients. Encourage your patient to write down questions that they want answered and that you know them as well to help facilitate questions. If the patient can not ask them, then ask the questions for your patient.

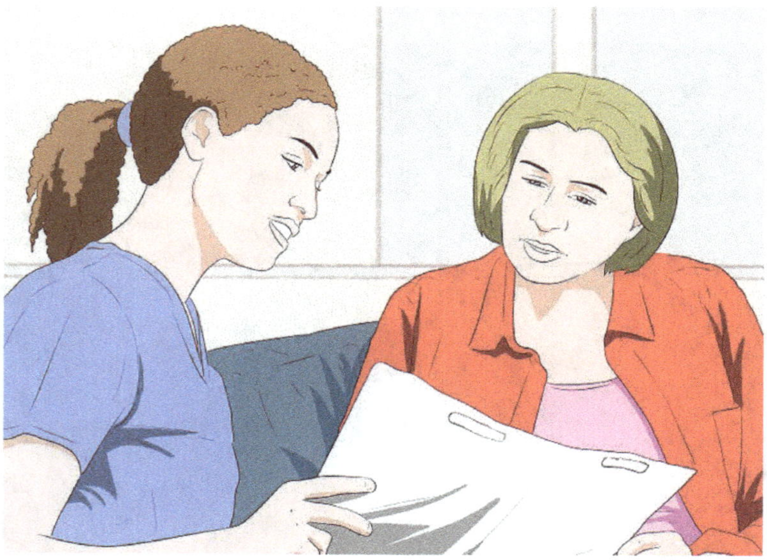

3. Be detail-oriented. Being detail-oriented means you pay attention to both the big stuff and the small stuff. When dealing with a patient, even the smallest anomaly or symptom can be a big deal, so you need to always be paying attention. Being detail-oriented means you ensure all your patients get the exact treatment they need, when they need it.

- While not exactly the same, being detail-oriented has a lot to do with being organized. It's easier to pay attention to the details when you are organized.
- Detail-oriented also means being accurate. In the medical field you can't estimate or guess at the amount of medication you give a patient, you need to be accurate. Your patient's life may depend on it.
- Being detail-oriented also means paying attention. Getting distracted or allowing your mind to wander will likely result in you missing something important. Because all details regarding your patient's care are critical, you need to remain focused and on task at all times.

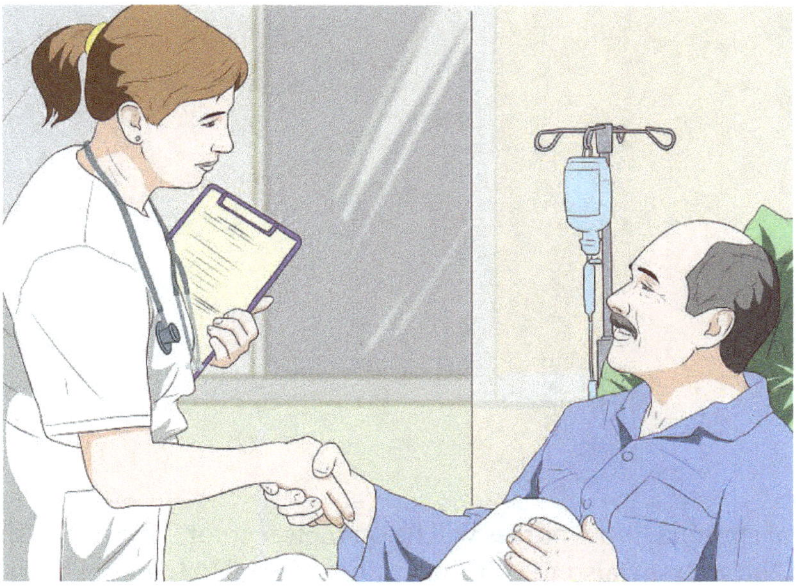

4. Organize efficiently. Nurses, especially those working in a hospital, need to deal with multiple patients at the same time. Each patient has their own personal requirements that are critical to their well-being. Each patient also has his or her own personality and emotional needs. As a nurse you need to be able to organize yourself to keep track of who each of your patients are, what their treatments are, when they need their treatments, and the small details about the patient that will help them feel better (both physically and emotionally). Being able to organize yourself efficiently means being able to do the following things when needed:

- Learning to say no. While you may not be able to say no very often at work, you can certainly say no in your personal life. Sometimes being able to clear out all the stuff you don't really want to be doing will lower your stress level overall and help you become more focused when you're at work.
- Finding balance in your life. There is such a thing called caregiver burn out. Always ask yourself before accepting an extra shift: what the benefit it and what is the cost? If the cost is personal loss of perceived health, sleep, enjoyment, then the extra money is not worth it.
- Asking for help. If you are new to the nursing field, you are going to need to ask for help. Don't be afraid to ask, just ask. Once you've asked chances are you're going to be able to move forward with what you need to do, and understand how to efficiently carry out that task the next time.
- Prioritizing. Being organized means being able to prioritize all the tasks you have on your to do list. Knowing which ones are more important or which ones have the earliest due dates.
- Spending your time wisely. Think about all the things you need to do in the next little while, and carry those tasks out efficiently. If you need to go to the storeroom for one thing, think about all the things you need in there over the next little while so you only have to make one trip. Don't waste your time doing repetitive and unnecessary tasks.

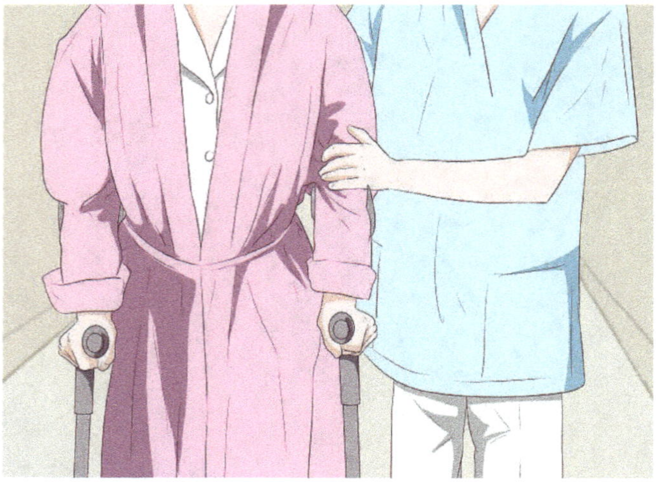

5. Maintain physical stamina. Most nurses will be on their feet for their entire shift, which can last 12 hours or more. Nurses may also need to restrain patients, help patients walk from one place to another, hold patients up, move patients to and from a bed or gurney, and other physically demanding tasks. If you aren't up to the physical requirements of the job, you will likely be in a lot of pain at the end of a shift.

- Personal health must be observed first — how can you advise health-related behavior if you do not observe it yourself?
- Physical stamina isn't just about being able to do physical activities, it's about being able to do them over a long period of time, over and over again.
- As a nurse you're allowed to wear scrubs and comfortable shoes — take advantage of this. There is nothing worse than being on your feet for 12 hours in shoes that are really painful.

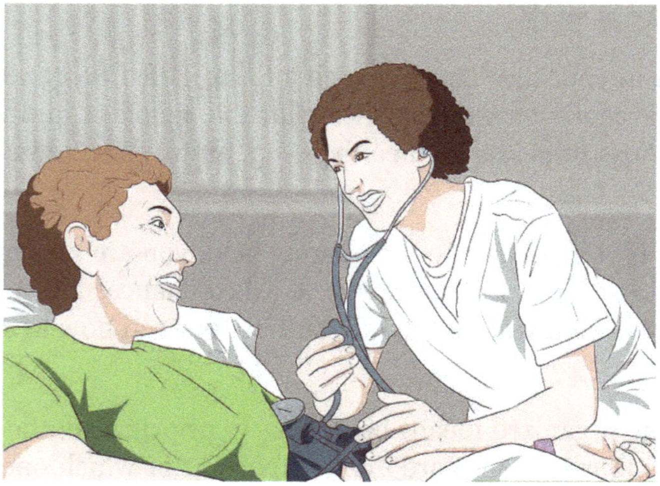

6. React and think quickly. The medical profession in general isn't the type of profession where you can always just sit back and "wait and see." In many cases, as a nurse, you'll notice something and need to react to it quickly. You won't always get the chance to pause and evaluate all the options and debate back and forth with another nurse as to the best course of action — sometimes you just need to act.

- Being able to think and react quickly comes with experience and confidence. The more experience and confidence you gain, the faster your ability to react will become.
- Thinking and reacting quickly can also include knowing when it's time to get help from someone else ASAP. Don't worry if you may be overreacting or if someone will have a bad opinion of you because you bothered them, those things aren't important. Keep in mind that your patient's well-being is always the most important thing and react quickly when that well-being is in jeopardy.
- Reacting quickly doesn't mean forgoing critical thinking; it means going through the critical thinking process quickly and carrying out your decision immediately.

Method 2

Learning on the Job

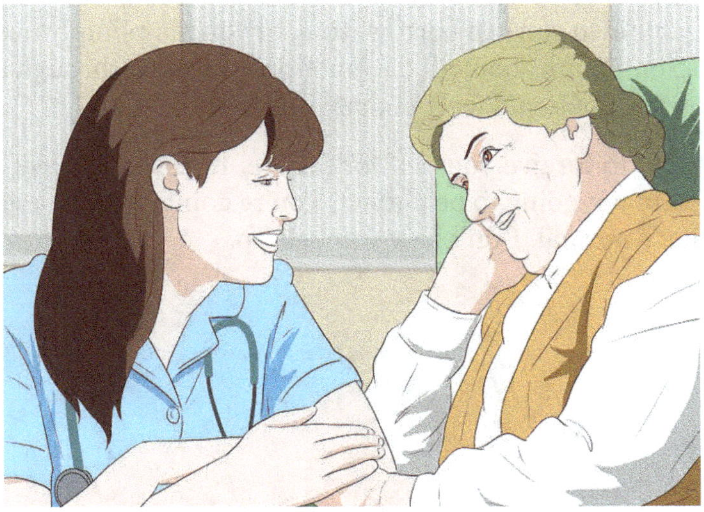

1. Understand and have the ability to be compassionate. One of a nurse's main jobs is to take direct care of patients. You'll likely see these people at their worst. Nurses need to understand that their patients are human beings that are probably stressed, scared, depressed, upset, in pain, and confused. This understanding requires the ability to be compassionate and empathetic. Being able to put yourself in your patient's shoes will help you understand what she's going through, and what she needs from you.

- Often times, because a patient sees nurses most often, those nurses get the brunt of any anger the patient is feeling. Being compassionate and empathetic means you do not take this anger personally. Patients are likely sick or injured and not having a very good day! Understanding that some patients may need to release their anger in order to reduce their stress or fear is what being compassionate is all about.
- In addition to patients, nurses often deal with the family and friends of their patients. Being compassionate and empathetic means being able to show those family members and friends that you truly do care about your patient and are doing your absolute best to help her.

- The following six steps can help you learn to be a more compassionate person:
    - Step 1: Listen without judgement or formulating an immediate response. Try to understand the person's feelings, needs, and wants so that you can formulate a plan to best help her.
    - Step 2: Reply back to the speaker based on her emotions and not her words. For example, mean and angry words are likely a sign of someone who is scared or fearful.
    - Step 3: Make sure you have someone who is compassionate to you. This means having your own support system at or outside of work. If you have a million problems on your mind, it may be harder to care about the problems of others.
    - Step 4: Think about the whole person, not just who she is at that very moment. You're going to see many people at their worst, but that's not who they really are. Remember that there is much more to your patients than just what you see.
    - Step 5: Think about a time when you were in a similar situation. You may have an actual memory of your own you can borrow from, or you may simply need to imagine yourself in that situation. Think about all the emotions you went through (or would go through) and how you felt (or would feel) in that situation.
    - Step 6: Be able to forgive yourself for failure. In essence, have some compassion for yourself. You're not going to be perfect. You're going to make mistakes. But you're human, and that's normal. Don't beat yourself up.

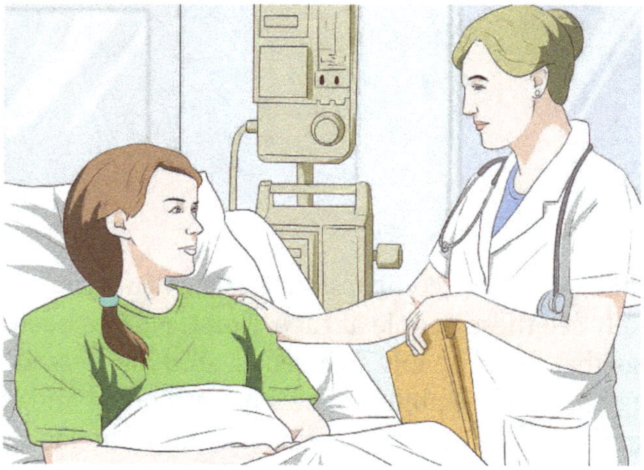

2. Have emotional stability. Being a nurse means you're going to see people at their very worst. You'll likely have to take care of patients who are about to die. You may need to take care of patients in an extreme amount of pain. You may need to take care of patients who have just been diagnosed with a life-threatening illness. Constantly being around people who are suffering can take an emotional toll on you. As a nurse you need to be able to control your emotions while you're on the job, and not allow those emotions to cloud your judgement or slow your reaction time.

- Being emotionally stable doesn't mean keeping all your emotions bottled-up forever. It means knowing when the time is right for letting those emotions out. And allowing yourself that emotional release on a regular basis. Try exercise, time with friends, yoga, reading, and developing hobbies.

- Emotional stability also doesn't mean developing an ice-cold personality where you do not allow yourself to care about anything. You need to allow yourself to care about your patients in order to provide them with compassion and empathy.
- Having, or being able to have, emotional stability may mean you have to do certain things outside of work so you're able to control your emotions at work. One helpful way to develop stable emotions and have better control over your mood is to practice mindfulness. This means being in the moment without thinking about the past, the future, or anything judgmental.

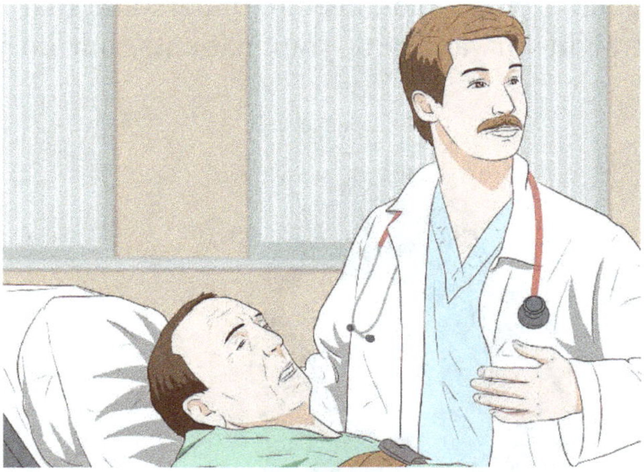

3. Take responsibility. Being a responsible nurse means not cutting any corners. Not allowing yourself to make an error, but if you do, making sure the proper people know about the error you made and making sure it's corrected as soon as possible. Being responsible also means using your best judgement when evaluating a patients' needs and making good decisions that are in the best interests of your patients.

- If you are a nurse that works in an emergency room or an operating room, or something similar, you also need to be responsible with your time. You need to understand that things do not always go as planed, and emergencies do not happen on a schedule that matches your shifts. A good nurse is prepared to work longer if necessary and understand that's just part of the job.

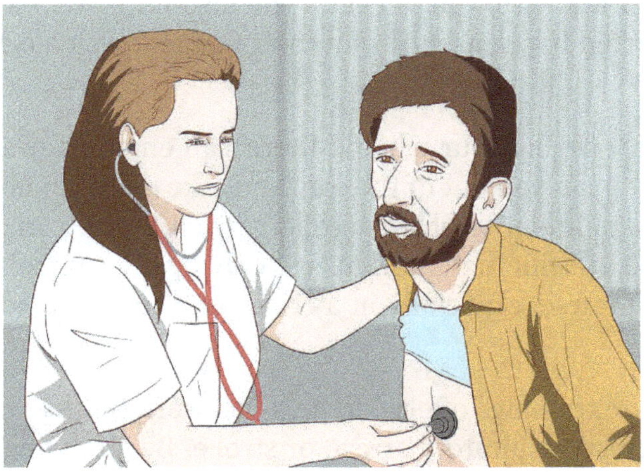

4. Respect everyone. In addition to being compassionate, empathetic, and sympathetic to your patients and their needs, you also need to be respectful and non-judgemental about the decisions

your patient has made in life. It is not up to you, as a nurse, to judge your patients. It is up to you to help them and make sure they leave you care in the best possible condition — regardless of how they may have ended up in your care in the first place. It also means not treating patients differently because of their backgrounds, ethnicity, or personality. A homeless man who is being treated for a drug overdose deserves just as much respect from you as a pregnant woman who has been hit by a car.

- Being respectful of your patients also means being truthful with them. When communicating news — good or bad — you need to understand that the patient has the right to honesty. Be straight-forward with your patients, but do it respectfully and with compassion.

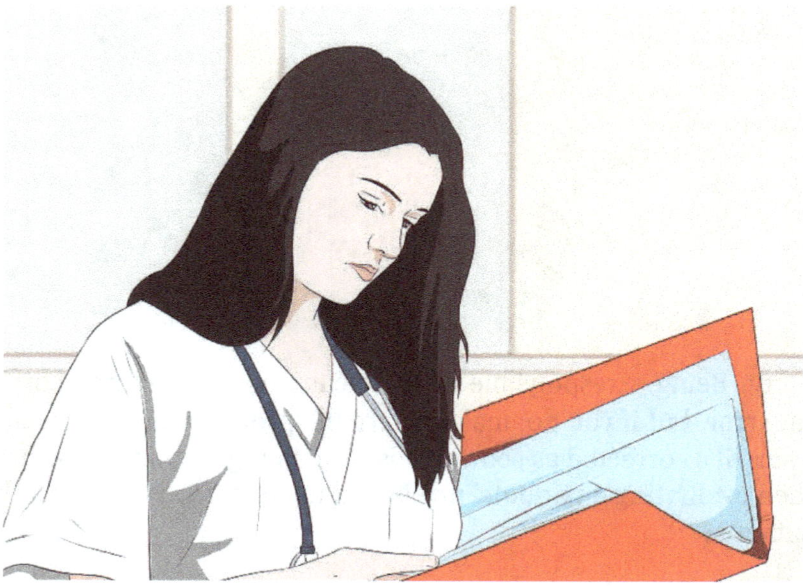

5. Keep calm under pressure and during a crisis. Keeping calm means maintaining your level-headedness. It means having confidence in what you're doing and the decisions you're making. Your confidence will grow not only throughout your education, but the longer you're on the job. And as such, your ability to remain calm will also improve. As a nurse, you can't panic when something unexpected happens, and you can't freeze up because you aren't sure what to do.

- When you're first learning your job and there's an emergency situation, a more experienced nurses may push you out of the way and take over. Do not take this personally or be upset. Use this moment to observe exactly what's going on, what the nurse is doing and how, and the specific details that are driving the nurse's decisions. Watching a more experienced nurse, especially in a crisis, can be one of your most useful learning experiences.
- Find out if there are trainings offered to help you work through specific scenarios such as sudden cardiac arrest, respiratory arrest, or stroke. By attending these trainings, you can practice going through these steps in a less intense environment so that in the real situation, you will be able to work through it easier.

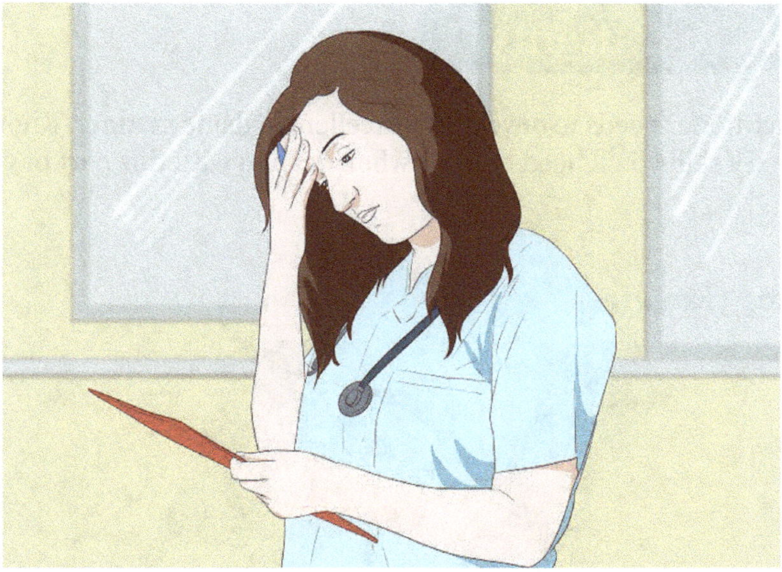

6. Adapt to new and constantly changing situations. As a nurse no two days will ever be the same. While you may have some routine, it is likely that that routine will also change every now and again. No two patients are going to behave the same, even when they're getting the exact same treatment. Nurses need to be adaptable and flexible. Nurses need to understand that their work environment and job requirements will change on a daily basis. Being flexible and adaptable, and just going with the flow, will not only help your day go smoother, it will help reduce the amount of stress you feel.

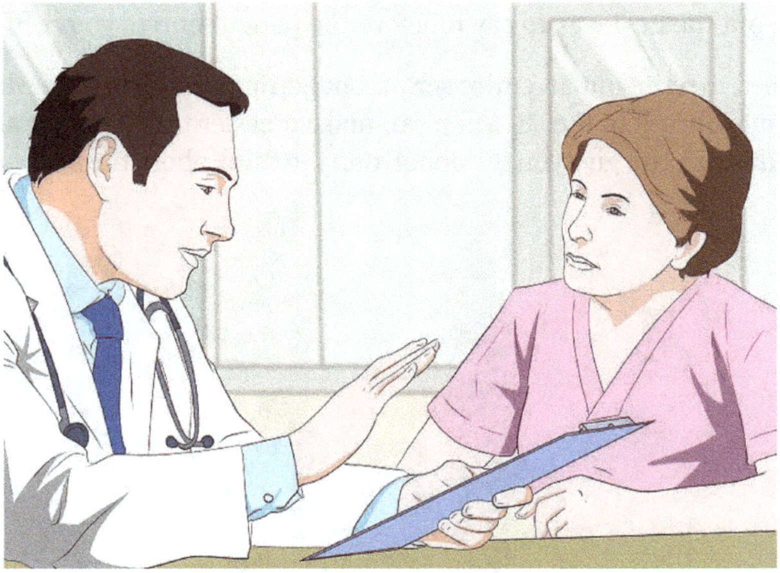

7. Improve your knowledge constantly. Nurses, just like many professions, are constantly learning. Whether they learn through a formal classroom environment, or simply by observing, doesn't matter. What matters is that you are constantly improving your knowledge and skills, and recognizing specific areas where you might need improvement. It also means receiving feedback from your peers and supervisors critically, and working with your supervisor and others to correct any deficiencies you have with your skills.

How to Talk to Patients

A good medical practitioner needs to develop an excellent bedside manner. Knowing how to talk to patients is the primary skill you'll need to hone when dealing with this part of your practice.

Part 1

Mastering Basic Strategies

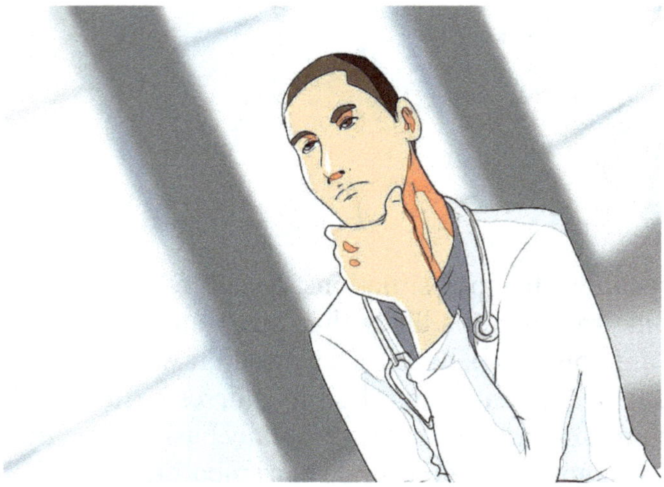

1. Think about what you want to say before saying it. When you already know what needs to be said, start planning out the best way to say it before the patient enters your office.

- You don't need to write out an entire script, but getting a basic idea of what needs to be said before you put yourself in the situation can make it easier to remember all the necessary details. Doing this can also give you the opportunity to think about the best way to phrase things.

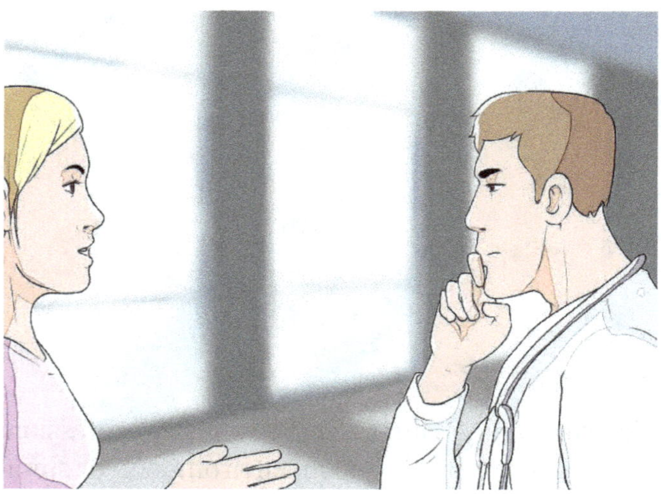

2. Become an active listener. Ask the patient plenty of open-ended questions about his or her concerns. Pay close attention to the patient's responses, and parrot those responses back to the patient.

- Watch for both verbal and nonverbal responses.
- Repeating your patient's replies can clarify the situation for you while assuring the patient that his or her concerns are being addressed.

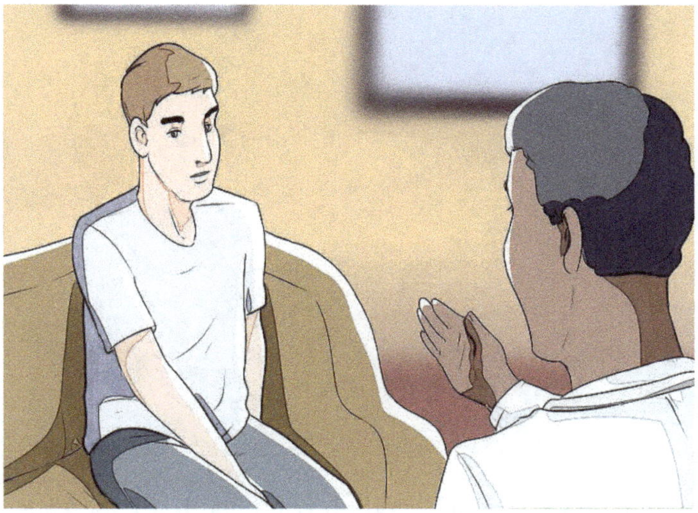

3. Address the needs of the whole patient. The patient is more than a medical specimen. You need to view the patient as a whole being with unique fears, beliefs, and circumstances.

- Respect all of the beliefs your patient holds, even if you disagree with them.
- Encourage the patient to ask questions and address those questions fully.

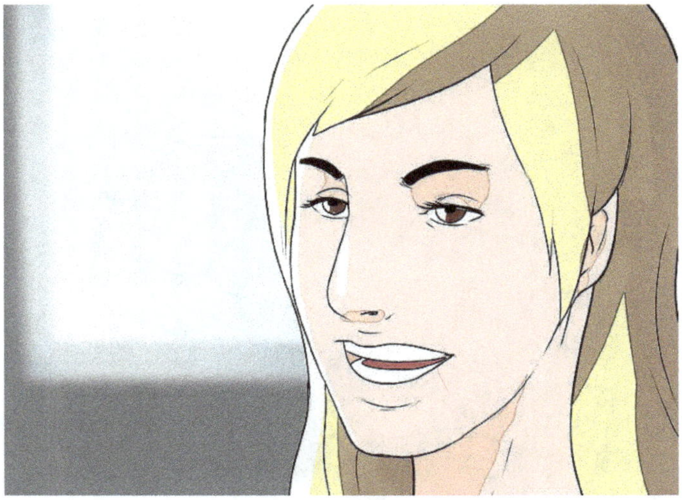

4. Speak in plain English. Abandon as much formal medical terminology as possible and speak to the patient in layman's terms. Speak slowly and clearly to avoid unnecessary confusion.

- When describing important information about a condition or treatment, separate that information into small chunks. Let each chunk sink in before continuing.
- Only provide technical details when asked. Too much complicated detail can overwhelm many patients.

- Some say that in the United States, the average person's reading comprehension is stuck at a sixth grade level. Try translating the words you would use to describe the situation to another doctor into words a sixth grader might use.

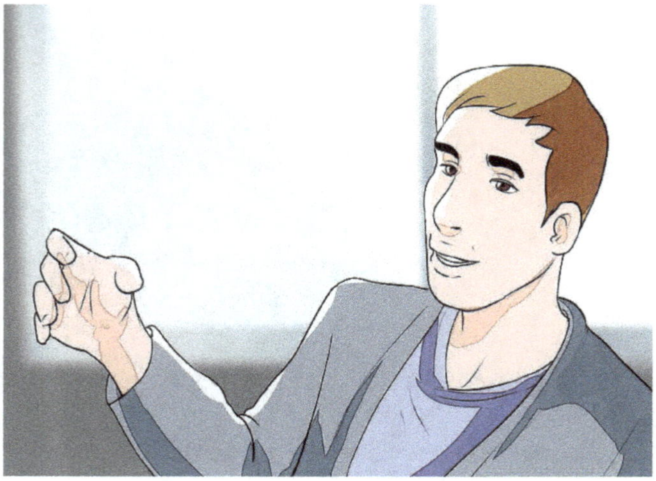

5. Base your discussion on past experiences. When you need to explain the significance of certain actions, try framing your explanation in past experiences the patient will understand.

- If the patient has recently been to the hospital, explain how neglecting a certain treatment plan may make hospitalization necessary again.
- When the patient's family or friends have experienced a similar illness, talk about the good and bad ways the loved one's illness was handled.

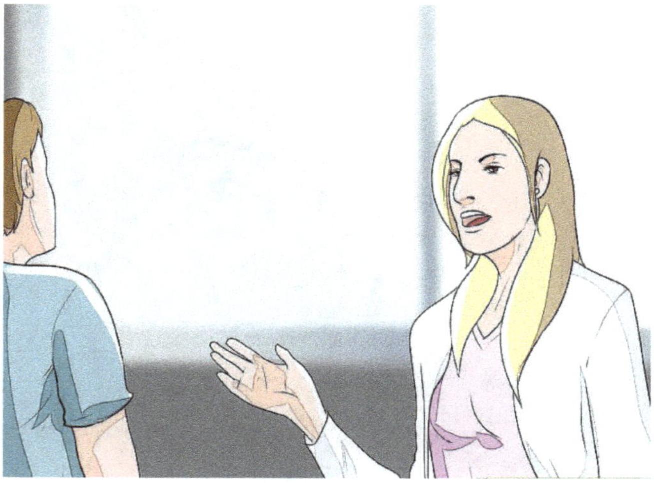

6. Accurately and thoroughly educate the patient. The information you disclose about illnesses, conditions, and treatments must be true and complete.

- Offer an understandable definition of the diagnosis. Spell out what it means for the patient's short-term and long-term wellness.
- Describe the expected course of treatment and the anticipated outcome. If there are alternative treatments, describe those, as well.

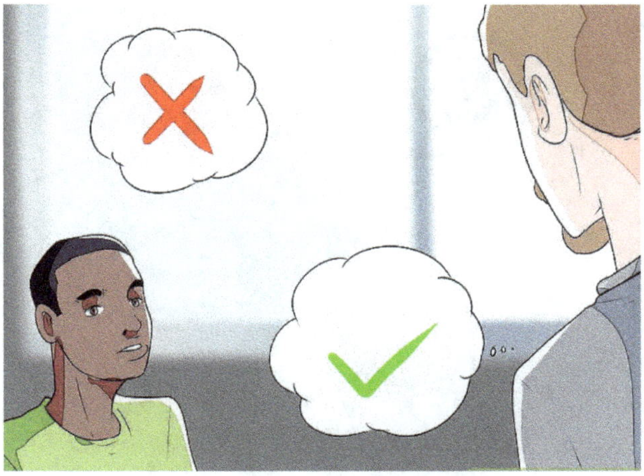

7. Verify comprehension. After telling the patient all he or she needs to know, ask the individual to repeat what you said. Doing so will let you know if your explanation was clear enough.

- Correct any misunderstandings immediately.
- You can also provide sources for additional information if the patient seems eager to learn more once he or she leaves.

Part 2

Meeting New Patients

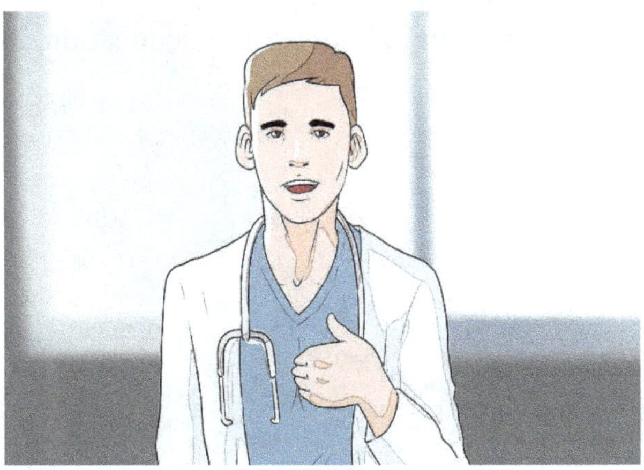

1. Introduce yourself carefully. When meeting a patient for the first time, you should introduce yourself by stating that, as a doctor, your primary concern is taking care of the patient in the best way possible.

- Let the patient know that you intend to listen to his or her concerns and beliefs, and to accommodate those ideas when determining treatment plans.
- Assure the patient that he or she can bring up anything without facing the fear of condemnation or ridicule.
- By introducing yourself as the patient's ally, it might be easier to establish a healthy doctor-patient relationship.

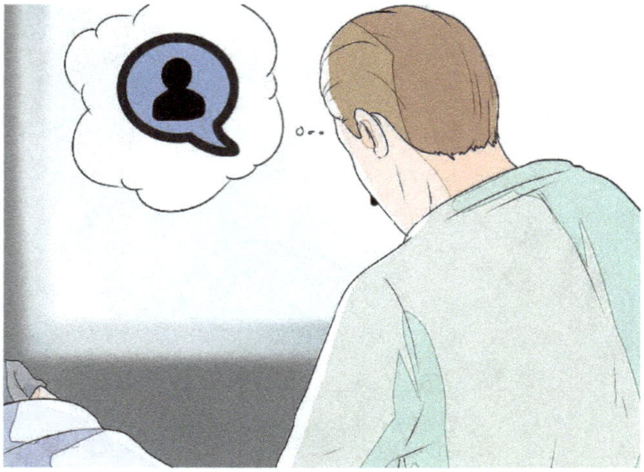

2. Break the ice with small talk. Small talk creates a relaxed, friendly environment that your patient may feel more comfortable in. You can lead in with a bit of small talk, weave it into the appointment when appropriate, and/or conclude on a lighthearted note.

- Small talk can be used when you first meet a patient and when you interact with that patient from then on.
- Impersonal topics of conversation may include the weather, the economy, recent medical news, or similar current events.
- If you think you'll be establishing a long-term professional relationship with the patient, personal topics of conversation might be appropriate. Talk about your family and ask about your patient's family. Discuss your patient's career, education, likes, and dislikes.

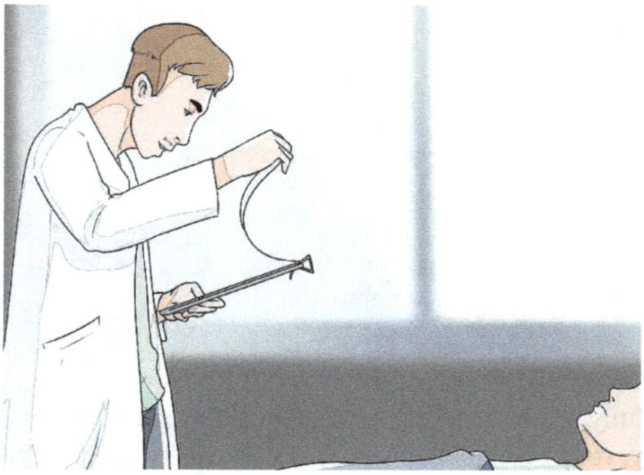

3. Double-check the patient's medical history. You should already have your patient's medical history in front of you, but when it may still be a good idea to ask for confirmation about critical points in the midst of discussion.

- Ask for clarification on any point that is not clear in your patient's records.
- Review the family medical history of your patient and ask if any illnesses related to the diagnosis run in the family line.

- Before prescribing a certain medication, ask if the patient has ever experienced any negative side effects to a medication in the past.

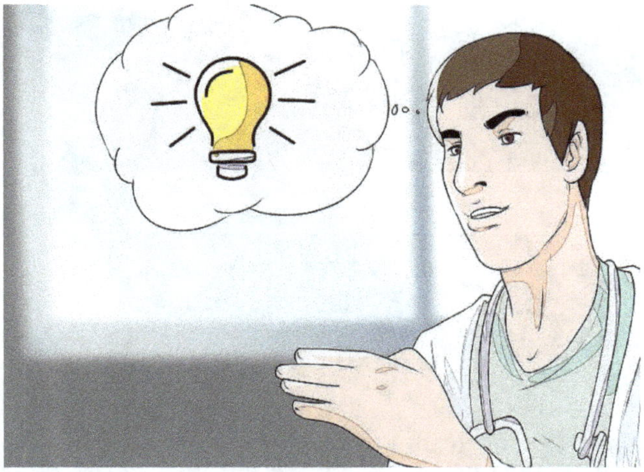

4. Ask about the patient's values and ideas. Ask the patient if there are any beliefs you should take into consideration from the start. Regardless of the answer, you should also gauge additional values and goals as you interact with the patient over time.

- Ask open-ended questions to determine what your patient believes. When dealing with a patient who has a deadly illness, you might ask, "What makes life worth living?" Depending on the response, you might be able to determine how far a patient is willing to go in order to survive.
- Keep asking questions until you have a fairly complete picture of the patient's perspective.

Part 3

Using Nonverbal Communication

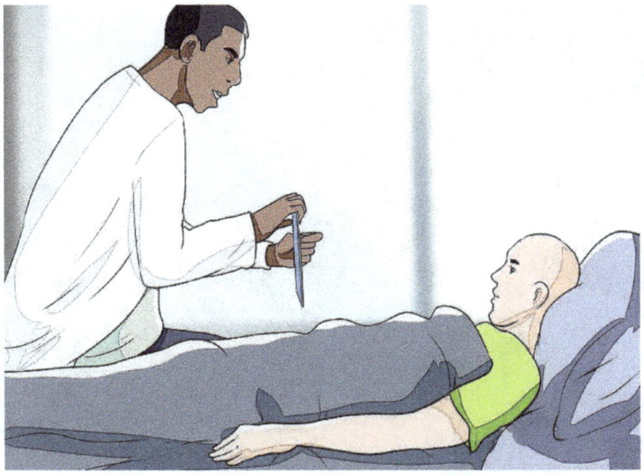

1. Use visuals. The use of visuals can help a patient understand concepts that would otherwise be hard to imagine.

- When possible, look for diagrams and charts that show the anatomy of the area you're dealing with.

- If you cannot find a diagram or chart, compare abstract concepts using concrete analogies and mental images.

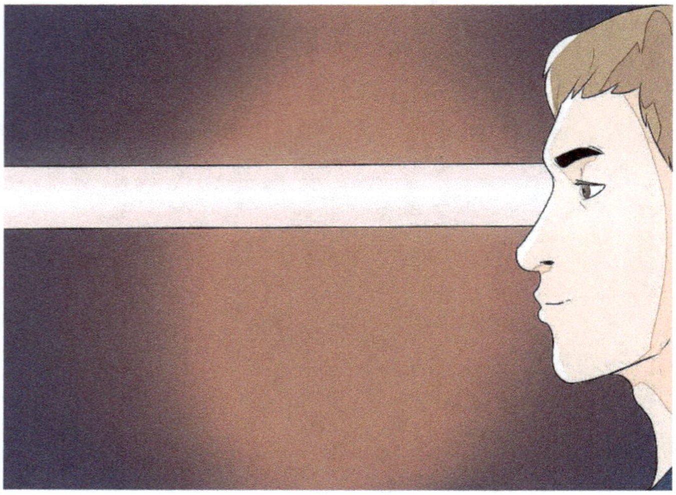

2. Be engaged. Let the patient know that you are actively engaged in the appointment by maintaining eye contact and being attentive.

- There may be times when you need to look over medical charts and equipment, but you should typically make eye contact with the patient during at least half of the appointment. It is especially important to maintain eye contact when listening to your patient's concerns and questions.
- Making eye contact also gives you the chance to observe the nonverbal communication your patient is using toward you.

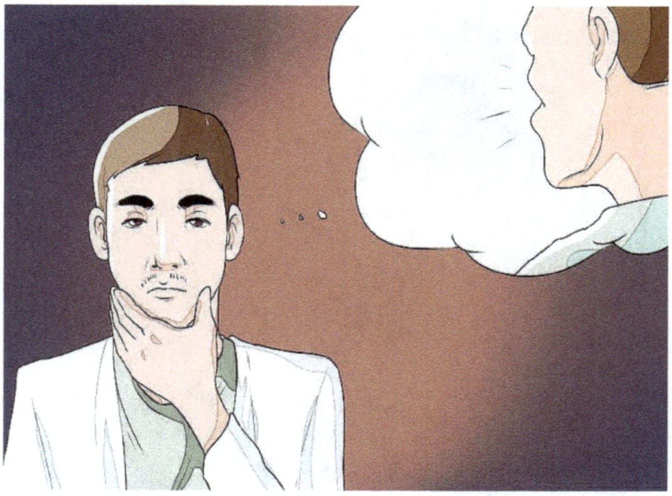

3. Monitor your tone of voice. Your tone should be firm and professional, but it should also be fairly friendly.

- The idea is to create a comfortable ambiance rather than one that feels cold or strict. Your patient also needs to feel confident in your abilities, though, so you should always maintain an air of certainty and professionalism.

Part 4

Discussing Difficult Topics

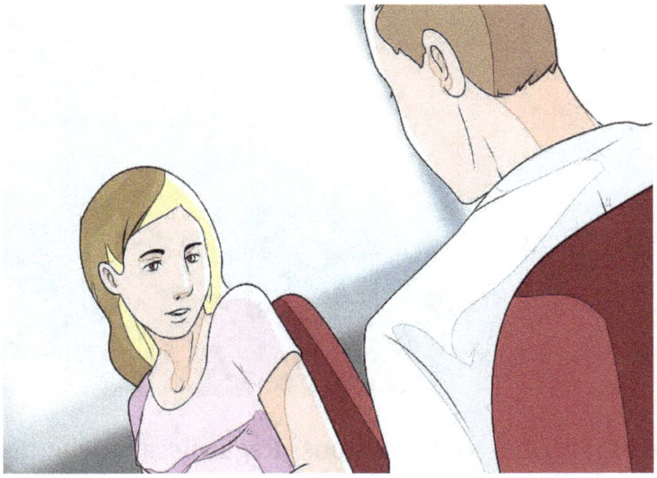

1. Bring up difficult topics before a crisis occurs. As soon as a patient is diagnosed with an illness or condition, or becomes at risk for developing such a disease, you should begin discussing some of the tough decisions that may need to be addressed.

- This can include anything from radical treatments to end-of-life care.
- The ideal place to discuss tough decisions is in your office, not in a hospital. Patients are more likely to make wise, calm decisions when in a low-stress environment.

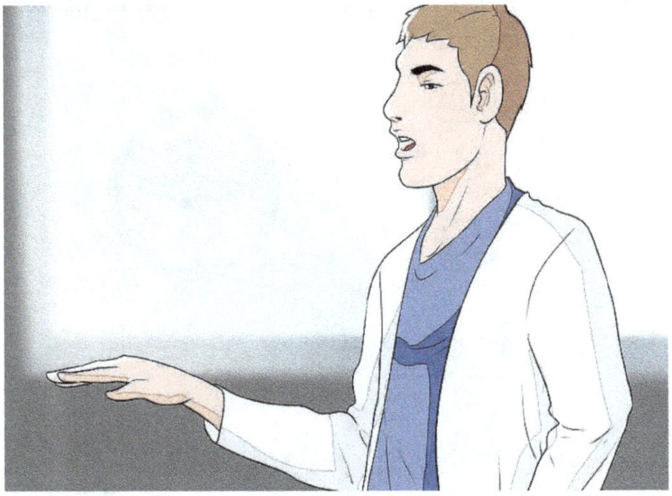

2. Take your time discussing major decisions. Some circumstances may require an immediate decision, but usually, a patient can afford to take a few days or weeks to think things over.

- Stress the urgency of making a decision, but back off and allow the patient to take as much time as possible when reaching that decision.
- Decisions made in haste are often regretted. One goal you should have is to limit your regrets and the patient's regrets.

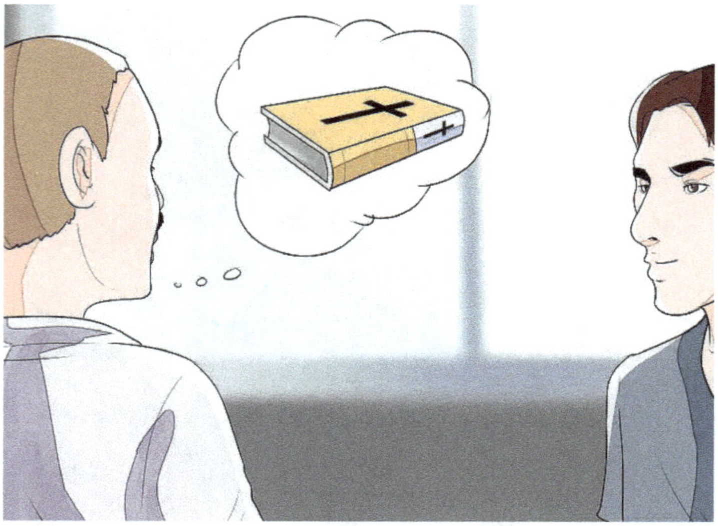

3. Understand the value of faith-based discussions. Regardless of whether or not you share your patient's faith and religious beliefs, there can be a lot of benefit to the patient if you encourage and respect those beliefs.

- If you have spiritual beliefs of your own and your patient asks about them, feel free to share your thoughts. Doing so can actually provide a good dose of comfort to the patient when things are tough.
- If you do not feel comfortable taking on this topic yourself, you can direct your patient to someone who can address it. Encourage the patient to seek pastoral counsel. Guide the patient to the chaplain at a nearby hospital or recommend a professional counselor who is equipped to discuss faith-based matters.

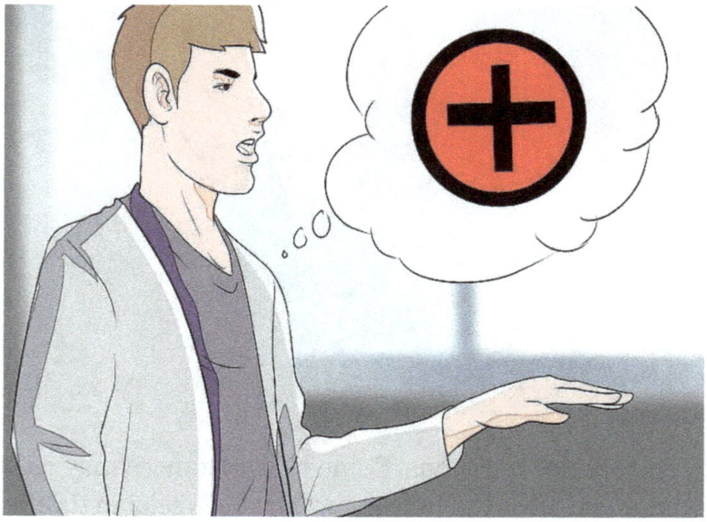

4. Affirm positive beliefs. Even when a situation looks grim from a medical perspective, you should affirm the patient's desire to hope and fight through the condition or illness.

- This doesn't mean giving false hope, however. When the odds of recovery are low, you should be honest about that fact.

- This does mean allowing for the existence of hope. Do not completely rule out the possibility of something positive happening, even when a full recovery is out of the question.

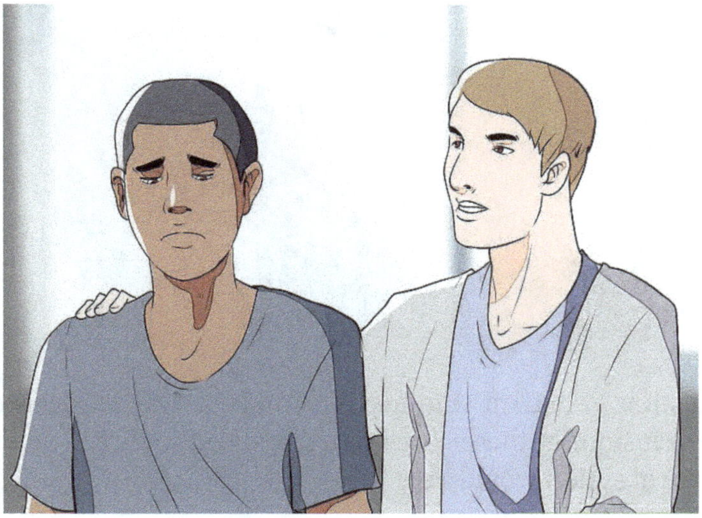

5. Take your dialogue to the place your patient is at. Regardless of how hopeful the patient or family feels, you need to take your dialogue to their level.

- When a patient is praying for a miracle, you can say that you pray or hope for one, too.
- If the patient has accepted the inevitability of succumbing to his or her illness, you do not need to pressure the patient into acting more hopeful. You should, however, discuss different ways to make the patient's current life more pleasant in spite of the illness.

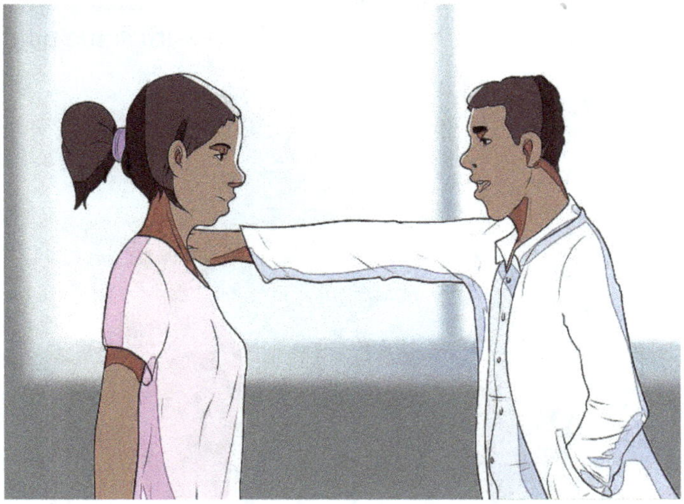

6. Reassure the patient about your commitment. Tell the patient that you will stick with him or her throughout the duration of the illness and treatment. When someone receives frightening news, a knowledgeable ally can be a source of great comfort and support.

- If most of the treatment will be performed by other doctors, you should still assure your patient that you will continue to stay updated and are more than willing to discuss your patient's concerns and treatment as time continues to pass.

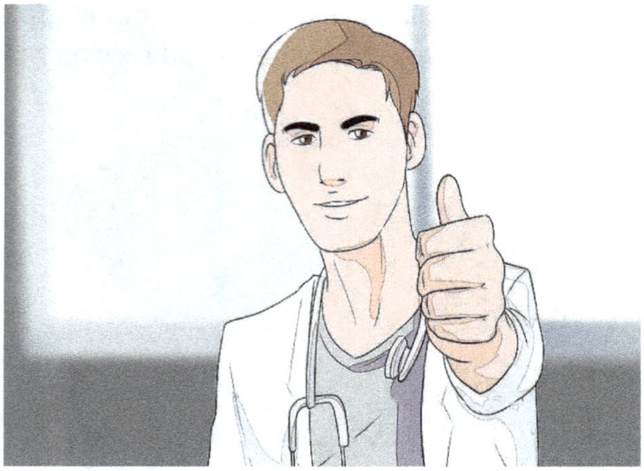

7. Make the best suggestion. A patient who needs to make a difficult decision may feel too overwhelmed to reach a conclusion. In these cases, you may need to directly tell the patient what you believe the wisest course of action would be.

- Present your recommendation as a suggestion and explain why you believe it to be the best option. Do not pressure your patient into accepting that suggestion, though.

How to Deal with the Elderly

No one wants to face the fact that their parents and other family members are aging. It's scary and stressful, and it can seem like a daunting task to plan for or take on their care. However, you can make sure that your elderly loved ones are healthy, happy, and safe with some planning and assistance.

Part 1

Managing Difficult Behavior

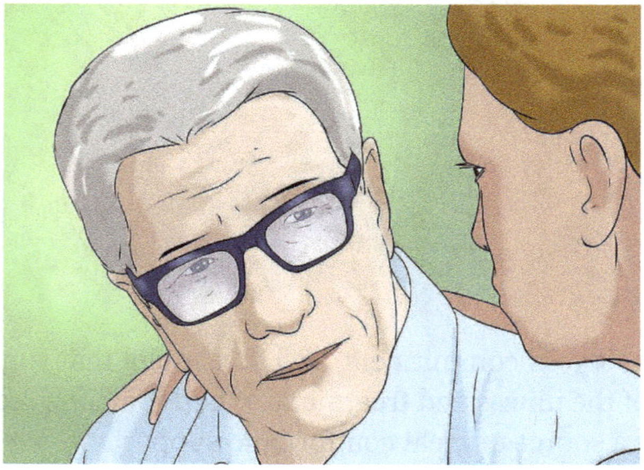

1. Examine old dynamics. If your relationship has had the same power structure for a long time, old patterns will begin to emerge. If you are caring for someone who has always been controlling or critical, this dynamic will continue.

- If the behavior is very old, changing it is unlikely. Ask yourself what is and is not acceptable. If you feel that the behavior is abusive toward you, then you will need to either have a discussion about boundaries, or enlist someone to help you with caregiving.
- Sometimes difficult behavior is new and unrelated to old dynamics. If this is the case, you should try to determine a cause.

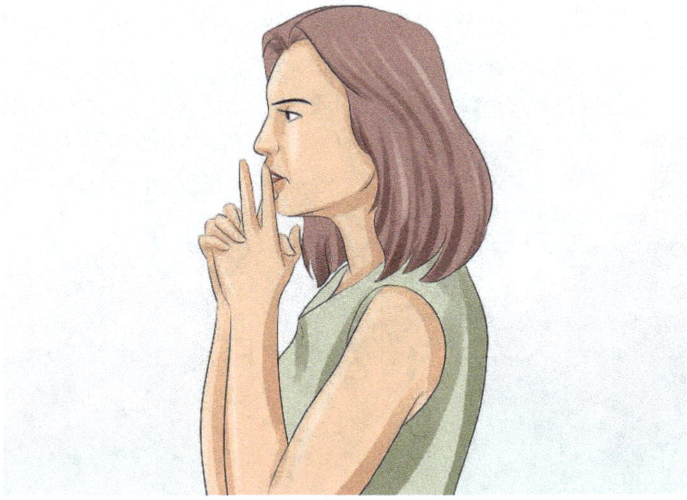

2. Understand the cause of the behavior. If difficult behavior is a big break from old patterns of behavior, it is usually caused by the traumas of aging. Have a discussion about what might be bothering them.

- It's not a good idea to bring up what might be bothering them while they are having an outburst. Try to wait until they are calmer.
- Do not blame them. Say, "I notice some things have been bothering you more. What can I do to help you out when you're dealing with them?"

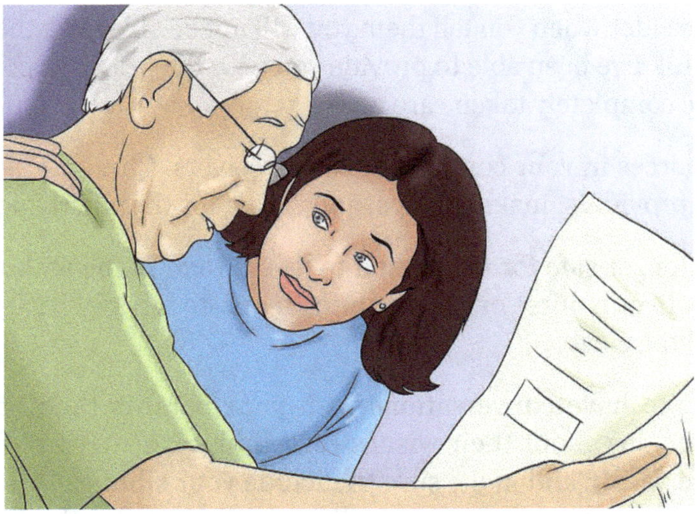

3. Set boundaries. If an elderly person has become too controlling or aggressive, you may start to dread visiting. When it begins to significantly impact your quality of life, it is time to confront them about it.

- When confronting them, make sure that you stress that you love them. Say, "I am always going to love you, no matter what, as long as you live."
- Then tell them why you are having trouble. "If you continue this behavior, though, I am not going to want to spend as much time around you or visit you as often."
- Finish by appealing to their dignity. "I am telling you this because I want you to help me by ending this behavior. That way we can make the most of this time we have together."

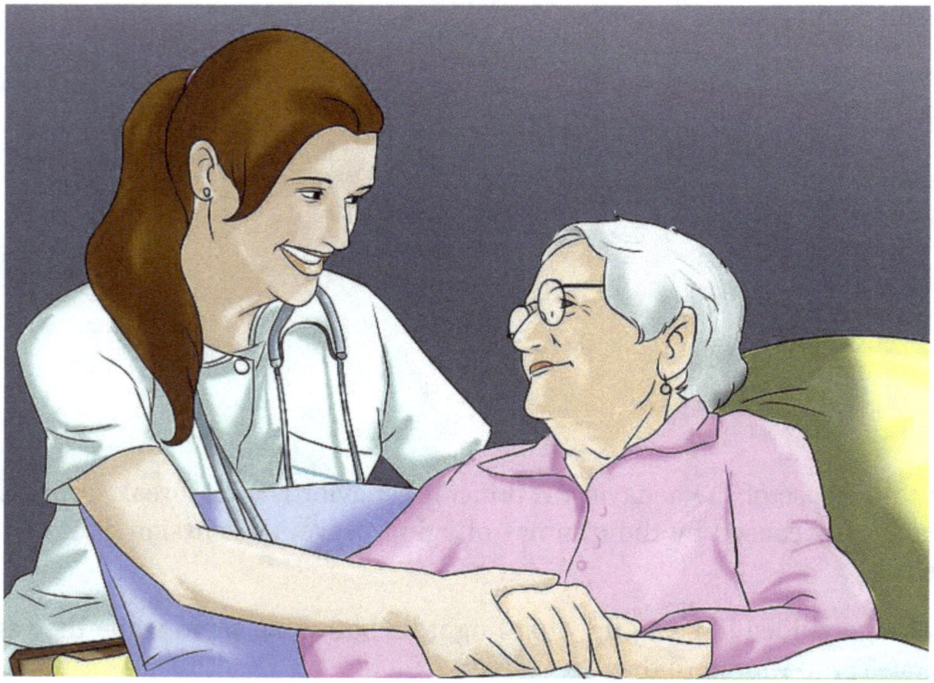

4. Utilize other sources of care. If an elder's difficult behavior is driving you to depression, you may have to distance yourself.

- Don't blame the elder when you tell them you will not be able to be the sole provider of care. Say, "I don't think I've been able to provide you with the best care possible. I want to make sure that you're completely taken care of."
- Search for resources in your community for caregivers. Check for advice and guidance in finding service providers, making plans, and caring for the elderly person in your life.
- If it is truly no longer safe for the person to live in their home without outside assistance, suggest either a live-in nurse or moving into an assisted living situation where staff will be present around the clock.
- It is important to have conversations with your parents (and other elderly relatives who depend on you) about their wishes regarding care later in life. Start having these conversations early on and make sure to include your siblings. Ask your loved one what their wishes are regarding care late in life and be sure to obtain all of the necessary legal documents to provide them the care that they have requested, such as a power of attorney.

Part 2

Helping them Cope with Changes

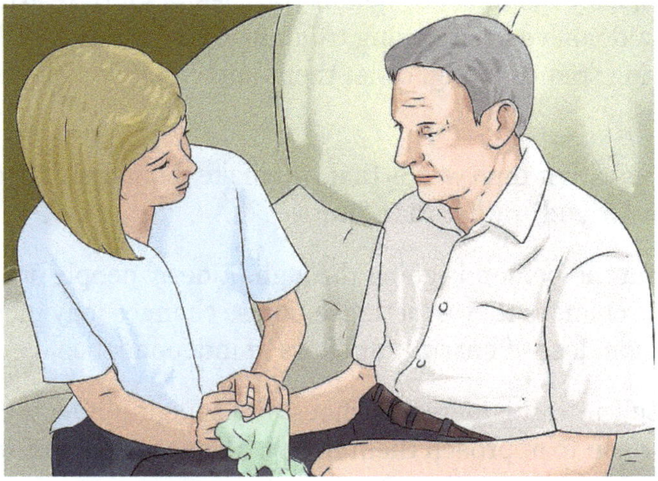

1. Determine what sort of care they need. Figure out what their preferences are, and what your availability to help is. If you go into a conversation armed with the facts, you can pre-empt any complaints that they might have. You might consider asking your family doctor for resources and information about things like home health care, physical therapy, occupational therapy, and social workers.

- Try discussing all of the care options available with your loved one. This will give them an opportunity to consider their options and choose the one that is the most appealing. For example, your loved one may be more comfortable with having a home health care aide some to visit them a few days per week than moving into a nursing home.
- Be sure to check the references for any eldercare services you consider hiring.
- You might also explain that accepting some care early on may prolong independence in the long term.

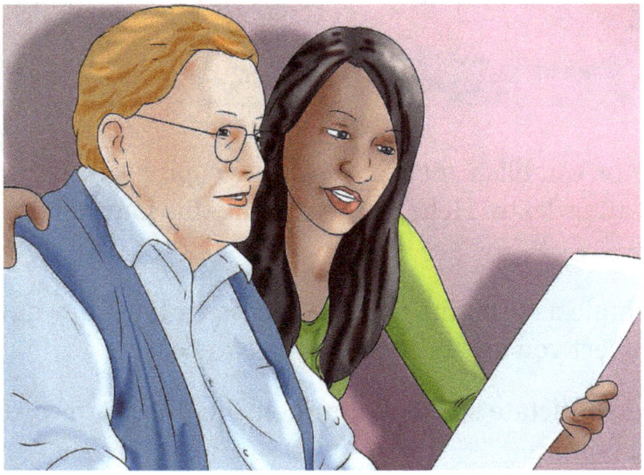

2. Prepare them for care. Some elderly people will be resistant to receiving care. Aging people are losing independence, mental agility, and physical ability, so they may fight to keep some control.

- Choose a time when you are both relaxed. It will be easier to have an honest conversation if there are no other tensions.
- Use friends and family members to help if you meet a lot of resistance. Do not say things like "So and so said you've been having trouble with x", as this will cause miscommunications. Rather, bring friends along, or let them know that you've started having these conversations.
- Use positive words rather than words that will make them feel like invalids-- "client" rather than "patient", or "friend" rather than "nurse".

3. Show empathy for what the person is going through. Elderly people are especially prone to depression as a result of the changes they experience. These changes may include incontinence, pain from arthritis, loss of vision, loss of hearing, and loss of independence.

- Try to put yourself into this person's shoes and imagine how they are feeling. This will make it easier for you to approach them from a place of compassion and love.

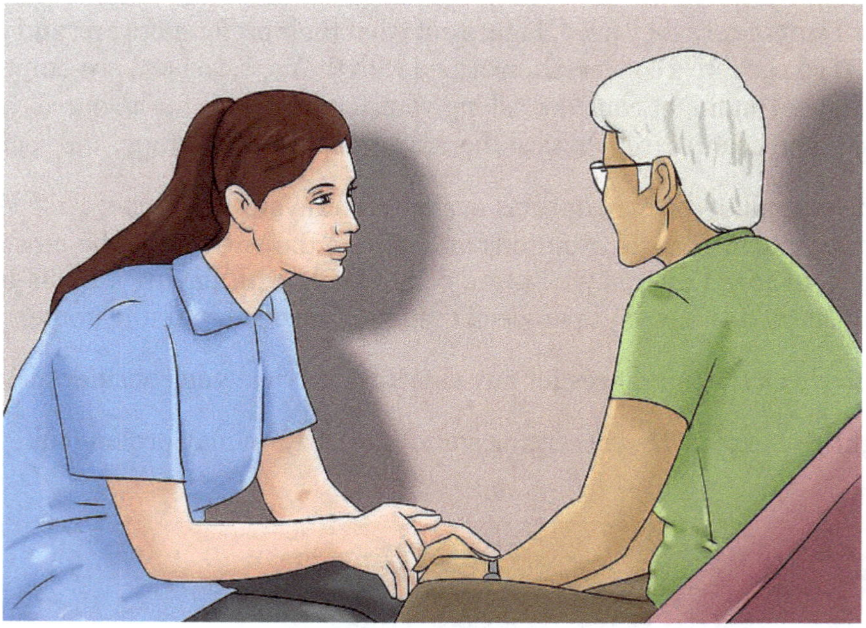

4. Help them determine or establish their legacy. One coping process for aging is determining how an elder will live on after death. Helping them along this journey can be healing for everyone involved.

- This may be as simple as bringing up and discussing how they have impacted lives: "Your children really respect you and take your advice to heart."
- Ask them to write or dictate stories from their life. Keep a recording of what they say, or have their writing bound.
- If asking them is unfruitful, you may want to get them involved in activities that will bring them into contact with people. You can keep a record of what happens there.

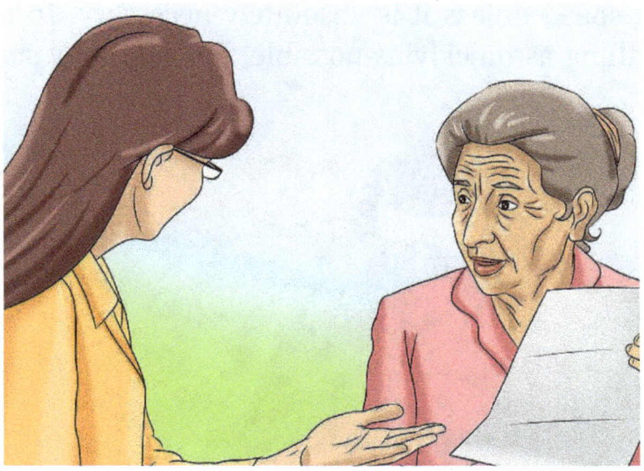

5. Allow them to be autonomous. Allowing them to make their own decisions will keep them from feeling out of control and lashing out.

- Even though it may not be the most efficient way to do something, it will mean a lot to an elder to be able to make even small choices. Call and ask how they want something done, whether it be a doctor's appointment or a trip to the park.
- "When do you want to get there?" and "Who should I invite?" are both good questions that may go ignored if you are too concerned with making decision quickly.
- If they have trouble making decisions, you can present them with a few choices. This way, they still get to be the deciding factor.

Part 3

Giving Respect and Affection

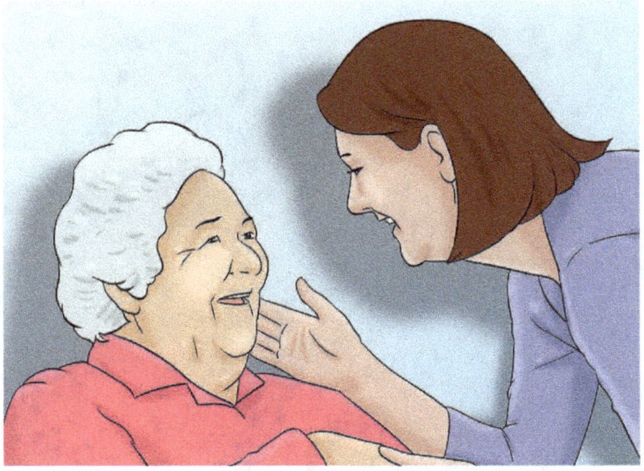

1. Be patient and treat them kindly. Elderly people often forget things or ask the same questions over and over. They can be slow-moving or even obstinate. Keep in mind that they usually can't help it and aren't deliberately trying to be difficult or cause you stress.

- Don't try to rush them. Use gentle reminders if they are getting distracted, but do not force them to move faster.

- Don't worry about speed unless it is absolutely necessary. In today's world, we've been taught to do everything as quickly as possible, but that may simply not be necessary for older people.

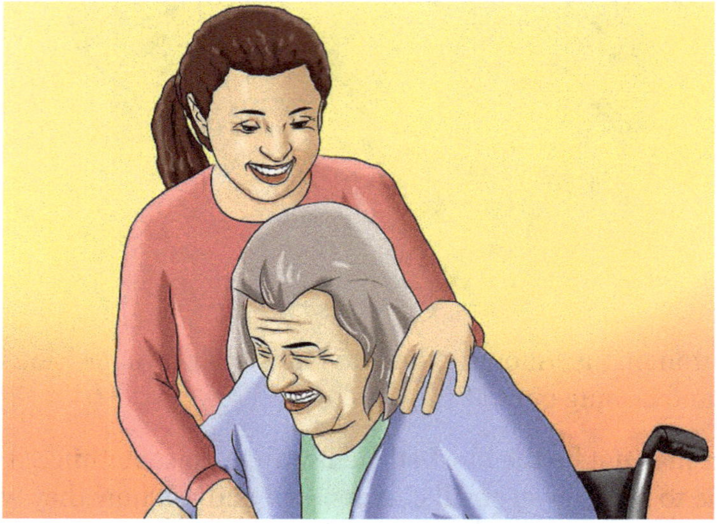

2. Respect their opinions and feelings. As their abilities change, elderly people may begin to feel ignored. Often they feel as though they lose the respect that they fought for all their lives.

- Ask them their opinions about skills that they are knowledgeable about, like gardening or cooking. For example you can say, "I've been trying to make that casserole you always used to make for potlucks, but I can't seem to get it right. What's the secret?"
- Update them on how their advice worked. This will make them feel both respected and useful. "Your advice worked great! Everyone loved it. I told them it was your help that made it so good."

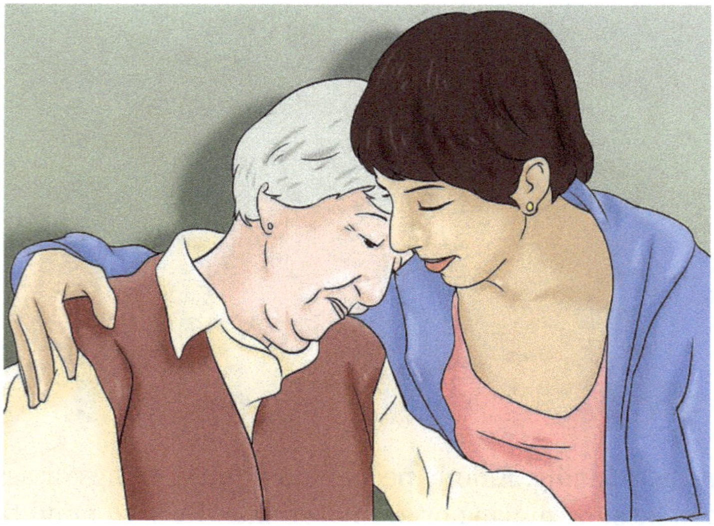

3. Provide physical contact. Contact is important in maintaining mental health and happiness. As people age and their friends and spouses pass away, they receive less physical contact, which can deepen depression.

- Give them hugs, hold their hand, or hold their arm as you walk together. Small touches during everyday interactions can go a long way to counteracting the social isolation that elderly people often endure.
- Touch can lower blood pressure, and even help reduce physical pain.

Part 4

Taking Care of yourself

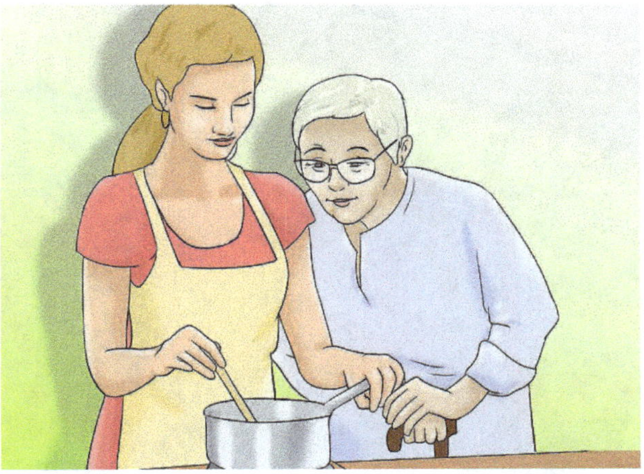

1. Allow for new dynamics. If you are taking care of a family member, you have likely been creating a relationship that has taken shape over years. As your roles reverse, this may change.

- Aging family members may become angry that they've lost the authority that they used to have over you. Allow them to work through this anger. Things are changing, but eventually everything will settle down.
- You may expect that your relationship will deepen or improve with increased contact, but also be aware that old emotions and ways of interacting may not work in your new role. Don't let your expectations get too high.

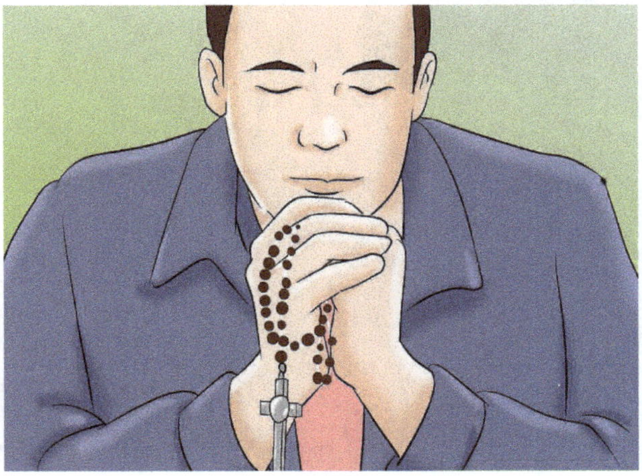

2. Meditate or pray. You may need to open yourself up to spirituality to get through rough patches. If this works for you, make sure that you keep up some sort of routine when times are easy as well.

- Meditation particularly is a long-term practice. If you meditate, try to do at least a few minutes each morning. The most simple form of meditation is just sitting with eyes closed, counting breaths up to ten. As your mind wanders, you just bring your thoughts back to the breath.
- Spiritual practices are about forgiving yourself. It is an opportunity to examine your feelings without guilt or shame, and just be okay with yourself.

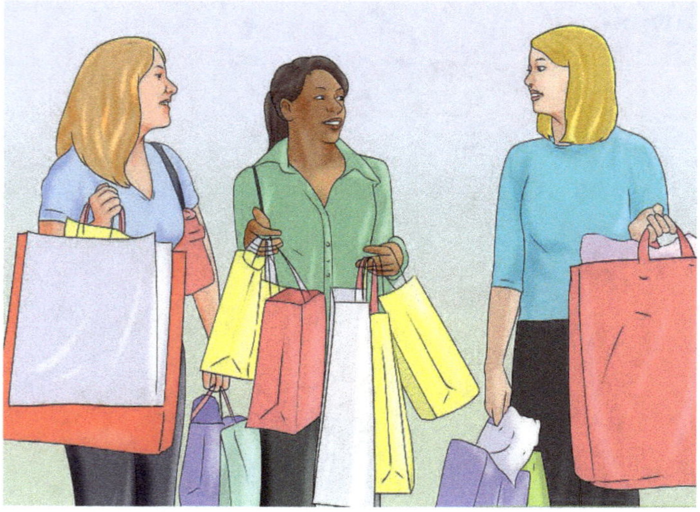

3. Wind down and have fun. Take time to visit friends, go to the movies, or have a glass of wine. This may seem difficult, but it's just as important as any other part of your life.

- It might be too hard to be spontaneous. Try to work a fun activity into your schedule, or just schedule some free time for yourself a few times a week.
- Having free time built into your schedule will reduce confusion from your elder about why you are unavailable.

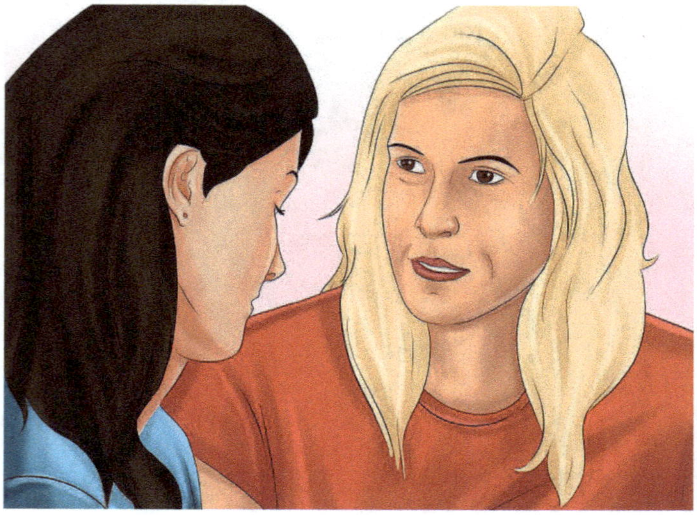

4. Talk to friends and family. Your support system will become even more important as you take on extra burdens. Make sure to talk out any difficult experiences with the people who matter most to you.

- Don't overload any one person. Your spouse probably understands you the best, but you won't want all of your conversations to revolve around caregiving. Talk to friends that even seem a little bit outside of your inner circle. Sometimes you will find people who have gone through similar experiences.
- Make it clear whether or not you want advice. Sometimes you just need to get something off your chest, but the person you are talking to thinks that you want a concrete solution. Let them know if you just want to rant, or if you're asking their advice.

Part 5

Encouraging Social Interaction

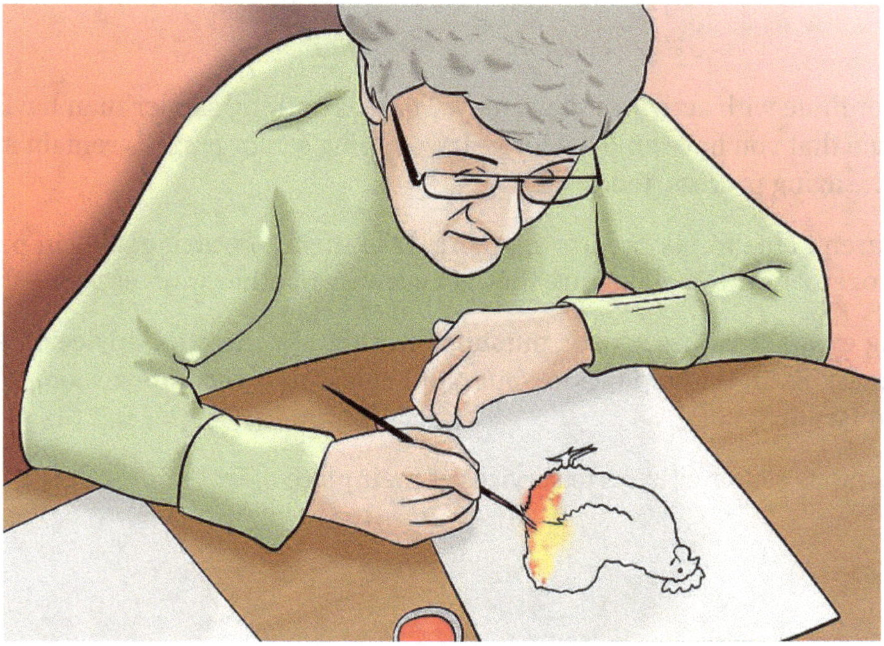

1. Take them to a senior center for activities. Getting older and becoming less mobile can be very isolating, so making sure that the elderly person in your care has ample opportunity to interact with others in their age will provide entertainment and comradery, which will have both physical and mental health benefits.

- Many of the activities at senior centers, like bingo, music, exercise, and games are designed to boost brain-power. Encourage them to join in on these activities, and accompany them if they are reluctant.
- Make sure they have whatever they need, like a hearing aid, in order to remain part of the conversation around them.
- Look into transportation options for seniors in your area. Some senior centers have their own shuttles to transport people to and from the senior center. There may also be a special senior shuttle in your area that will take people to and from their destination at a low cost.

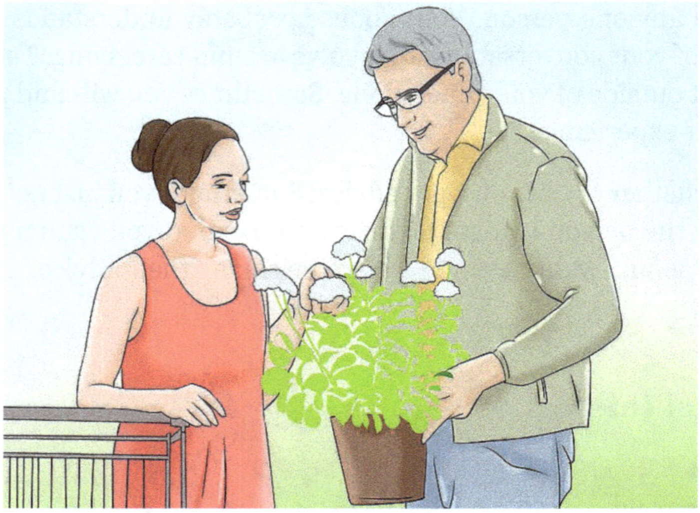

2. Help them continue with activities they enjoy. There is nothing sadder than having to give up a hobby or pastime that you have enjoyed for years. Helping senior citizens remain active can actually help slow the aging process, too.

- If they aren't able to play sports anymore, take them to watch games in person or watch games together on TV. Make sure they get exercise in other ways as well.
- If failing eyesight makes artistic pursuits difficult, ask them for advice on a quilt you are making, ask them for help picking out paint colors to redecorate a room, or take them to an art museum.
- Take religious senior citizens to services at their place of worship.

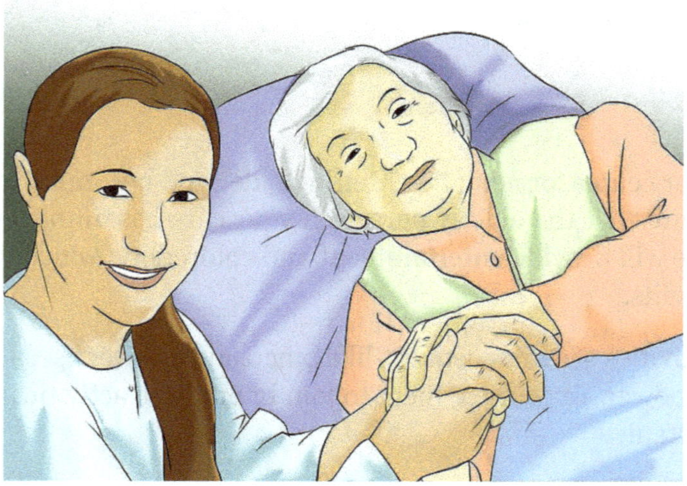

3. Visit regularly. Put regular visits to your elderly relatives or friends on your calendar so they are part of your regular routine. Showing up, even for a brief visit, will show them that you are thinking of them and will provide something for them to look forward to.

- Elderly people need to see family or friends a minimum of three times per week to ward off depression and loneliness. Unfortunately, emailing doesn't really help.

Part 6

Ensuring Health and Safety

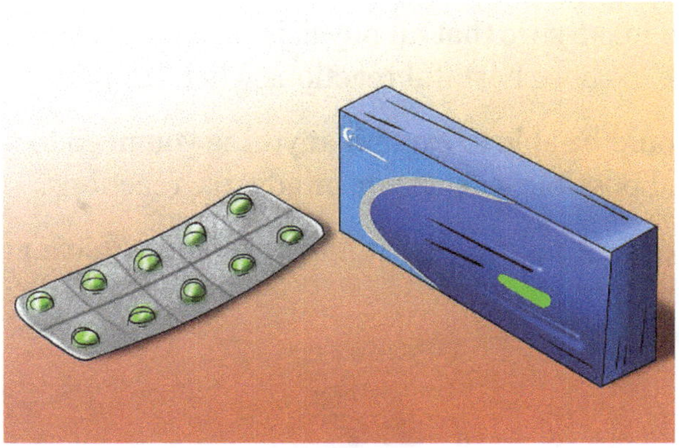

1. Keep track of their medications. Elderly people often have health problems that require multiple medications including pills, diabetic testing, and even injections. If keeping track of these medications becomes too much for you or for the elderly person, then talk with their doctor. You may be able to arrange for a registered nurse to visit their home once or twice per week to help with medication management.

- Sort pills into a pill box marked with the days of the week. If they need different medications in the morning and evening, sort morning pills into a pill minder designated with a specific color, and the afternoon or evening medications into a different pill minder designated with a different color, or use one box with multiple rows for medications to be taken at different times of the day.
- Keep a log book of medications taken, doctor's appointments, and any medical problems they experienced for each day. If something goes wrong or they end up in the hospital, the records will help doctors figure out what happened and what to do.
- The log book will also be helpful for reminding your elderly friend if they have already taken their medications for the day, so they won't be confused and double-dose themselves.

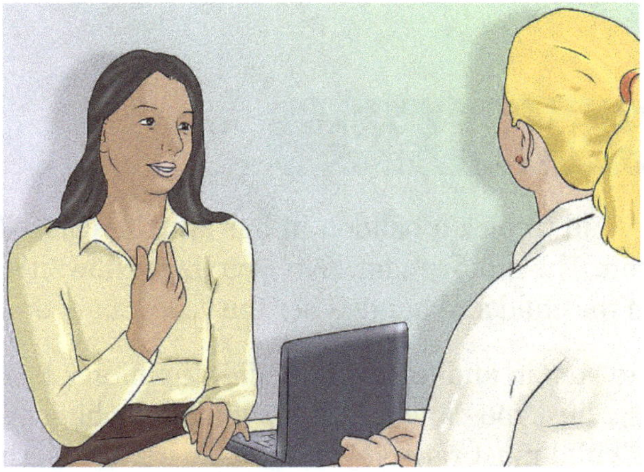

2. Talk to their doctors and pharmacists. Sometimes elderly people end up being over-medicated

and take so many pills a day that it is too confusing and may be unnecessary. Regularly going through each of the medications with the doctor and pharmacist can help prevent this problem.

- If the person has more than one doctor because they are managing multiple health problems, it is crucial to make sure that all physicians are aware of all of the drugs in their regimen. Some drugs can cause harmful reactions when combined.
- The pharmacist should be able to explain anything you need to know about timing for taking medications and possible side effects or adverse reactions.
- Contact their doctor and pharmacist right away if they have any adverse reactions after starting a new medication.

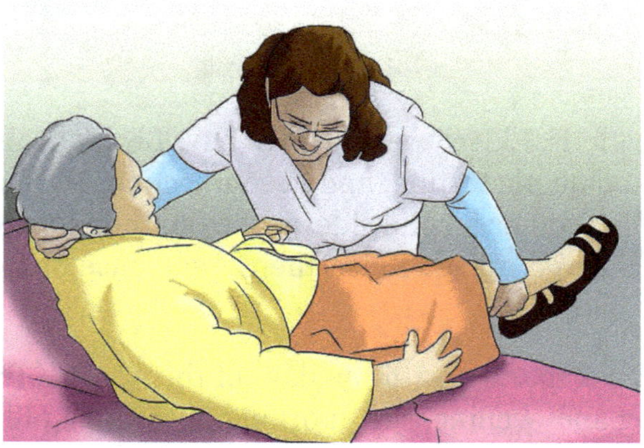

3. Protect their physical safety. Making sure that their environment is modified prevents falls and other accidents. People usually prefer to remain living independently in their own home as long as possible instead of moving in with relatives or into a nursing home. You can help make this possible by assessing the how the features of the home may present hazards, and fixing them to be safer when possible.

- If the elderly person in your life still lives in their own home, consider hiring an aging in place expert to help you make modifications like handrails in the shower.
- If climbing up and down stairs is difficult or impossible, you may want to have a chair lift installed to prevent falls. Or, ramps can be installed to accommodate wheelchairs.

How to be Patient with Kids

A mother once asked her child to pick a balloon in her favorite color. The child said "pink" and reached for the pink balloon. The mother said, "No, you like yellow, it's better". Then the mother took the pink balloon from the child and handed her the yellow balloon.

Do you ever feel the urge to step in and form your child's opinions, tastes, and to complete tasks that they seem to be doing "just too slowly"? If so, you're teaching your child a few unhelpful lessons, including that the child must rely on you to make decisions, that impatience is a virtue, and that the child's carers will always fix things rather than having to take on personal responsibility. Ultimately, impatience with a child risks lessening their independence and understanding.

Learning to let go despite the messes, frustration, and mistakes that will inevitably arise is a vital skill when caring for or being with children. Whether you're raising children, or working or volunteering with them, a little patience goes a long way.

Steps

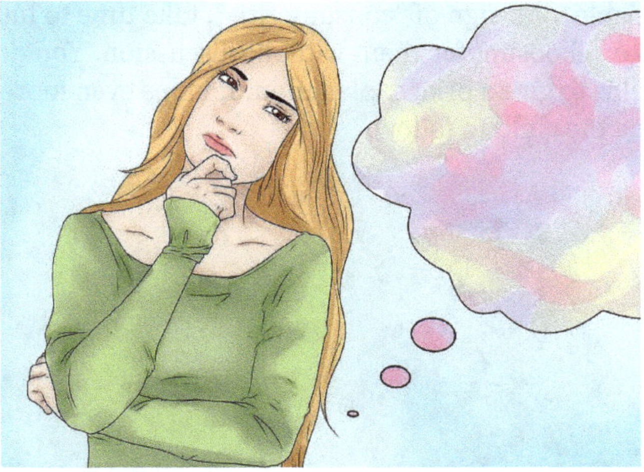

1. Take a little time to think about the purpose and beauty of patience. Patience gives us time to reflect, to slow down and think about the world and the things we're doing. It's a way of enjoying what we're experiencing rather than always rushing toward an end just to make room for the next rush. Patience allows us to enjoy the process of living. Patience also enables others to accept us into their lives through our faithful, continued presence and enduring respect for them. When we accept the importance of patience in our lives, it becomes easier to be patient with others too. Through respecting the rhythm of ourselves and others, being patient presents an opportunity to give of ourselves rather than expecting others to conform to our wants.

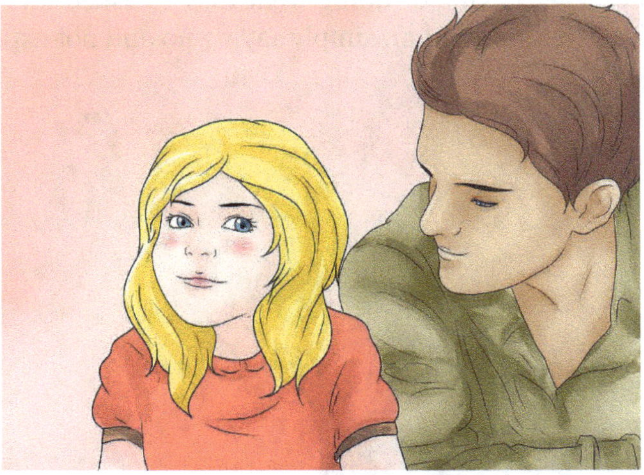

2. Ask the child what he or she wants to have, do, or be. Resist the impulse to have things the way you'd like them to be. Even a very young child can indicate their likes and dislikes; allowing these to express themselves at appropriate occasions is important. As part of asking for the child's preferences, be sure to show that you've heard the answer; aim to paraphrase the child's response so that it's clear you understand.

- Resist the temptation to change the child's mind about a future occupation. If little Johnny says he wants to be a window washer when he grows up, let it be. If you constantly interrupt with something like "Oh he's just saying that. We all know he'll be a doctor when he grows up", he'll start to resent the implications of being pushed toward a designated career.
- Balance the wants with realities. If you think that what the child is asking for is unreasonable, unaffordable, or a sign of "consumeritis", take time to talk it through rather than simply saying no or choosing for them without discussion. You don't have to reason with the child but it helps to give a brief explanation. It helps even more if you show by example what you're asking the child to follow.

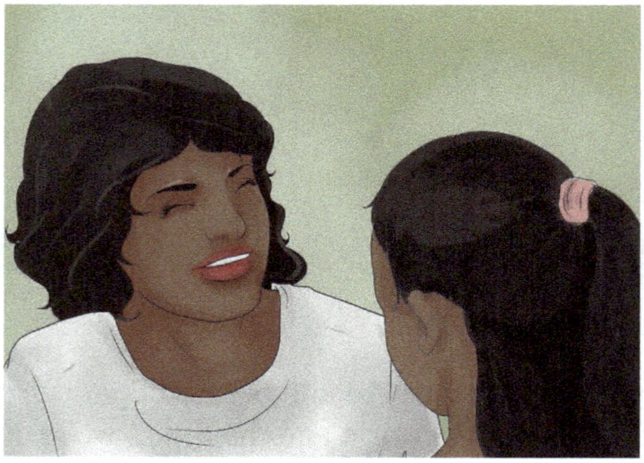

3. Show goodwill and interest in children. Where possible, try to please them. This isn't about being a doormat for the child's commands. It's about respecting the wants and requests of the child within the appropriateness of the situation. Help the child to learn the difference between making a request and making a demand and what the consequences are. It is also important to help them understand the importance of delayed gratification, teaching them that when you do say no, sometimes this is about waiting, rather than never having or doing what they've asked for. Helping them to understand this time perspective is far kinder than simply saying no and not explaining any further.

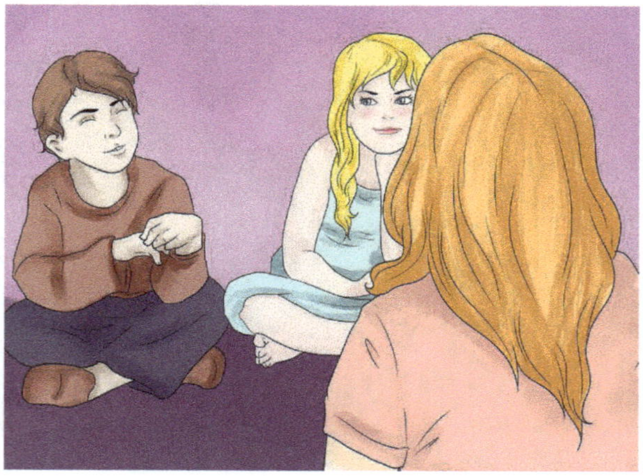

4. Be grateful for your children and for all children. When the daily chores mount up and everyone is rushing about, sometimes it's easy to take one another for granted. Taking time now and then to express your gratitude for your children will help you to respect them for the unique, individual beings they are, and helps them to see the importance of valuing others openly.

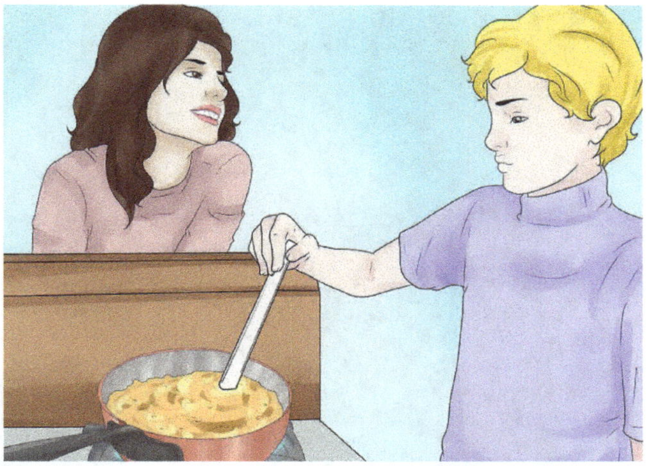

5. Humble yourself. Be willing to do things the child's way when possible. While their attempts might sometimes cause you frustration and worry, it is important to allow children to show you their way of doing things. If your child offers to help with making dinner, don't think of the mess they'll make. Accept that there will be a mess but realize that they're learning how to do something that will one day be of great importance as a skill (and eventually, they'll be making some of the household meals, relieving you of the burden occasionally). In watching and learning from your child or from other children, you will learn their character better, and see both their strengths and their weaknesses, giving you an opportunity to help them nurture the best talents and to learn to manage their weaknesses.

- If you do not allow children to do things their way, this takes away their autonomy and potentially stunts their ability to discover things for themselves. Allow a child to try new things often, so as to give them a sense of self-trust and personal responsibility.
- Naturally, keep safety and propriety in mind; it is entirely appropriate to step in and change the course of a child's behavior or activities where safety or appropriateness have been compromised; this is simply part of being responsible guardians.

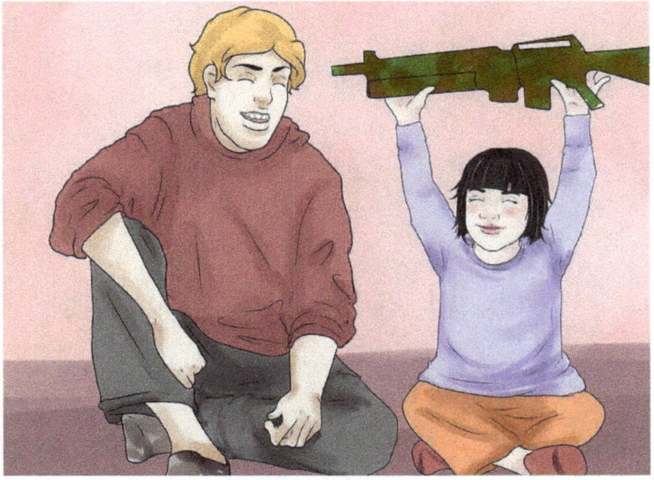

6. Remember that children are human too. Remember that children have feelings, likes, dislikes, favorite foods, colors, etc. Honor these things when possible.

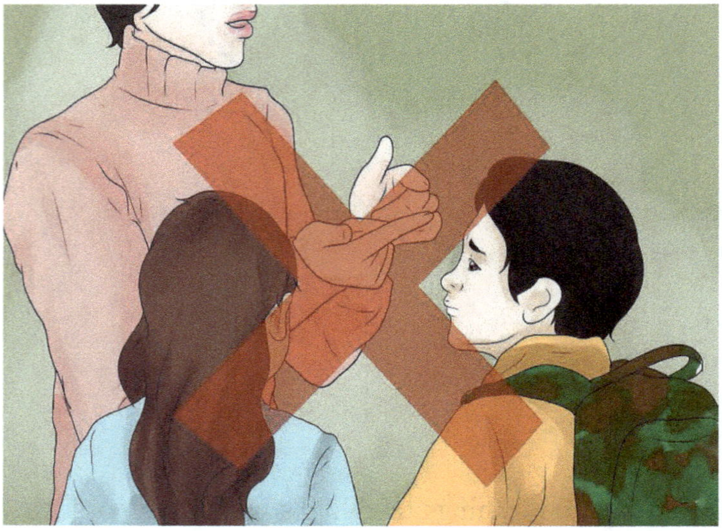

7. Resist the temptation to control children. Children are ready to trust and soak up information from the people who care for them and spend time with them. Trying to control children lacks respect for their own self and is a way of trying to insert your way of thinking and preferences onto them. Give them space to grow into the individual that they are.

- Patience allows you to be the ideal teacher. Instead of seeking to control, patience allows the child to grow at their own pace, rather than being pushed into doing things before being ready. For example, Dino de Laurentiis did not speak until he was 5. Despite the worries of others, his mother took this in her stride, believing he'd speak more than enough when he was ready. And so he did.
- Try this: see if you can say "yes" to the child, before you say "no". If your first instinct is to say "no", question this. Actually, why not? Are you just being controlling, or is there a good reason to deny their request?

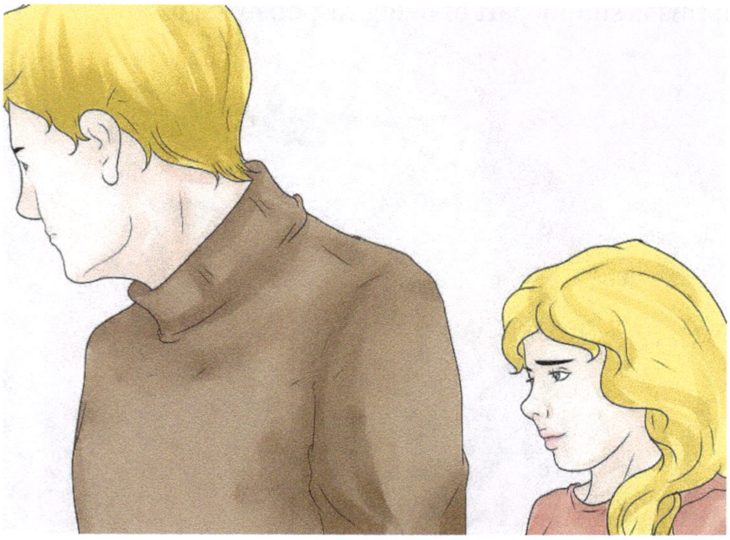

8. Pick your battles carefully. Most choices are not a life and death situation. Give children a rope long enough for them to safely learn on their own. Mistakes are a learning experience.

- If you feel that a situation is getting out of hand with a child, take a step back and create space between you and the child. This breathing space is important for both of you, after which you can express your thoughts and establish boundaries when you are collected, rather than channeling your concerns through frustration.

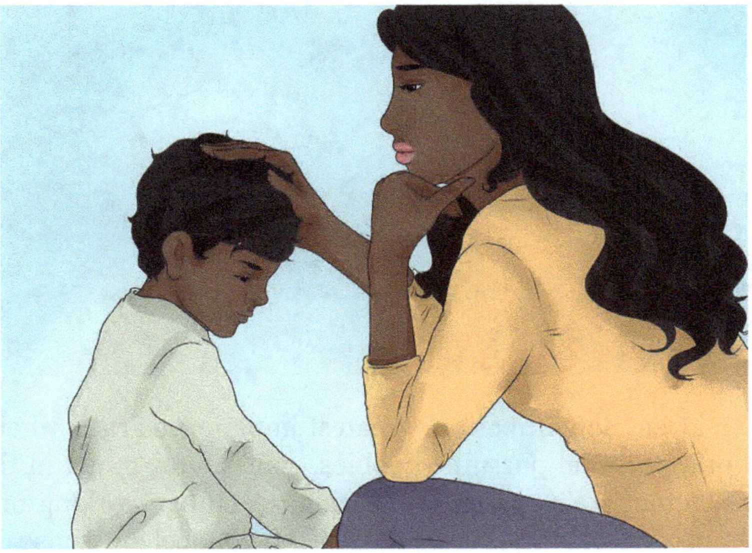

9. Be kind to your children and they will learn to treat you and others kindly by your example. Your example will be helpful to your children throughout their life. They will also have learned to make wise choices by the choices you allowed them to make. Now they will be kind to their children and teach them to make wise choices.

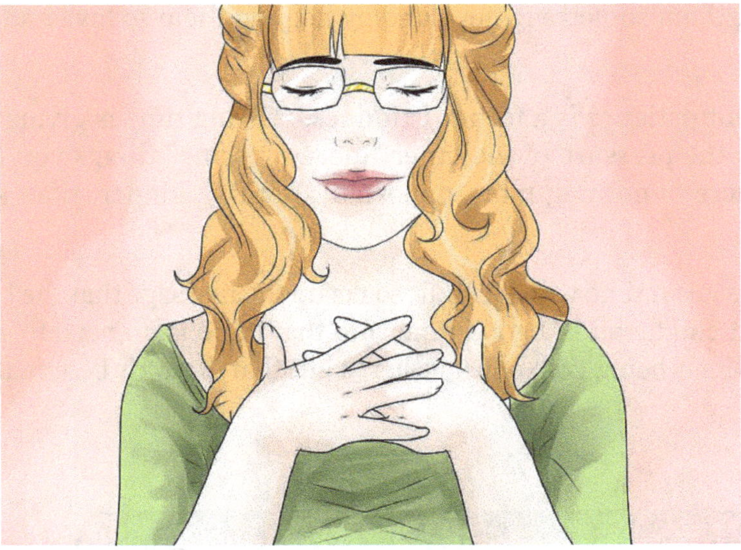

10. Be kind to yourself. It can be very hard to be patient sometimes in a world where teaching Mozart in the womb and expectations of exemplary behavior from preschool are considered the norm. No matter what the competitive approach insists upon, patience gives you a means for remaining calm within yourself, to give you the perspective to recognize the readiness of a child at their own developmental pace, independent of external standards. Rushing can cause you to lose sight of your guiding role, and of the precious essence of the child.

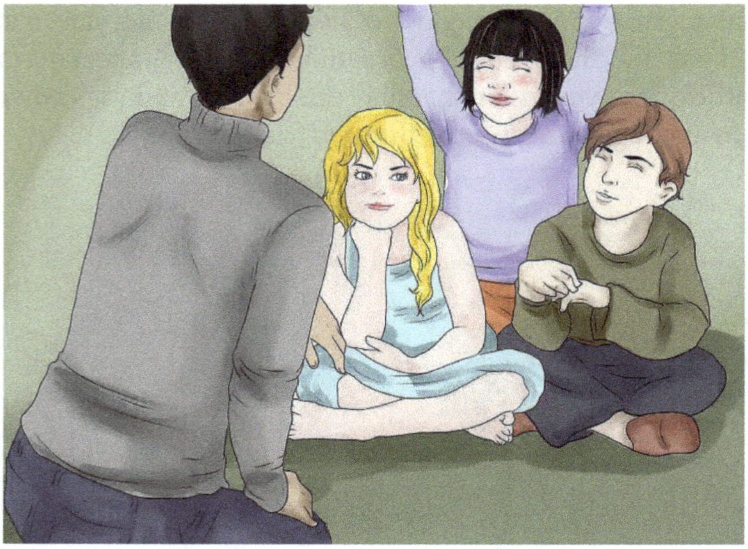

11. Love being with children. Sometimes our greatest impatience arises when we allow our own endeavors such as work, personal pursuits, hobbies, sports, etc., to get in the way of spending time with children. Whether we're parenting, caring, teaching, working or volunteering with children, nobody is immune from impatience at times. If you feel any sense of resentment when being around children for "holding up" the things you want to do, or you find yourself "half present" instead of giving your full attention, then being patient can restore your joy of spending time with children. Let go of the impatience and realize that time spent with children is precious. It is a time during which you can learn a great deal about seeing the world through fresh eyes. It can also be a time when you realize that you can make a big difference in the life of a child by teaching or showing them something new, and by helping them to love and respect themselves all the more.

- Recognize that patience is a form of kindness. Giving time is giving kindness a chance. By removing the pressure of the other "more pressing" things you feel, you show your child that there is nothing more important, nothing kinder, than spending time with them.
- A child who is given time with an adult soaks up the message that the busyness of adult life can wait, that childhood is a good time, and that there is no need to grow up too quickly. The point of life is being with one another, a gift that can only be imparted to a child in the doing.

How to Develop Emotional Intelligence

Emotional intelligence (EQ) is the ability to tap into your emotions and use them to make your life better. Being in touch with your feelings allows you to manage stress levels and communicate effectively with other people, two skills that enhance your life both personally and professionally. Unlike IQ, which remains constant throughout your life, EQ can be developed and honed over time.

Part 1

Tapping into your Emotions

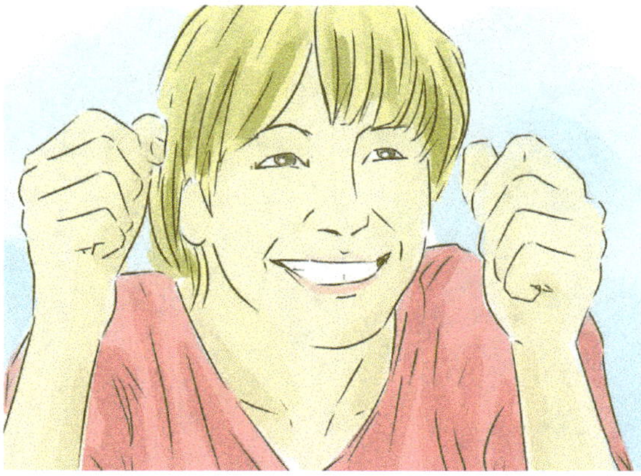

1. Note your emotional reactions to events throughout the day. It's easy to put your feelings about what you experience throughout the day on the back burner. But taking time to acknowledge how you feel about experiences is essential to improving your EQ. If you ignore your feelings, you're ignoring important information that has a big effect on your mindset and the way you behave. Start paying more attention to your feelings and connecting them to experiences.

- For example, say you're at work and you get cut off during a meeting. What emotions arise when this happens? On the other hand, how do you feel when you get praised for good work? Getting into the practice of naming your emotions as sadness, embarrassment, joy, contentment, or any other number of feelings will start raising your EQ right away.
- Get in the habit of tapping into your emotions at certain times every day. What are your first emotions upon waking? Your last before you fall asleep?

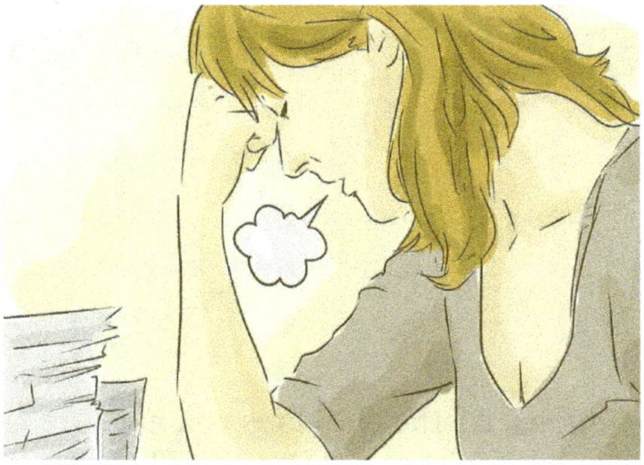

2. Pay attention to your body. Instead of ignoring the physical manifestations of your emotions, start listening to them. Our minds and bodies are not separate; they affect each other quite deeply. You can raise your EQ by learning how to read physical cues that clue you in to what emotions you're feeling. For example:

- Stress might feel like a knot in your stomach, tight chest, or quick breathing.
- Sadness might feel like waking up with slow, heavy limbs.

- Joy, pleasure or nervousness might feel like butterflies in your stomach, a racing heart or increased energy.

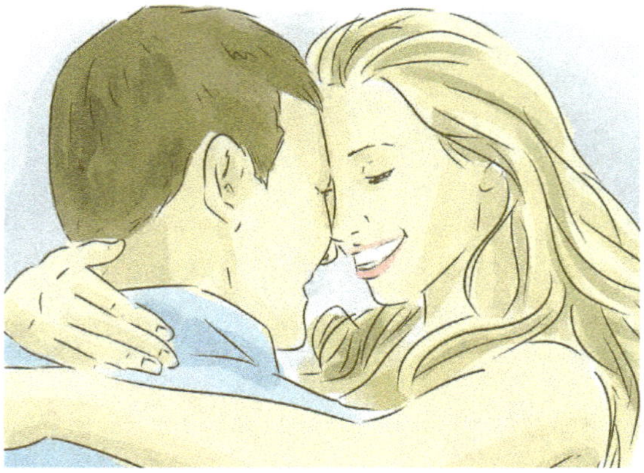

3. Observe how your emotions and behavior are connected. When you feel strong emotions, how do you react? Tune into your gut responses to situations you face every day, instead of just reacting without any reflection. The more you understand what spurs your behavioral impulses, the higher your EQ will be, and you'll be able to use what you know to actually change your behavior in the future. Here are some examples of behaviors and what's behind them:

- Feeling embarrassed or insecure might cause you to withdraw from conversation and disconnect.
- Feeling angry might cause you to raise your voice or angrily stomp away.
- Feeling overwhelmed might cause you to panic and lose track of what you were doing, or cry.

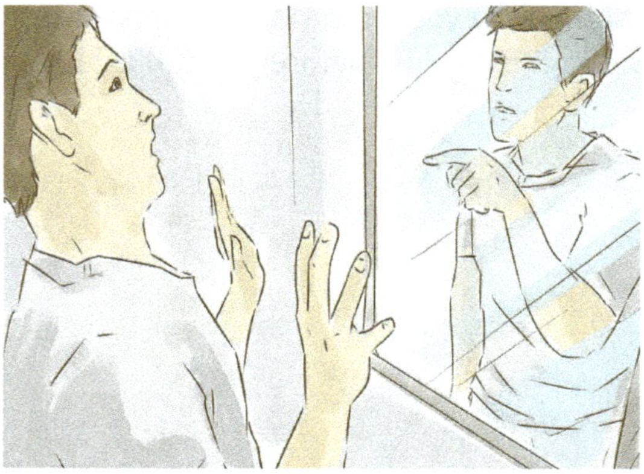

4. Avoid judging your own emotions. All the emotions you have are valid, even the negative ones. If you judge your emotions, you'll inhibit your ability to fully feel, making it more difficult to use your emotions in positive ways. Think of it this way: every emotion you have is a new piece of useful information connected to something that's happening in your world. Without this information, you'd be left in the dark about how to adequately react. That's why the ability to feel your emotions is a form of intelligence.

- It's hard at first, but practice letting negative emotions surface and connecting them to what's happening. For example, if you feel bitterly envious, what is that emotion telling you about your situation?

- Fully experience positive emotions, too. Connect your joy or satisfaction to what's happening around you, so you can learn how to feel them more often.

5. Notice patterns in your emotional history. It's another way to learn as much as you can about your own feelings and how they're connected to your experiences. When you have a strong emotion, ask yourself when you last felt like this. What happened before, during and after?

- When you see patterns, you can exert more control over your behavior. Observe how you handled a certain situation before, and how you'd like to handle it next time.
- Keep a journal of your emotional reactions, or how you feel from day to day, so you can clearly see how you tend to react.

6. Practice deciding how to behave. You can't help what emotions you feel, but you con connected to something that's happening in your world. Without this information, you'd be left in the dark about how to adequately react. That's why the ability to feel your emotions is a form of intelligence.

Part 2

Connecting with other People

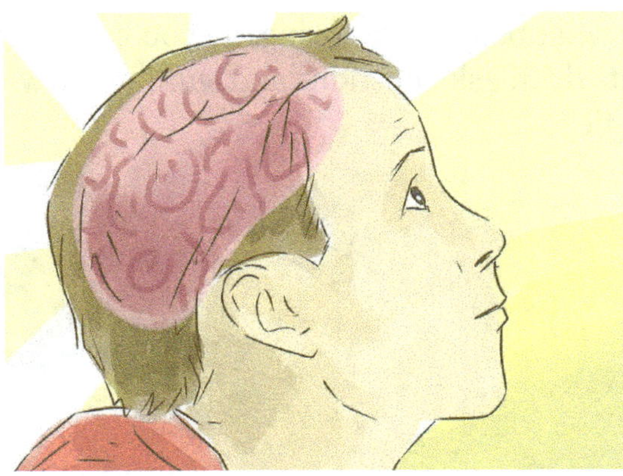

1. Be open-minded and agreeable. Openness and being agreeable go hand-in-hand when it comes to emotional intelligence. A narrow mind is generally an indication of a lower EQ. When your mind is open through understanding and internal reflection, it becomes easier to deal with conflicts in a calm and self-assured manner. You will find yourself socially aware and new possibilities will be open to you. To strengthen this element of your EQ, consider:

- Listening to debates on television or the radio. Consider both sides of the argument, and look for the subtleties that require closer inspection.
- When someone does not react emotionally the same way you would, consider why this is, and try to see it from their point of view.

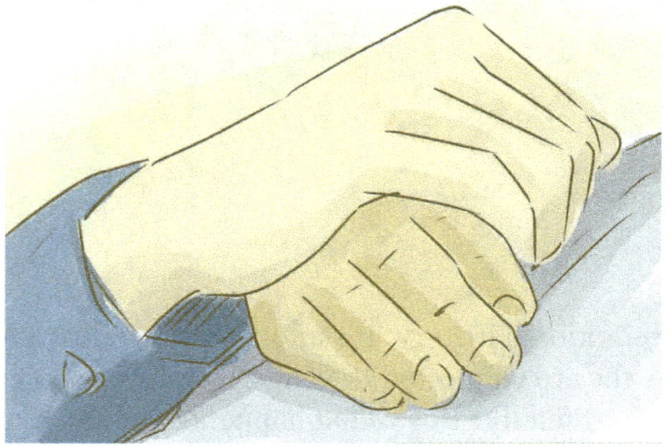

2. Improve your empathy skills. Empathy means being able to recognize how other people are feeling, and share emotions with them. Being a more active listener and really paying attention to what people are saying can help you get a better sense of how they're feeling. When you can use that information to inform your decisions and improve your relationships, that's a sign of emotional intelligence.

- To improve empathy, put yourself in other people's shoes. Think about how you would feel if you were in their situation. Actively imagine how it must be to go through the experiences they're having and what might alleviate some of their hardship in terms of support and care.
- When you see someone experience a strong emotion, ask yourself, "How would I react in the same situation?"
- Be truly interested in what people are saying, so you can react in a sensitive way. Instead of letting your thoughts drift, ask questions and summarize what they're saying so it's clear you're in the conversation.

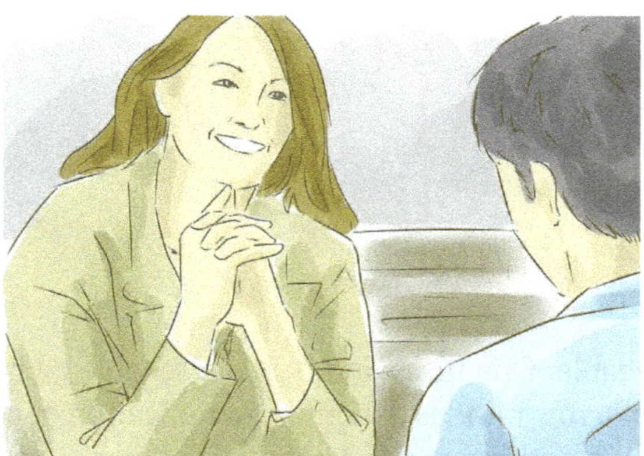

3. Read people's body language. Make a point of trying to read between the lines and pick up on

people's true feelings by observing their facial expressions and other body language. Often people say one thing when the look on their face reveals that there's a deeper truth. Practice being more observant and picking up on the less obvious ways that people communicate their emotions.

- If you're not sure that you're skilled at interpreting facial expressions, try taking a quiz to telling. A higher tone of voice indicates that someone's stressed.

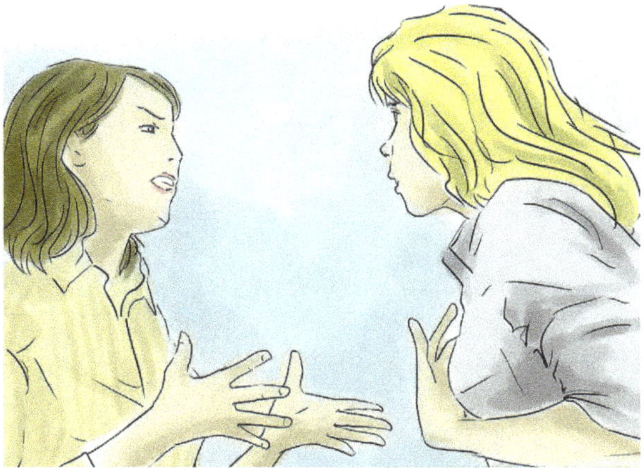

4. See the effect you have on others. Understanding other people's emotions is only half the battle when it comes to EQ; you also need to understand the effect you're having on other people. Do you tend to make people feel nervous, cheerful or angry? What happens to conversation when you walk in the room?

- Think about what patterns you might need to change. If you tend to pick fights with your loved ones, your girlfriend cries easily during conversations, or people tend to close up a bit when you come around, you might need to change you attitude so that you have a better emotional effect on people.
- Ask trusted friends or loved ones what they think about your emotionality where you have room for improvement.
- A person's tone of voice can also be of impact. You may have trouble recognizing the effect you have on others, and they can help.

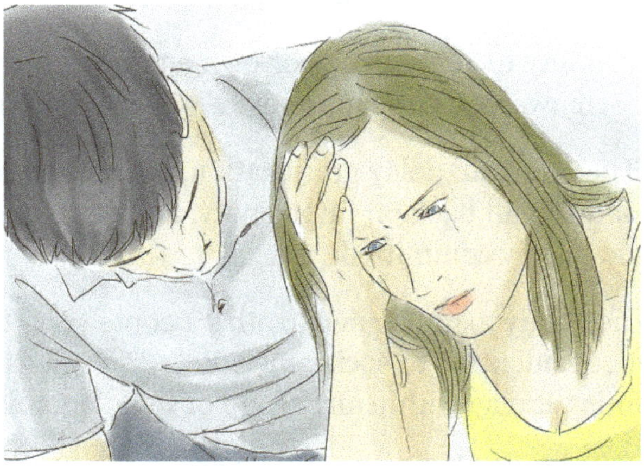

5. Practice being emotionally honest. If you say you're "fine" and have a scowl on your face, you're

not communicating honestly. Practice being more physically open with your emotions, so people can read you better. Tell people when you're upset, and share happiness and joy as well.

- Being "yourself" helps other people really get to know you, and they'll trust you more if they see where you're coming from.
- However, understand that there's a line: control your emotions so as not to hurt others with them.

Part 3

Putting EQ to Practical Use

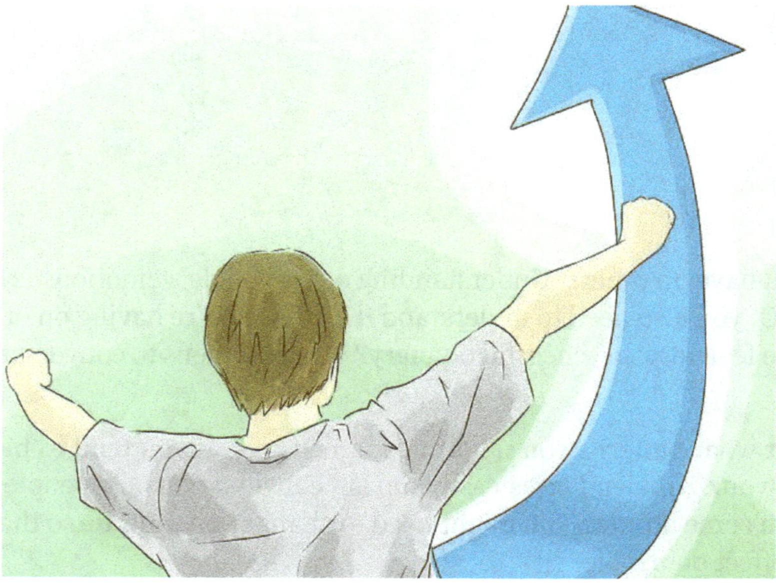

1. See where you have room for improvement. Being intellectually capable is important in life, but being emotionally intelligent is just as essential. Having high emotional intelligence can lead to better relationships and job opportunities. There are four core elements to emotional intelligence that help you lead a balanced life. Read this over and decide where you might have room for improvement, then take steps to practice your skills in that area:

- Self awareness: The ability to recognize your own emotions for what they are and understand their origins. Self awareness means knowing your strengths and limitations.
- Self management: The ability to delay gratification, balance your needs with those of others, take initiative and to pull back on impulsivity. Self management means being able to cope with change and to stay committed.
- Social awareness: The ability to be attuned to other people's emotions and concerns, as well as being able to notice and adapt to social cues. Being socially aware means being able to see the power dynamics at play within any group or in an organizational context.
- Relationship management: The ability to get along well with others, manage conflict, inspire and influence people and to communicate clearly.

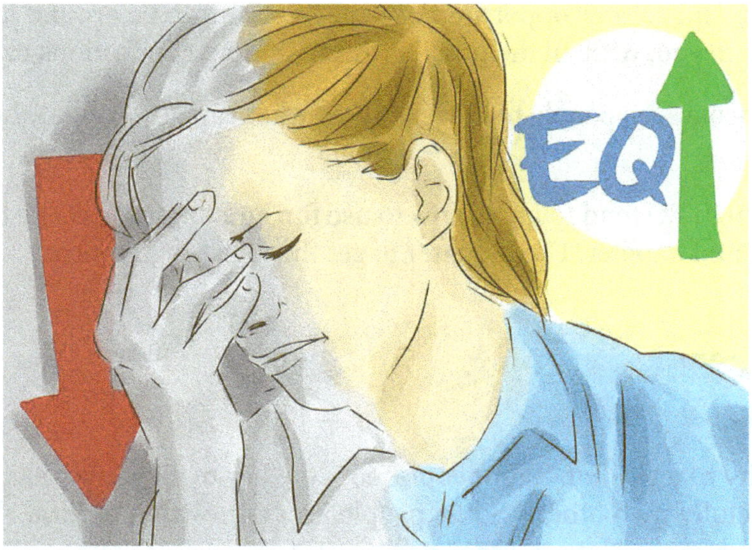

2. Lower your stress level by raising your EQ. Stress is a catchall word for feeling overwhelmed by a variety of different emotions. Life is filled with difficult situations from relationship breakdowns to job loss. In between, there are myriad stress triggers that can make any daily issue seem much more challenging than it probably is. If you're stressed a lot, it's difficult to behave in the way you want to. Having a good plan for relieving stress improves all aspects of your EQ.

- Figure out what triggers your stress, and what helps relieve it. Make a list of effective forms of stress relief, like hanging out with a friend or taking a walk in the woods, and put it to good use.
- Get help if you need it. If your stress feels too overwhelming to deal with alone, seek the help of a therapist or psychologist who can give you tools to cope (and help you raise your EQ in the process).

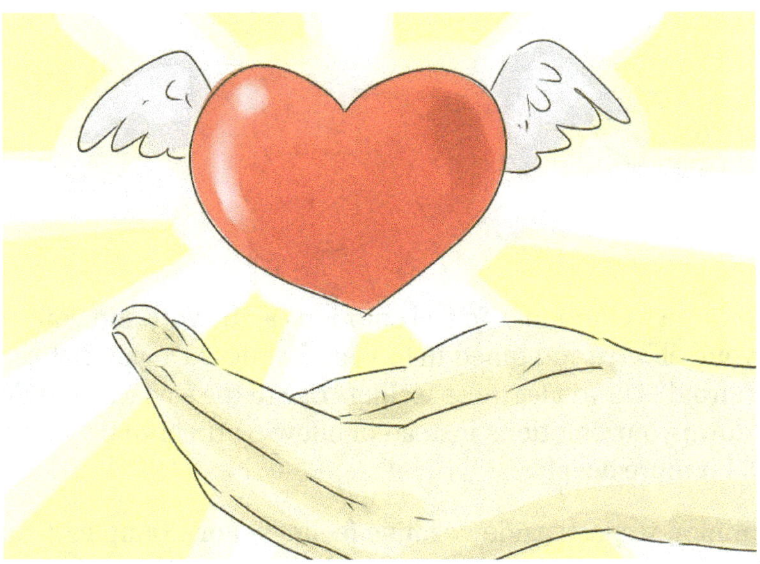

3. Be more light-hearted at home and at work. When you're optimistic, it's easier to see the beauty in life and everyday objects and spread that feeling to those around you. Optimism results in

emotional well being and greater opportunities – people want to be around an optimistic person and this draws them to you, with all the possibilities that more connections bring you.

- Negativity encourages people to focus only on what can go wrong rather than building resilience.
- People with high EQ tend to know how to use fun and humor to make themselves and others feel safer and happier. Use laughter to get through tough times.

How to Empathize

Empathy is the ability to feel what other people feel - the key to forming meaningful relationships and coexisting peacefully with others. Some people are born with a natural ability to empathize, and others find it harder to relate to other people. But if you feel your ability to put yourself in other people's shoes is lacking, there are many things you can do to deepen your sense of empathy. This topic discusses the meaning of empathy and steps you can take right away to become a more empathetic person.

Part 1

Tapping into your Empathy

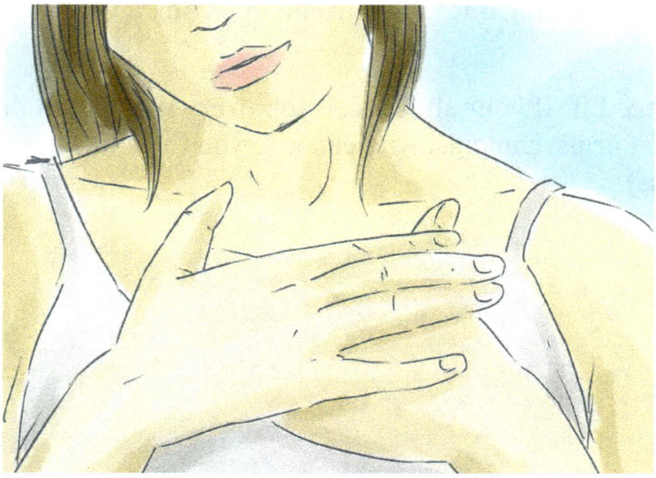

1. Get in touch with your own emotions. To feel emotions along with someone else, you've got to be able to feel them in yourself. Are you tuned in to your feelings? Do you notice when you're feeling happy, sad, angry or afraid? Do you let these feelings rise to the surface, and do you express them? If you tend to tamp down your emotions instead of allowing them to be part of your life, work on letting yourself feel a bit more deeply.

- It's pretty common to push aside negative feelings. For example, it's more fun to distract yourself with TV or go to the bar than it is to sit down and think about something upsetting that happened. But pushing feelings aside creates a disconnect, a lack of familiarity. When you can't express your own sadness, how can you expect to feel someone else's?

- Take time every day to let your emotions surface. Instead of hurriedly blocking out negative feelings, think them through. Be angry and afraid, and deal with the feelings in a healthy way, like by crying, or writing your thoughts down, or discussing how you feel with a friend.

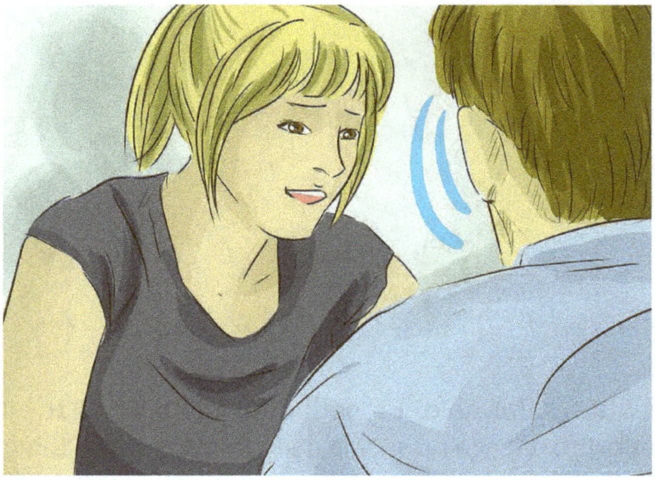

2. Listen carefully. Hear what the person is saying, and notice the inflection in their voice. Observe all the little clues that belie a way that someone is feeling. Maybe her lip is trembling and her eyes are glistening. Maybe it's more subtle - she's looking down a lot, or she seems vacant. Put yourself aside and absorb the person's story.

- Set aside judgement while you listen. If you find yourself remembering a disagreement you had, or feeling critical about the person's choices, or feeling anything that takes you out of the moment, struggle to reorient yourself into listening mode.

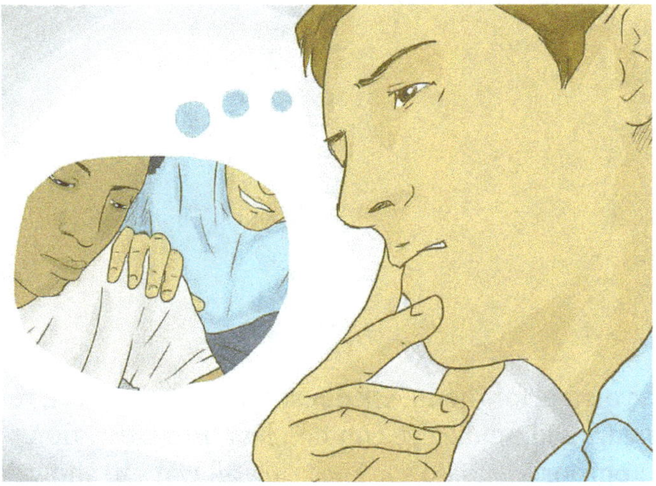

3. Pretend that you're the other person. Have you ever read a moving story that was so engaging, you forgot yourself? For a few minutes there, you became that character, and you knew exactly how it would feel to see your father for the first time in 10 years, or lose your love to someone else. Feeling empathy in person isn't so different. When you're listening to someone and really trying to understand, a moment will come when you start feeling what the other person is feeling. You'll see a glimpse of what it means to be them.

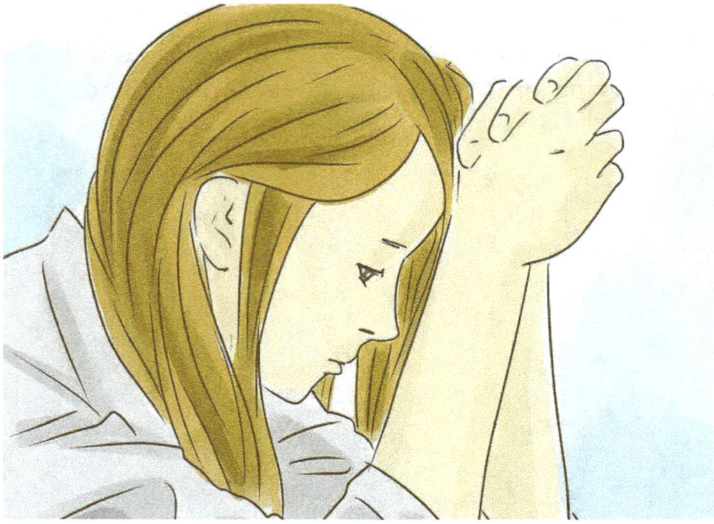

4. Don't be afraid to feel uncomfortable. Empathy can be painful! It hurts to absorb someone else's pain, and it takes effort to engage on such a deep level. Perhaps that's why empathy is on the decline - it's just easier to keep conversations light, to stay safely self-contained. If you want to be more empathetic, you can't shy away from people's feelings. Realize that they're going to have an effect on you, and that you might come away feeling different. But you'll have a deeper understanding of the other person, a foundation on which to build a more solid connection.

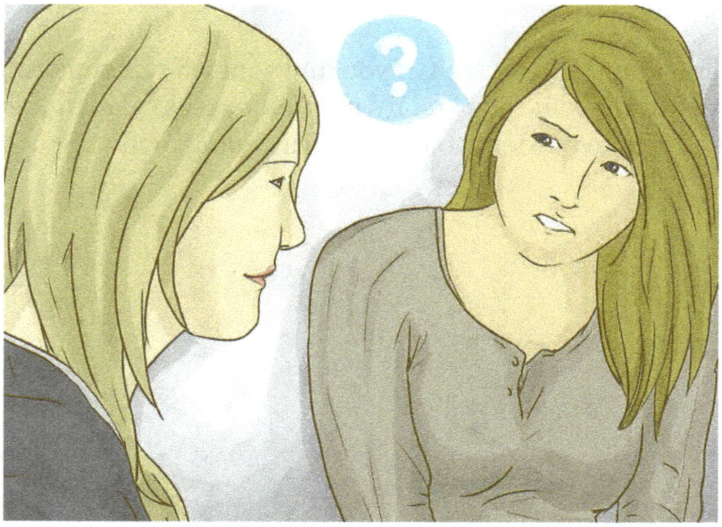

5. Show the other person you feel for them. Ask questions that show you're listening. Use body language that shows you're engaged: make eye contact, lean in a little, don't fidget. Nod, shake your head, or smile when it's appropriate to do so. These are all ways to show your empathy in the moment, to build trust with the person who is sharing feelings with you. If you seem distracted, look away, or give other cues that you're not listening or you aren't interested, the person will probably close up and stop sharing.

- Another way to show empathy is to share yourself, too. Making yourself as vulnerable as the other person is can build trust and mutual connection. Let down your guard and get into the conversation.

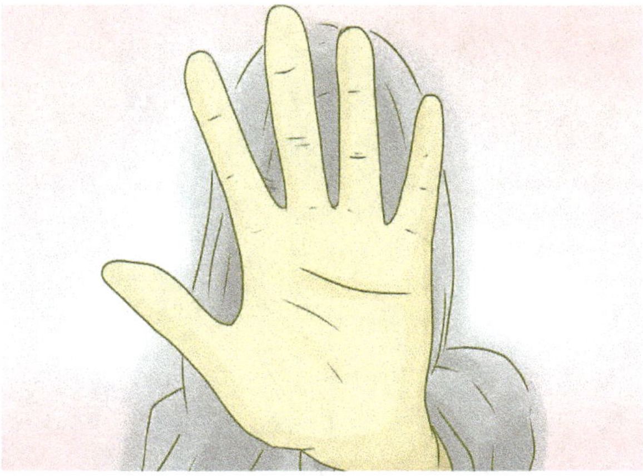

6. Use your empathy to help other people. Being empathetic toward someone is a learning experience, and it's good to let the knowledge you gained influence your future actions. Maybe that means standing up for someone who gets bullied a lot, because you understand him better now. It might change the way you behave next time you meet someone new, or your views on certain social or political issues. Let empathy influence the way you move through the world.

Part 2

Developing Greater Empathy

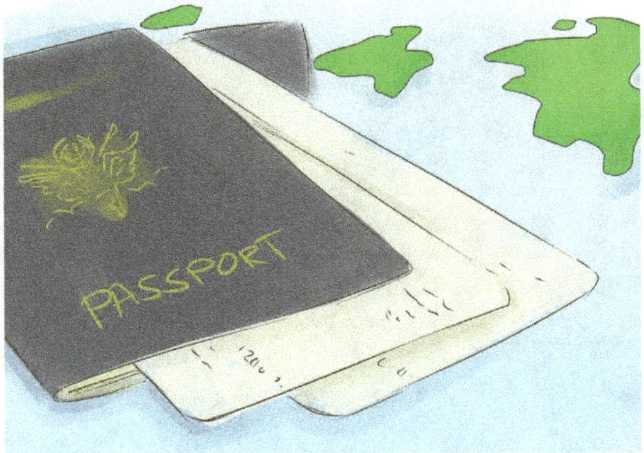

1. Be open to learning more about what you don't understand. Empathy stems from the desire to know more about other people, other experiences. Get curious about what life is like for people who aren't you. Make it a point to learn as much as you can about other things every day. Here are a few ways to act on your curiosity:

- Travel more. When you go to places you've never visited, make a point of spending time with people who live there and getting to know more about the way of life.
- Talk to strangers. If you find yourself sitting next to someone on a bus, strike up a conversation instead of burying your nose in a book.
- Get out of your regular routine. If you tend to hang out with the same people and go to the same places all of the time, mix it up and start meeting new people. Expand your world a little.

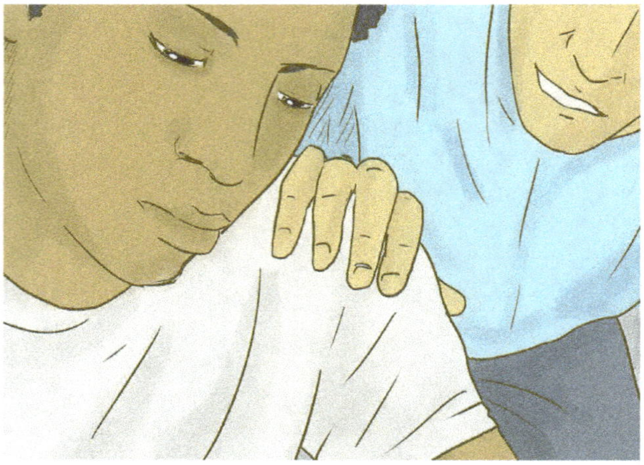

2. Try harder to empathize with people you don't like. If you notice areas where your empathy is lacking, make it a point to change how you feel, or at least gain a greater understanding of people and groups you don't like. The moment you feel repelled by someone, ask yourself why. Decide that instead of avoiding or badmouthing that person, you're going to put yourself in their shoes. Find out what you can learn by being empathetic toward people you don't like.

- Remember that even if you don't reach some kind of agreement, you can still feel empathetic. It's possible to feel empathy for someone you actively dislike. And who knows, once you open yourself up a bit, you might find reasons to change your mind about the person.

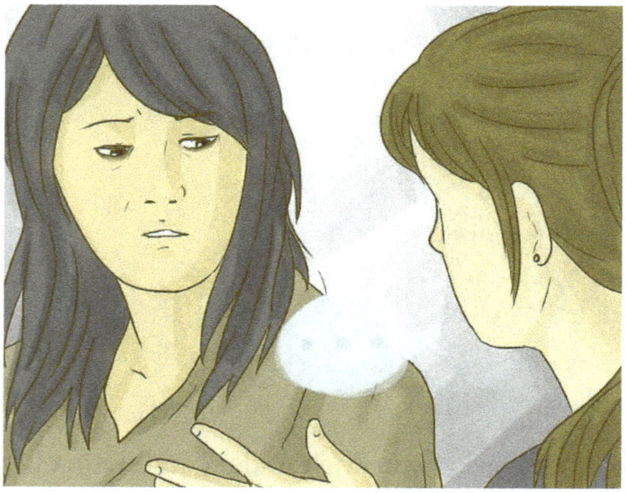

3. Make a point to ask people how they feel. This is a simple way to generate instances of empathy on a daily basis. Instead of considering emotional talk off limits, ask people about their emotions more often, and really listen to their responses. This doesn't mean that every conversation has to get deep, solemn and philosophical. But asking people how they feel can help you engage more fully, and really *see* the person you're talking to.

- The other side of the coin is to respond more truthfully when someone asks you how you feel. Instead of saying "Great!" when you actually feel down, why not express the truth? See what happens when you put your emotions out there a bit more instead of keeping them contained.

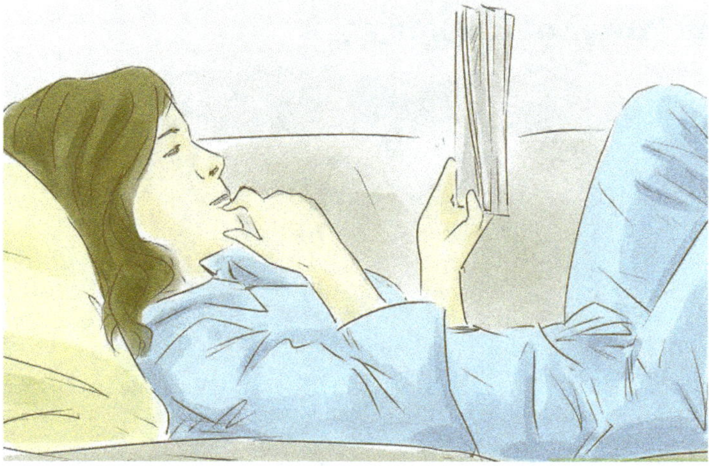

4. Read and watch more fiction. Absorbing a lot of stories, in the form of novels, films, and other media, is a good way to develop your sense of empathy. Studies show that reading literary fiction actually improves your ability to empathize in real life. It helps you get in the habit of imagining what life would be like if you were someone else. The catharsis of laughing or crying along with character can help you be more emotionally open with people.

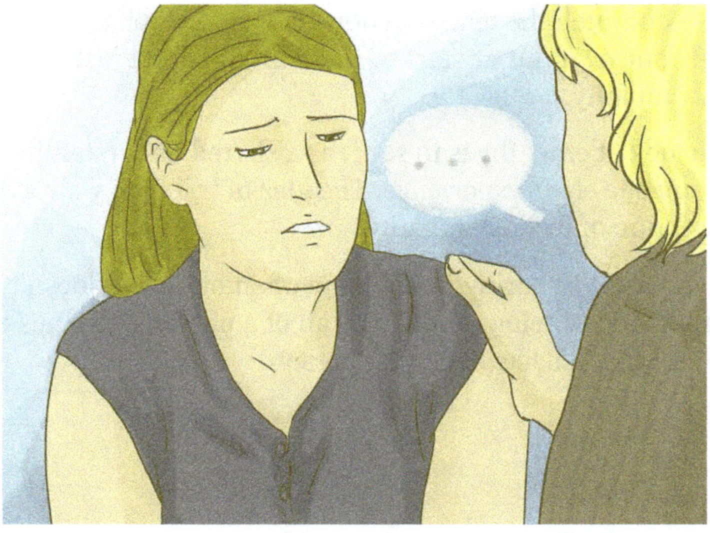

5. Practice empathy with someone you trust. If you're having trouble knowing whether you're empathetic, try practicing empathy with someone else. Make sure the person knows that you want to work on this, so they'll understand if you don't hit just the right note. Ask the person to tell you how they feel, and practice all the steps above to feel along with them. Then tell the person how you feel as a result of what they told you.

- See if the feelings matched up. If the person expressed sadness, and you felt sad when they were talking, then you read their emotions correctly.
- If the feelings didn't match up, you may need to spend more time getting in tune with your own emotions and practice recognizing emotions in other people.

Part 3

Understanding the Power of Empathy

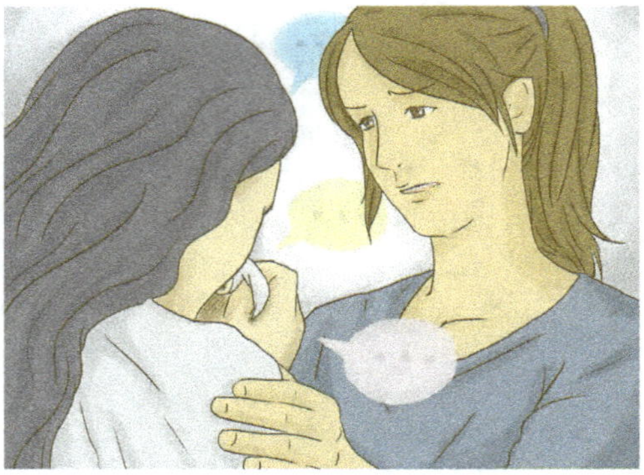

1. See it as sharing someone's emotions. Empathy is the ability to feel with someone. It requires you to go below the surface and experience the same emotions someone else is experiencing. It's easy to get empathy mixed up with sympathy, which is when you pity someone for their misfortune, and perhaps act on that feeling to try to help. But empathy runs deeper: rather than feeling *for* someone, you feel *with* them.

- For example, let's say your sister begins to cry as she tells you that her boyfriend just broke up with her. As you watch the tears roll down her face and listen to her describe what happened, you feel your own throat start to tighten. You don't just feel sorry for her, you feel sad, too. That's empathy.
- Another way to look at empathy is to see it as a shared understanding, an ability to project yourself into someone else's experience. The idea of trying to walk a mile in someone else's shoes is a description of feeling empathy.
- Being empathetic means sharing in any kind of emotion - it doesn't have to be a negative one. Being empathetic is being tuned in to all of a person's feelings and emotions, so that you get a sense of what it's like to be that person.

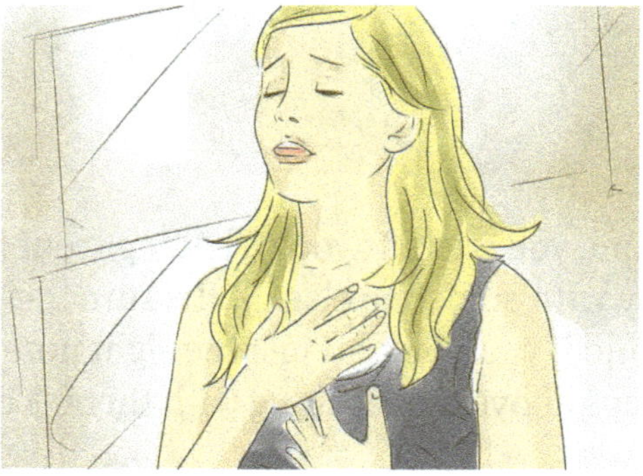

2. Realize you can feel it for anyone. You don't have to have a similar background to someone else to feel empathy for them. It's not about having a shared understanding because you've been there, too. In fact, you can feel empathy for people with whom you have nothing in common. Being empathetic is about experiencing what someone else is feeling - whatever it is. It doesn't have to be something you've felt before.

- This means you can feel empathy for anyone. A young person can empathize with an elderly person in a nursing home, even though she has clearly never had that experience. A rich person can empathize with someone who is homeless, even if he has always been privileged to have a roof over his head and plenty to eat. You can feel empathy for a stranger on the train you're watching from across the aisle.
- To put it another way, being empathetic doesn't mean imagining what life must be like for someone - it means actually feeling what life is like for that person on an emotional level.

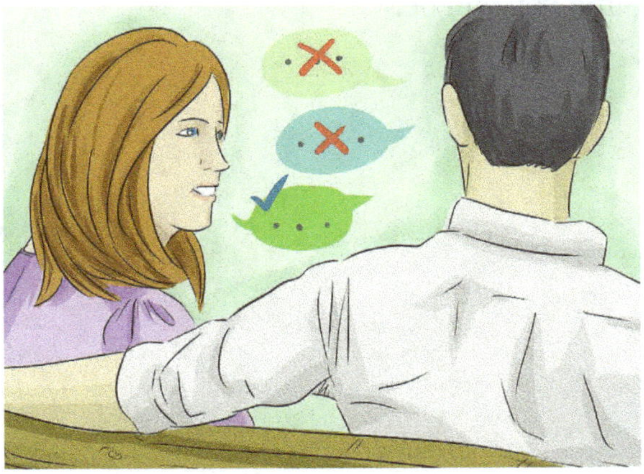

3. See that you don't have to agree with someone to empathize with them. In fact, it's still possible to be empathetic toward someone if you completely disagree with their views and don't even like them very much. The person you don't like is still human, and has the same range of emotions as you. It might not be easy to do, but you can still empathize with that person's pain and suffering, just as you would for someone you love.

- For example, let's say your neighbor is on the opposite end of the political spectrum from you, and he brings up views you think you are completely wrong at every opportunity. But if you saw him get hurt, you'd come to his aid.
- It might be even more important to develop the ability to empathize with people you don't like. Empathy helps us see each other as people in need of love and consideration, no matter what. It creates the possibility of peace.

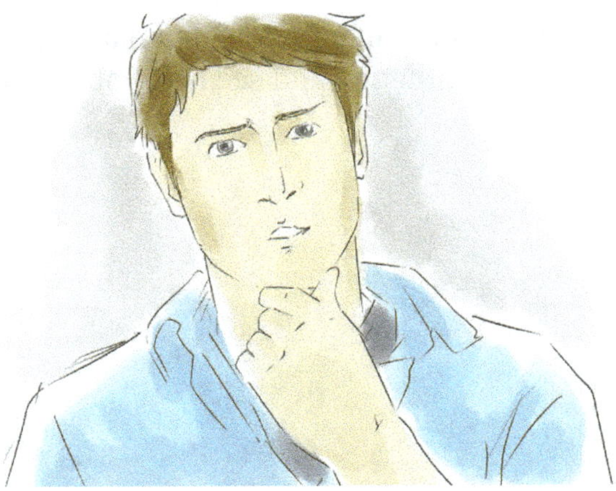

4. Forget the "do unto others" rule. George Bernard Shaw said, "Do not do unto others as you

would have them do unto you—they might have different tastes." The "Golden Rule" doesn't really apply when it comes to empathy, because it doesn't help you understand what it's like to be someone else. Being empathetic means opening yourself to someone else's point of view, someone else's "tastes," instead of imposing your own experiences and ideas.

- Thinking about how you'd like to be treated can serve as a good starting point for respectful and conscientious, but to be empathetic, you have to go a little deeper. It's difficult to do, and it might even feel uncomfortable. But the more you do it, the deeper your understanding of the people around you will be.

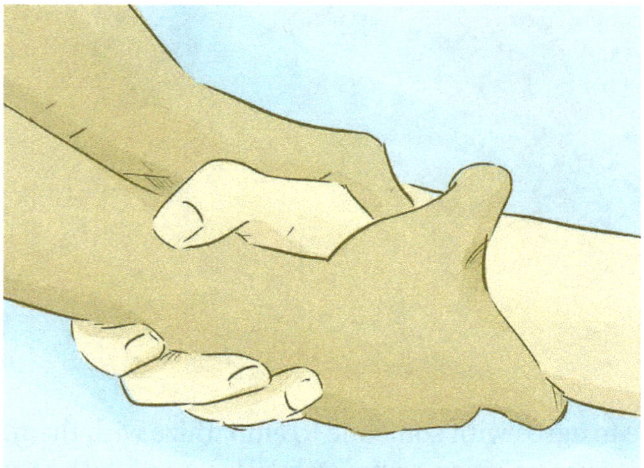

5. See why empathy matters. Empathy improves quality of life on both a personal and social level. It helps you feel more connected to the people around you and creates a sense of shared meaning. What's more, humans' ability to experience empathy for people different from them leads to big social gains. It helps individuals and groups get past racism, homophobia, sexism, classism, and other social problems. It's the foundation of social cooperation and mutual aid. Without empathy, where would we be?

- A recent study showed that the empathy level among college students has dropped 40% over the last 20 - 30 years. This suggests that empathy is, at least in part, something that can be learned or unlearned.

- By getting in touch with your sense of empathy and making it a priority every day, you can improve your ability to be empathetic - and see how your life improves as a result.

Chapter

4 Basic Nursing Tasks

Tasks such as checking an individual's temperature and blood pressure, providing patients with bedpans, sponge baths, clean linen are basic nursing skills. It also includes ensuring that the patients have their medication in time. The major nursing tasks are discussed in this chapter.

How to take Blood Pressure Manually

If you or someone you know is at risk for high or low blood pressure, you may want to invest in a manual blood pressure kit for home use. Learning how to take your blood pressure manually may take a little practice, but it is actually quite easy once you learn how. You'll need to know what to wear, when to take your blood pressure, how to take it accurately, and how to interpret the results. With a little practice you'll know how to find your systolic and diastolic pressure readings and what those numbers *actually* mean.

Part 1

Preparing to Check your Blood Pressure

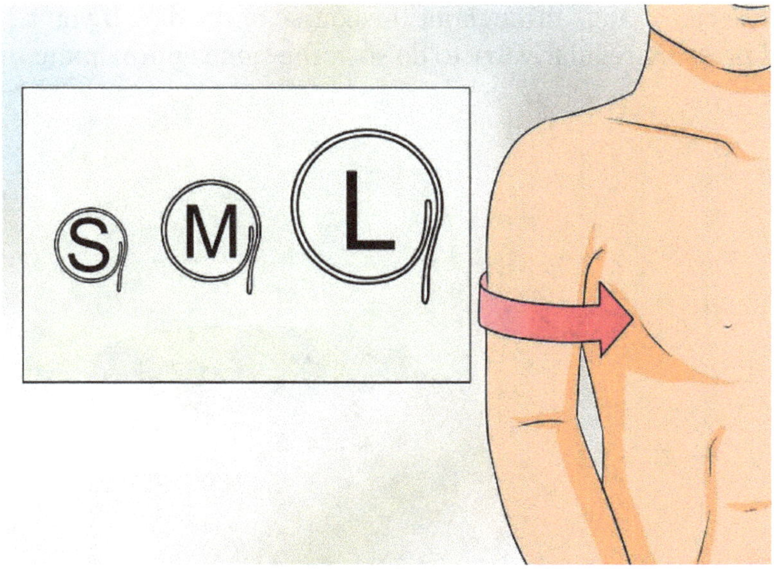

1. Verify that you have the right cuff size. A standard size blood pressure cuff purchased from a drugstore will fit around the arm of most adults. However, if you have an especially narrow or wide arm, or if you plan to take the blood pressure of a child, you may need a different size.

- Check the size of a cuff before buying it. Look at the "index" line. This is the range line on the cuff that tells you if it fits. Once it is on the patient's arm it will tell you whether or not the circumference of your arm fits within the "range" area of the cuff.

- If you do not use the proper cuff size, you may end up with an inaccurate measurement.

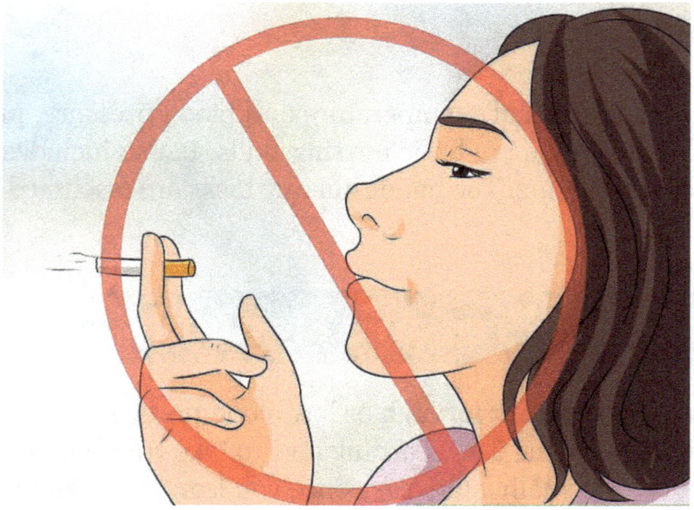

2. Avoid factors that can increase blood pressure. Certain conditions can cause blood pressure to spike temporarily. In order to get an accurate measurement, you or your patient should avoid these conditions before taking your blood pressure.

- Factors that can affect blood pressure include: stress, smoking, exercise, cold temperatures, a full stomach, a full bladder, caffeine, and some medications.
- Blood pressure can change throughout the course of the day. If you need to check the patient's blood pressure regularly, try to do so at the same approximate time each day.

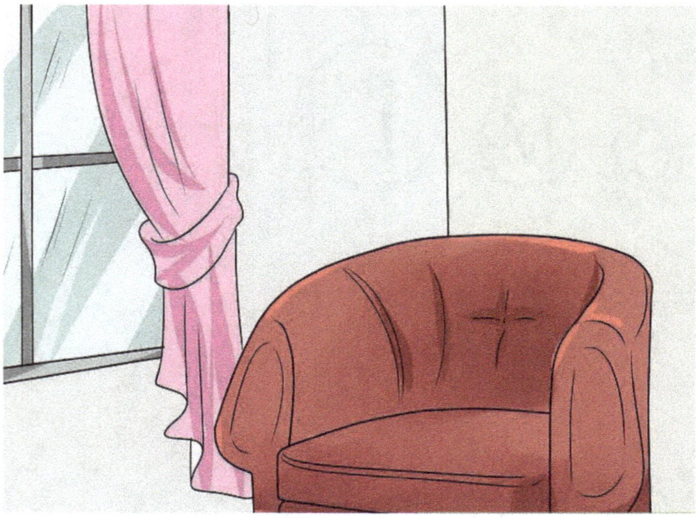

3. Find a quiet place. You will need to listen your, or your patient's heartbeat, so a quiet setting is ideal. A quiet room is also a calm room, so someone who rests in a quiet room while checking his or her blood pressure is more likely to feel relaxed, rather than stressed. Therefore you are more likely to get an accurate reading.

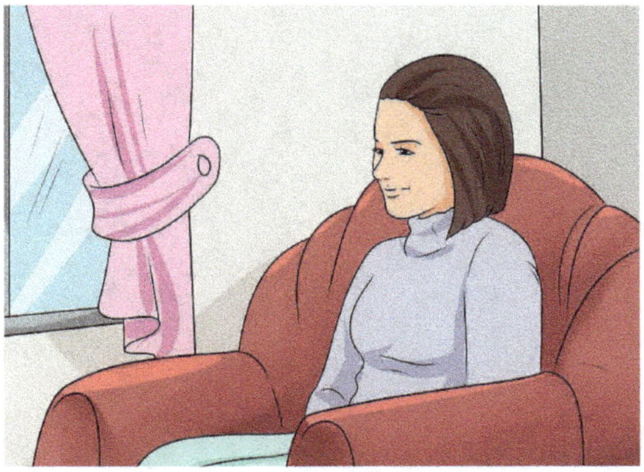

4. Get comfortable. Since physical stress can affect a blood pressure reading, you or the patient whose reading you take, should get comfortable. For example, use the bathroom before you have your blood pressure taken. It's also a good idea to keep yourself warm. Find a warm room, or if the room is chilly, wear an extra layer of clothing to keep warm.

- In addition, if you have a headache or body ache, try to reduce or relieve the pain before taking your blood pressure.

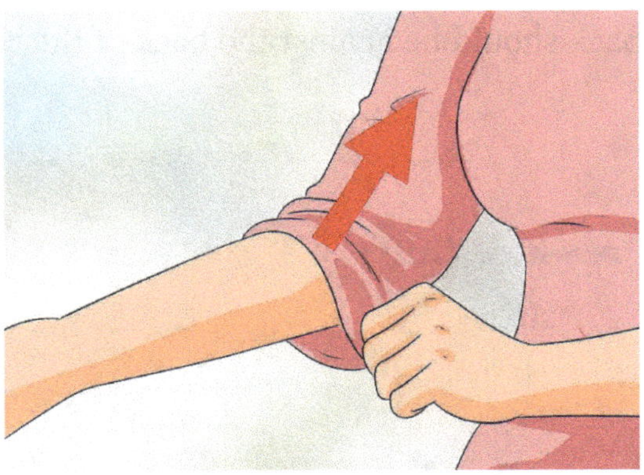

5. Remove tight sleeves. Roll up your left sleeve or, better yet, change into a shirt that exposes your upper arm. Blood pressure should be measured from the left arm, so the sleeve should be removed from the upper left arm.

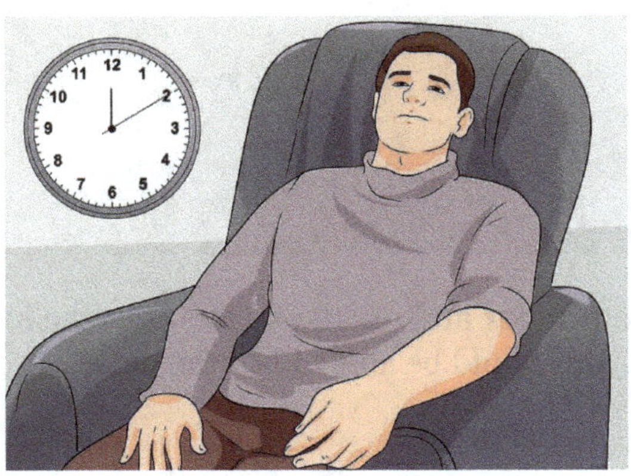

6. Rest for 5 to 10 minutes. Resting will assure that your heart rate and blood pressure have the chance to stabilize before the measurement is taken.

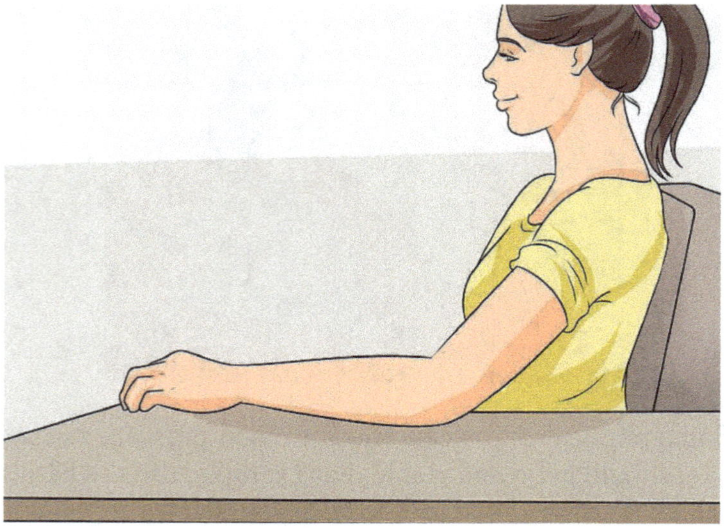

7. Find a comfortable and appropriate location to take your blood pressure. Sit in a chair next to a table. Rest your left forearm on the table. Position your left arm so that it rests at about heart level. Keep the palm of your hand facing up.

- Sit up straight. Your back should be against the back of the chair and your legs should be uncrossed.

Part 2

Positioning the Blood Pressure Cuff

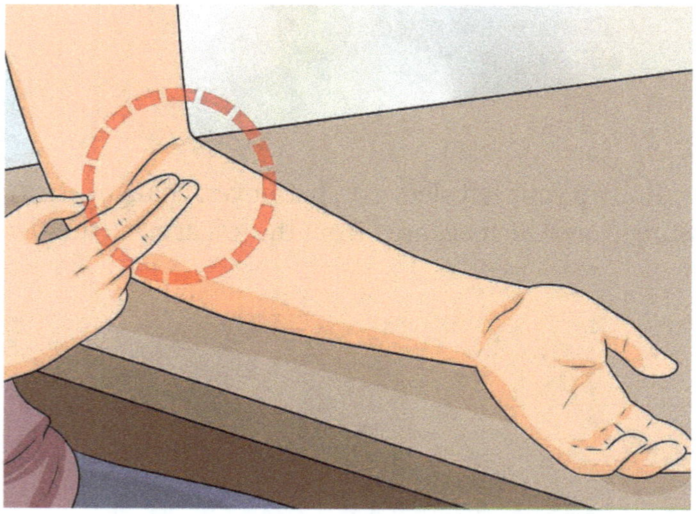

1. Locate your pulse. Place your index and middle fingers over the inside center of your inner elbow. When you press lightly you should be able to feel the pulse of your brachial artery from this position.

- If you have difficultly locating your pulse, place the head of the stethoscope (the round piece at the end of the tube) in the same general area and listen until you can hear your heartbeat.

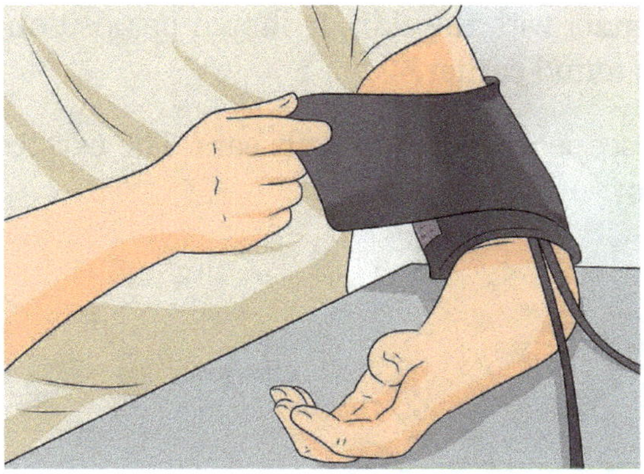

2. Wrap the cuff around your arm. Tuck the cuff end through the metal loop and slide it onto your upper arm. The cuff should be roughly 1 inch (2.5 cm) above the bend of your elbow and should be evenly tight around your arm.

- Make sure that your skin is not pinched by the cuff as you wrap it securely. The cuff should have heavy duty velcro on it, which will hold the cuff closed.

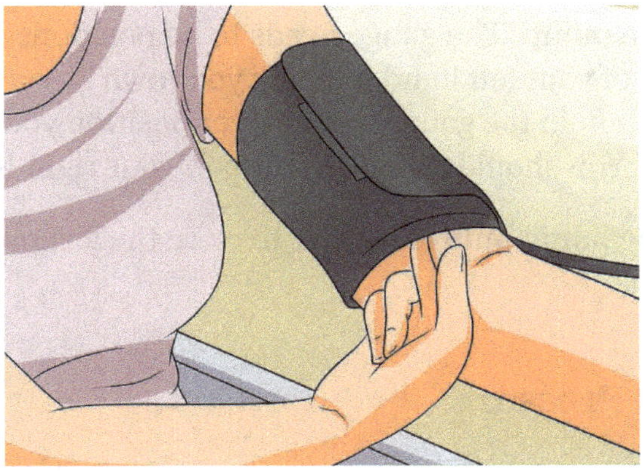

3. Check the tightness of the cuff by slipping two fingertips underneath. If you can wiggle the two fingertips under the top edge but cannot wedge your full fingers beneath the cuff, the cuff is tight enough. If you can wedge your full fingers under the cuff then you need to open up the cuff and pull it tighter before closing it again.

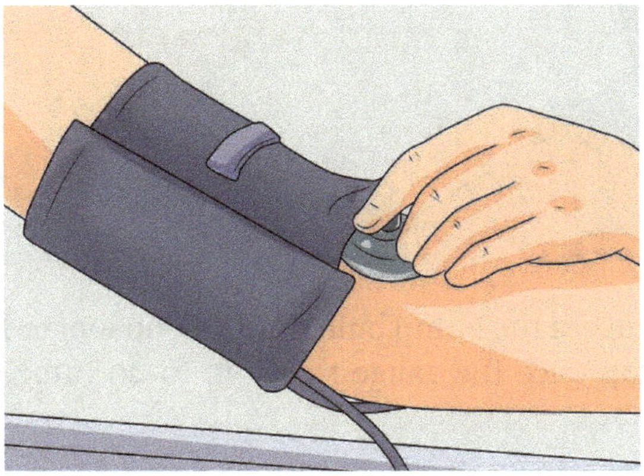

4. Slide the head of the stethoscope under the cuff. The head should be face down, with the wide

part of the chest piece in contact with the skin. It should be positioned directly over the pulse of your brachial artery that you found earlier.

- Also place the stethoscope earpieces in your ears. The earpieces should face forward and point toward the tip of your nose.

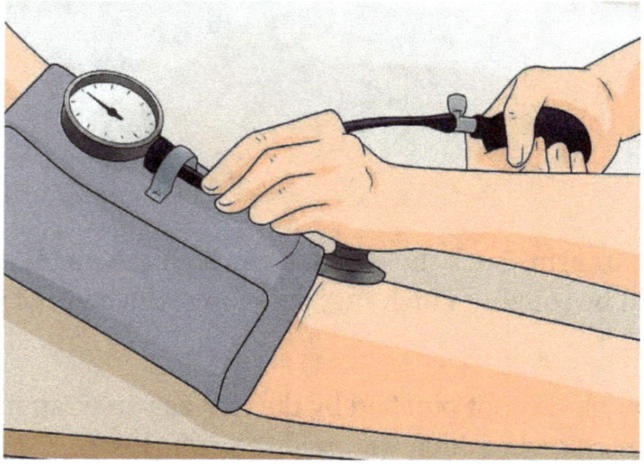

5. Position the gauge and the pump. The gauge needs to be positioned where you can see it. Hold the gauge lightly in the palm of your left hand if taking your own blood pressure. If taking someone else's blood pressure, you can hold the gauge in whatever position you want as long as you can see the face of the gauge clearly. You should hold the pump in your right hand.

- Turn the screw on the pump bulb clockwise to close the airflow valve, if necessary.

Part 3

Measuring your Blood Pressure

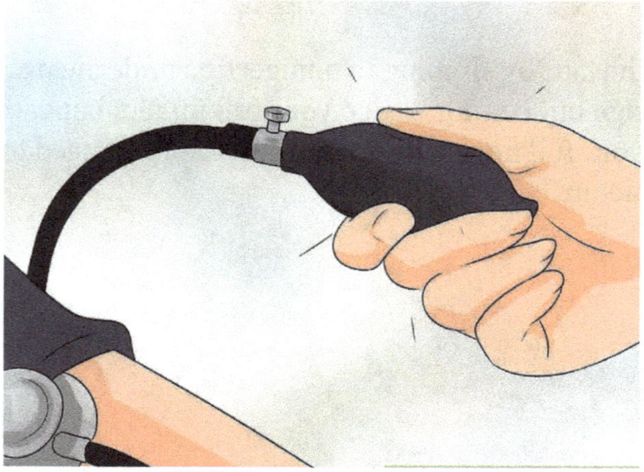

1. Inflate the cuff. Rapidly squeeze the pump bulb until you no longer hear the sound of your pulse through the stethoscope. Stop once the gauge reads 30 to 40 mmHg above your normal blood pressure.

- If you do not know your normal blood pressure, inflate the cuff until the gauge reads between 160 to 180 mmHg.

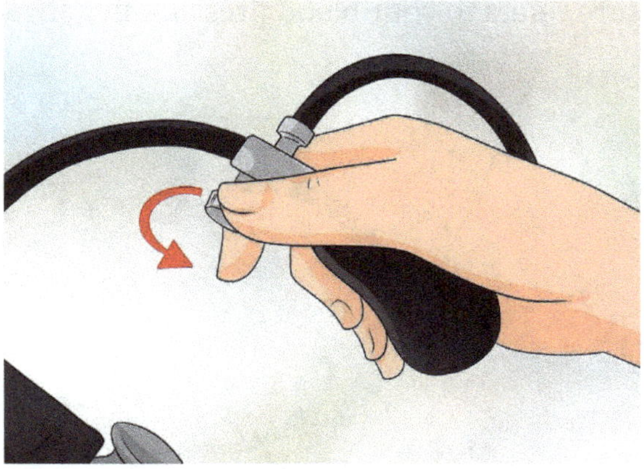

2. Deflate the cuff. Open the airflow valve by twisting the screw counterclockwise. Let the cuff deflate gradually.

- The gauge should fall 2 mm, or two lines on the gauge, per second.

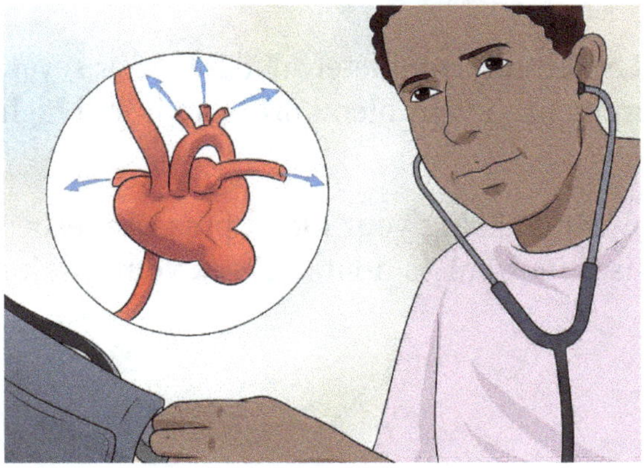

3. Listen for the systolic reading. Note the measurement on your gauge at the precise moment you hear your heartbeat again. This measurement is your systolic reading.

- Systolic blood pressure refers to the force your blood exerts against the artery walls as your heart pumps. This is the blood pressure created when your heart contracts.

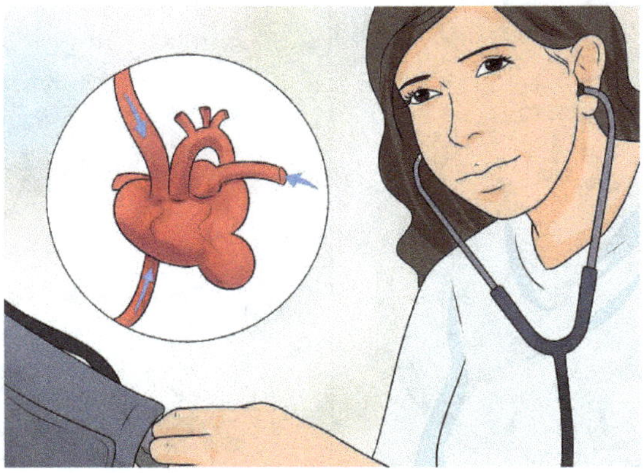

4. Listen for the diastolic reading. Note the measurement on your gauge at the precise moment the sound of your heartbeat disappears. This measurement is your diastolic reading.

- Diastolic blood pressure refers to your blood pressure in between heartbeats.

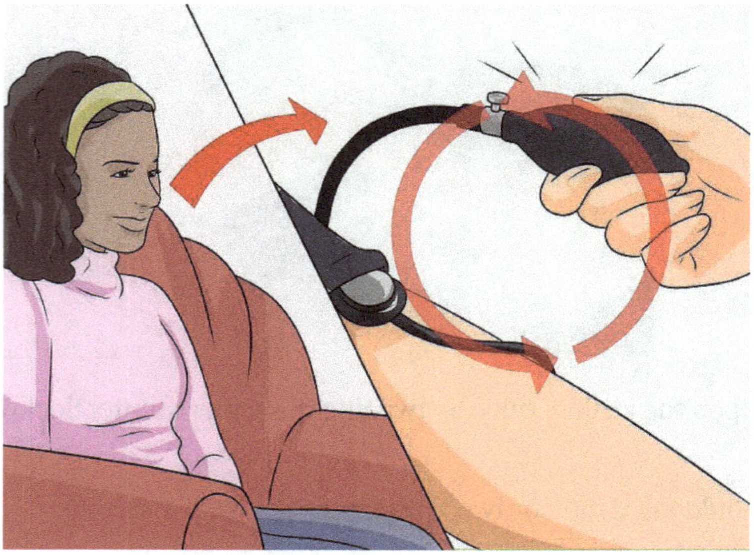

5. Rest and repeat the test. Let the cuff completely deflate. After several minutes, follow the same steps to take another measurement. If your blood pressure is still high, consider comparing readings with the other arm.

- Mistakes can happen while taking your blood pressure, especially if you are not used to doing it. As such, it is important to double-check your findings by taking a second measurement.

Part 4

Interpreting the Results

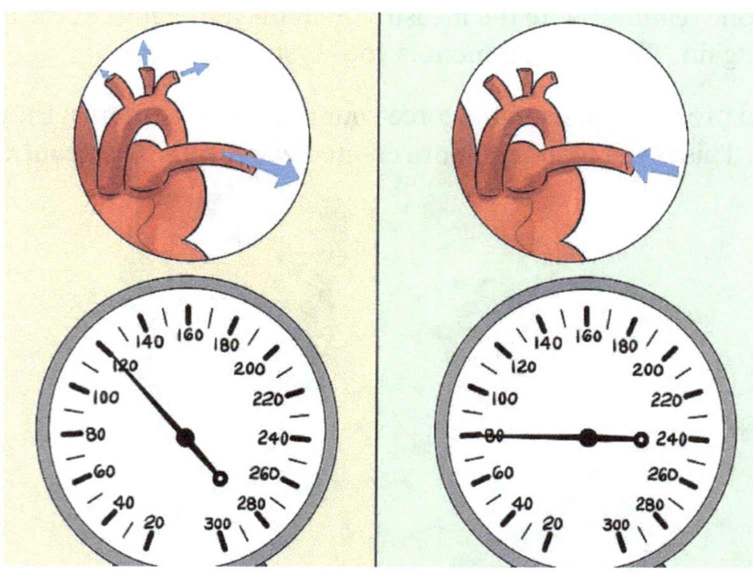

1. Know what normal blood pressure should be. For an adult, the systolic blood pressure should be less than 120 mmHg and the diastolic blood pressure should be less than 80 mmHg.

- This range is considered "normal." Healthy behaviors, including diet and exercise, should be maintained in order to maintain this blood pressure range.

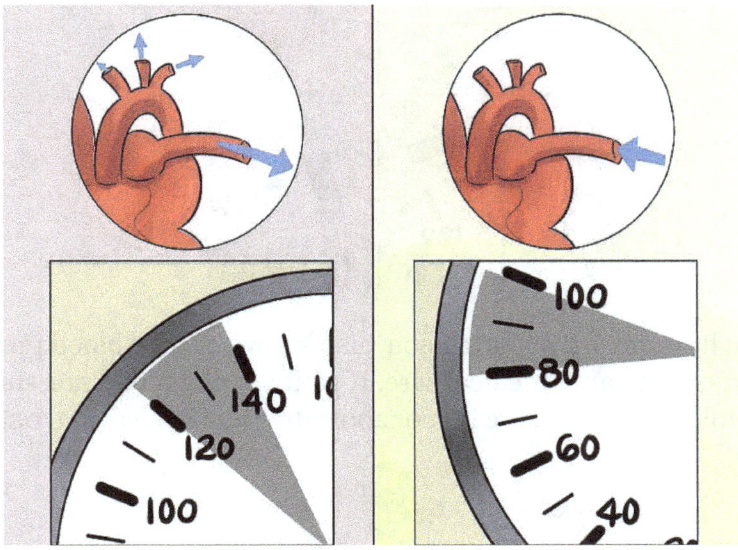

2. Catch signs of prehypertension. Prehypertension is not necessarily dangerous by itself, but someone with prehypertension is at risk of experiencing hypertension in the future. An adult in a state of prehypertension will have a systolic blood pressure between 120 and 139 mmHG and a diastolic blood pressure between 80 and 89 mmHg.

- Talk to a health care professional about making changes to your diet and lifestyle in order to drop your blood pressure.

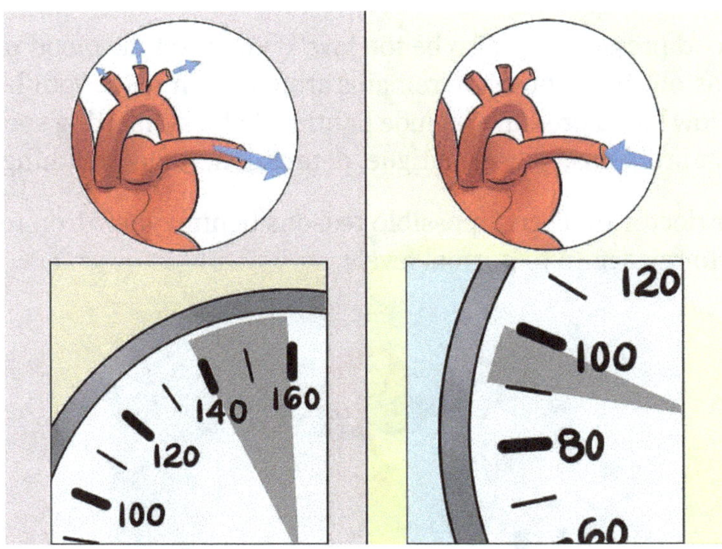

3. Detect signs of stage 1 hypertension. During state 1 hypertension, also known simply as high blood pressure, an adult's systolic blood pressure is between 140 ad 159 mmHg. The diastolic blood pressure is between 90 and 99 mmHg.

- Hypertension requires professional medical care. Schedule an appointment with your doctor so that he or she may prescribe an appropriate hypertension medication.

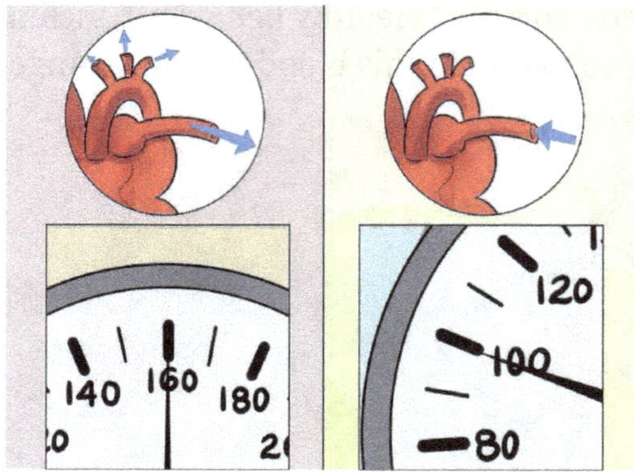

4. Assess whether you have stage 2 hypertension, also known as high blood pressure. This is a serious condition and requires prompt medical care. If your systolic blood pressure is at or above 160 mmHg and your diastolic blood pressure is at or above 100 mmHG, you have stage 2 hypertension.

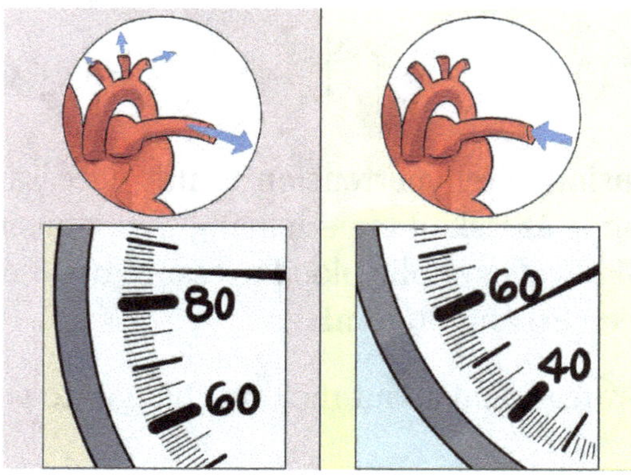

5. Understand that blood pressure can also be too low. If your systolic blood pressure stays around 85 mmHg and your diastolic blood pressure remains around 55 mmHG, your blood pressure may be too low. Symptoms of low blood pressure include lightheadedness, fainting spells, dehydration, lack of concentration, vision problems, nausea, fatigue, depression, rapid breathing, and clammy skin.

- Talk with your doctor to discuss possible reasons behind your drop in blood pressure and possible ways to raise it up to normal levels.

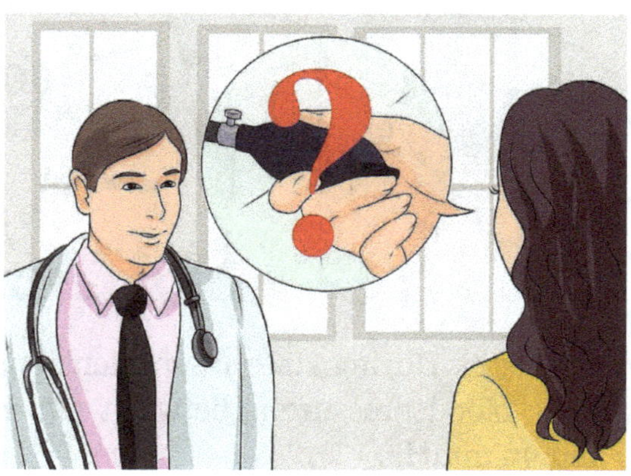

6. Consult a physician if you suspect you have any stage of hypertension or low blood pressure. Your doctor will retest your blood pressure to make sure your readings are accurate. If you do

have hypertension, or prehypertension, your doctor will make recommendations for lowering your blood pressure. This will include lifestyle changes, if you have prehypertension, in addition to medication if you have actual hypertension.

- The doctor may also test for other conditions that hinder normal blood pressure, especially if the patient is already on medication.
- If you are already on medication for your blood pressure, your doctor may suggest therapy or consider testing for additional health problems that prevent the medication from working properly.

How to take a Temperature

When it comes to taking someone's temperature, use the method that will give the most accurate reading. For babies and children under five years of age, taking a rectal temperature is most accurate. For older children and adults, taking an oral temperature is perfectly fine. As an alternative for people of any age, you may take an axillary (armpit) temperature, but this method is not as accurate as the others and should not be relied upon if you're worried the person has a fever.

Choose a Method

1. Oral: For adults or older children. Infants cannot hold the thermometer in their mouth.
2. Armpit: Too inaccurate for use on infants. Use for a quick check, then switch to another method if result is above 99 °F (37 °C).
3. Rectal: Recommended method for infants due to greater accuracy.

Method 1

Taking Oral Temperature

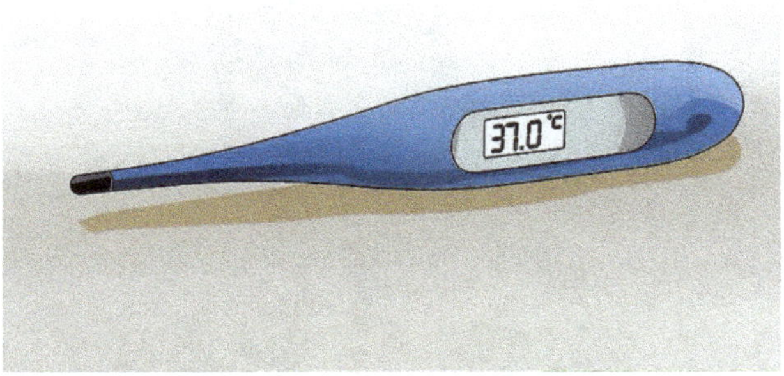

1. Use a multi-use or oral digital thermometer. Some digital thermometers are designed to be used either rectally, orally or in the armpit, while others are designed to be used specifically in the mouth. Either type of thermometer will give an accurate reading. You can find digital thermometers in the drugstore.

- If you have an old glass thermometer, dispose of it instead of using it to take a temperature. Glass thermometers are considered unsafe now because they contain mercury, which is poisonous to the touch.

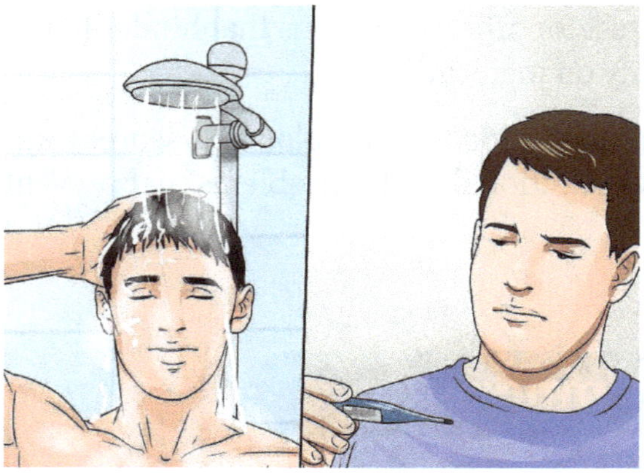

2. Wait 20 minutes after bathing. A warm bath or could affect the child's body temperature, so wait a good 20 minutes to make sure you get the most accurate possible reading.

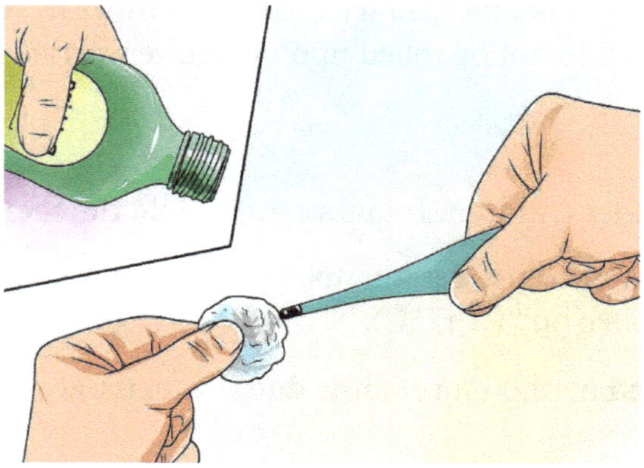

3. Prepare the tip of the thermometer. Clean it with rubbing alcohol soap and warm water, then rinse it with cool water and dry it thoroughly.

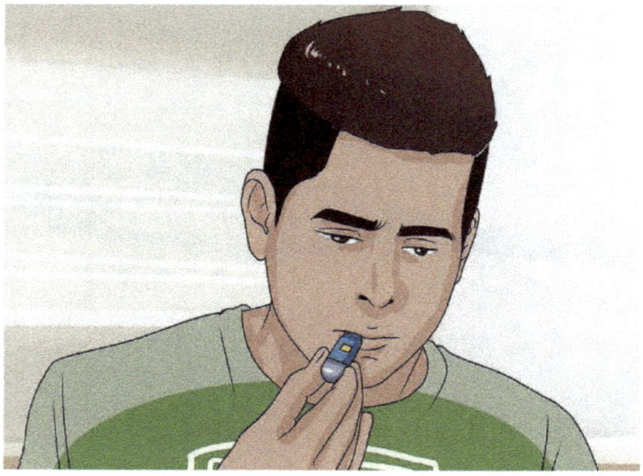

4. Turn on the thermometer and insert it under the tongue. Make sure the tip is completely in the mouth and under the tongue, not up near the lips. The person's tongue should completely cover the tip of the thermometer.

- If you're taking your child's temperature, either hold the thermometer in place or instruct your child to do so.
- Try to move the thermometer as little as possible.

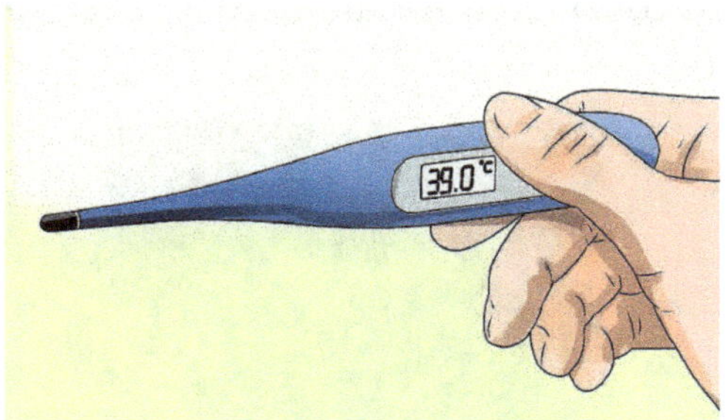

5. Remove the thermometer when it beeps. Look at the digital display to determine whether the person has a fever. Any temperature above 100.4 °F (38.0 °C) is considered a fever, but going to the doctor right away isn't necessary unless the fever is above a certain temperature:

- If the child is over 5 months old, call the doctor for a fever 101 °F (38 °C) or higher.
- If the person with the fever is an adult, call the doctor if it's 104 °F (40 °C) or higher.

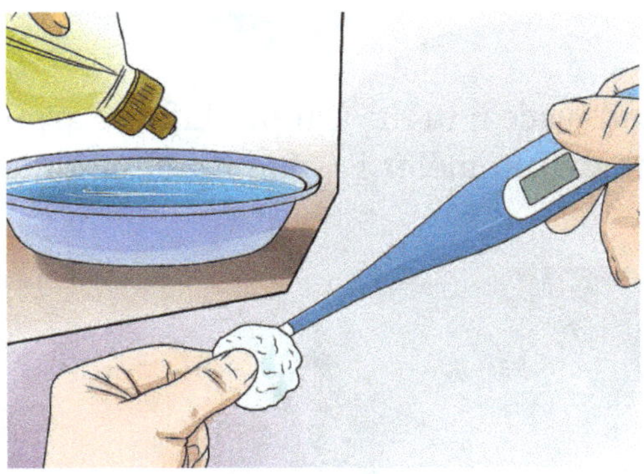

6. Wash the thermometer before putting it away. Use warm, soapy water and dry it thoroughly before putting it away for next time.

Method 2

Taking Axillary (Armpit) Temperature

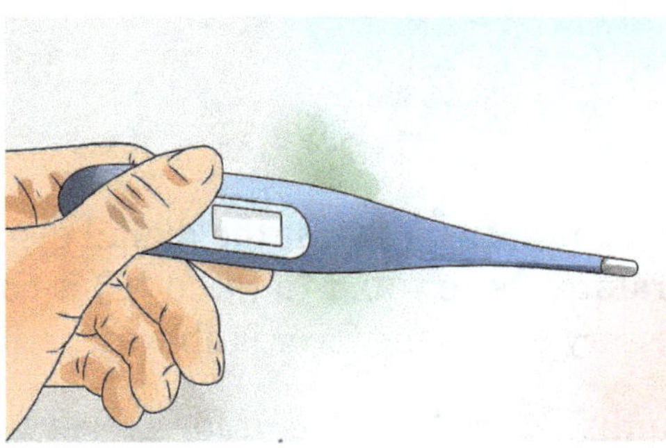

1. Use a multi-use digital thermometer. Look for a digital thermometer designed to be used either

rectally, orally or in the armpit. This way you can take the axillary temperature first, and if a high temperature is indicated, you can try a different method as well.

- If you have an old glass thermometer, dispose of it instead of using it to take a temperature. Glass thermometers are considered unsafe now because they contain mercury, which is poisonous to the touch.

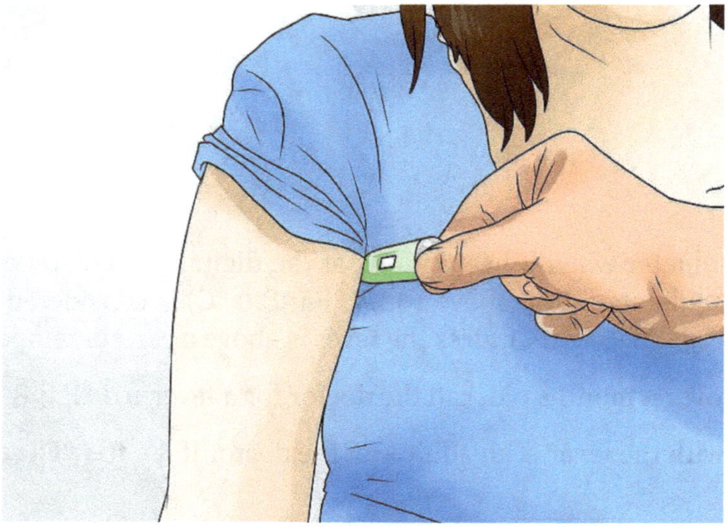

2. Turn on the thermometer and place it in the armpit. Lift the arm, insert the thermometer, then lower the arm so the tip of the thermometer is snug in the middle of the armpit. The entire tip should be covered.

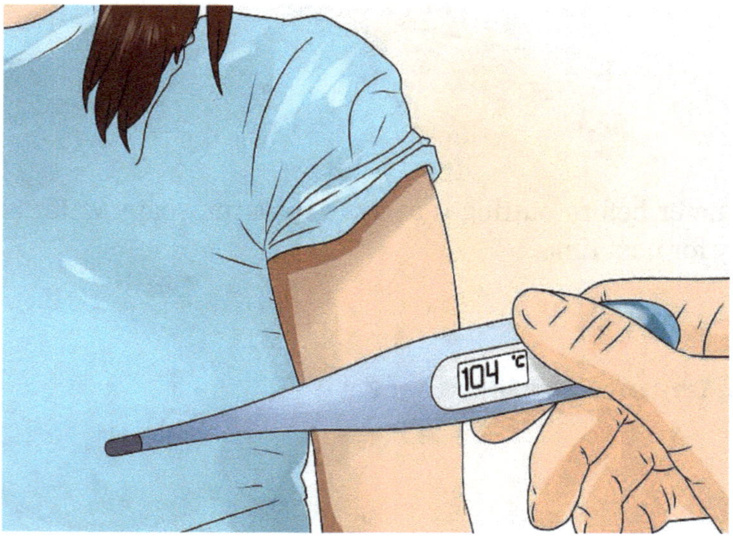

3. Remove the thermometer when it beeps. Look at the digital display to determine whether the person has a fever. Any temperature above 100.4 °F (38.0 °C) is considered a fever, but going to the doctor right away isn't necessary unless the fever is above a certain temperature:

- If the child is over 5 months old, call the doctor for a fever 101 °F (38 °C) or higher.
- If the person with the fever is an adult, call the doctor if it's 104 °F (40 °C) or higher.

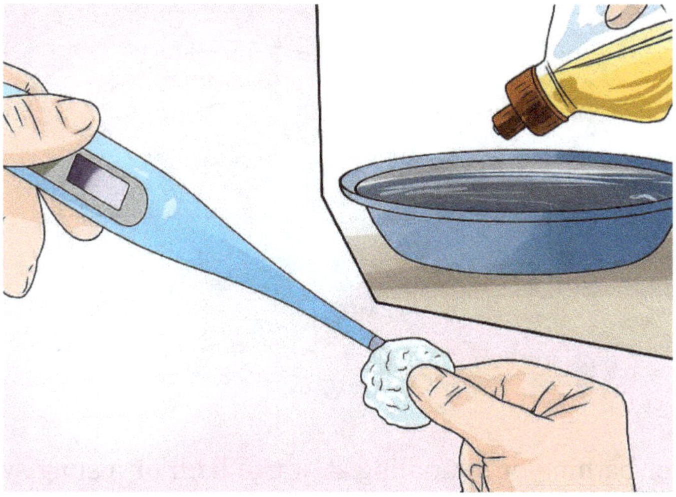

4. Wash the thermometer before putting it away. Use warm, soapy water and dry it thoroughly before putting it away for next time.

Method 3

Taking Rectal Temperature

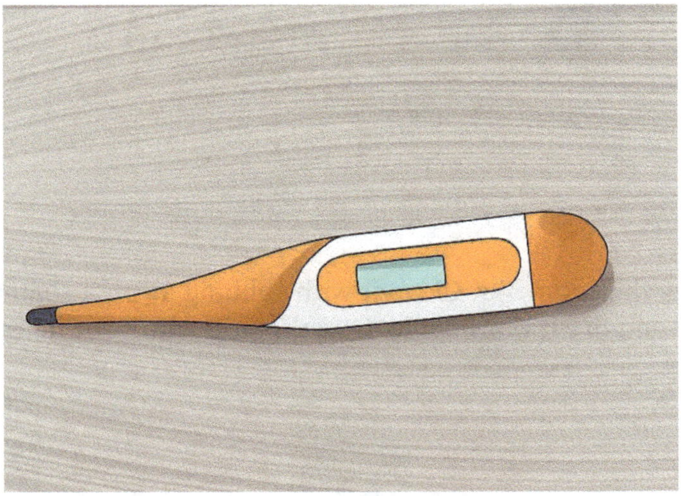

1. Use a multi-use or rectal digital thermometer. Some digital thermometers are designed to be used either rectally, orally or in the armpit, while others are designed to be used specifically in the rectum. Either type of thermometer will give an accurate reading. You can find digital thermometers in the drugstore.

- Look for a model that has a wide handle and a sip that can't be inserted too far into the rectum. This will make the process easier and help prevent you from inserting the thermometer too far.
- If you have an old glass thermometer, dispose of it instead of using it to take a temperature. Glass thermometers are considered unsafe now because they contain mercury, which is poisonous to the tough.

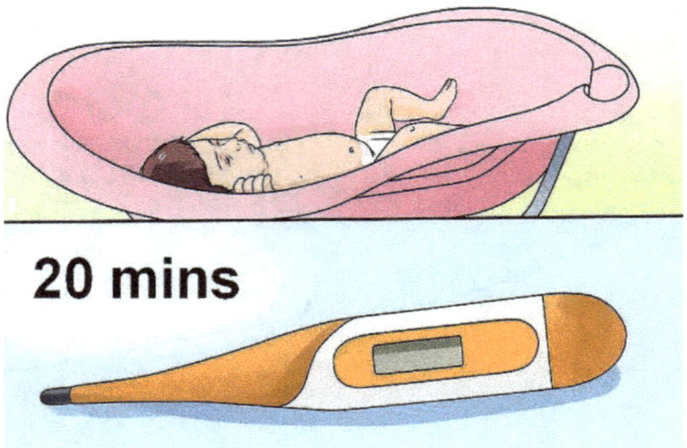

2. Wait 20 minutes after bathing or swaddling. A warm bath or a snug swaddling session could affect the child's body temperature, so wait a good 20 minutes to make sure you get the most accurate possible reading.

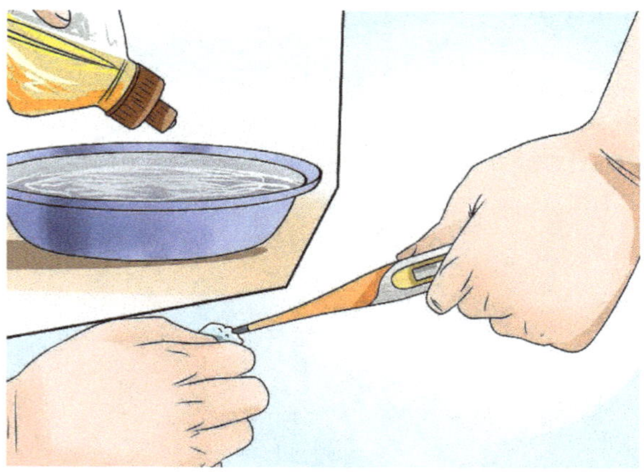

3. Prepare the tip of the thermometer. Clean it with rubbing alcohol soap and warm water, then rinse it with cool water and dry it thoroughly. Cover the tip with petroleum jelly to make it easier to insert.

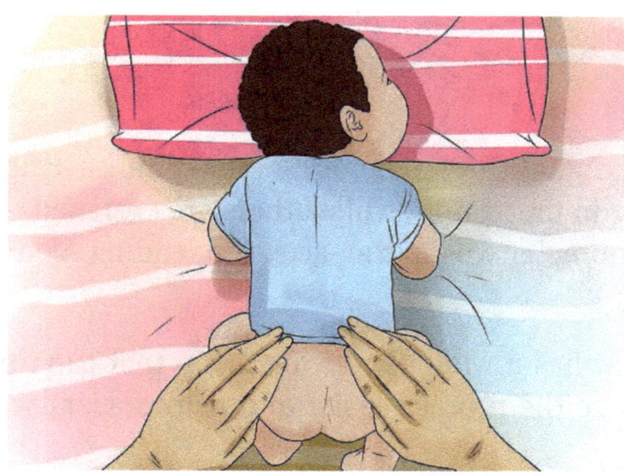

4. Position the child comfortably. Place the child either tummy down across your lap, or tummy up on a firm surface. Choose the position that's most comfortable for the child and makes it easiest for you to access the rectum.

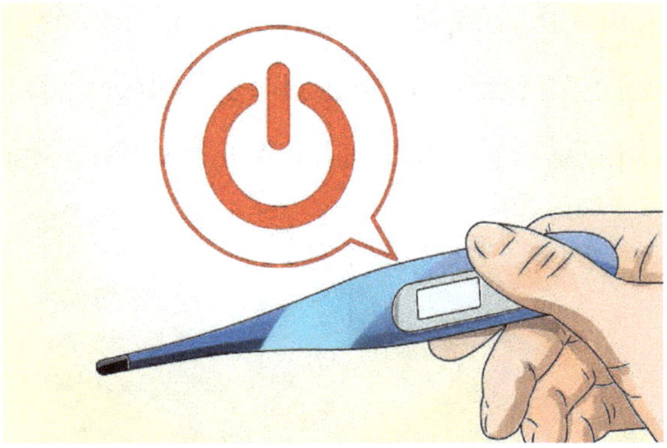

5. Turn on the thermometer. Most digital thermometers have a clearly labeled button you press to power on the device. Allow a moment or two for it to get set to take the temperature.

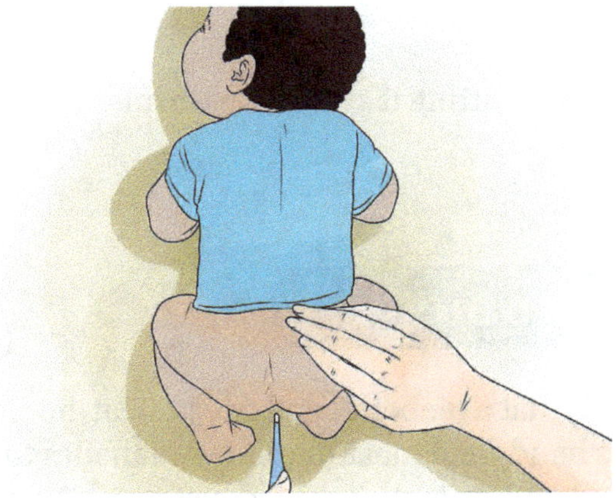

6. Hold the child's buttocks apart and gently insert the thermometer. Use one hand to hold the child's buttocks apart and the other to insert the thermometer about three quarters of an inch to once inch inside. Stop if any resistance is felt.

- Keep the thermometer in place by holding it between your first and middle fingers. Meanwhile, keep your other hand hand firmly but gently on the child's bottom to prevent squirming.

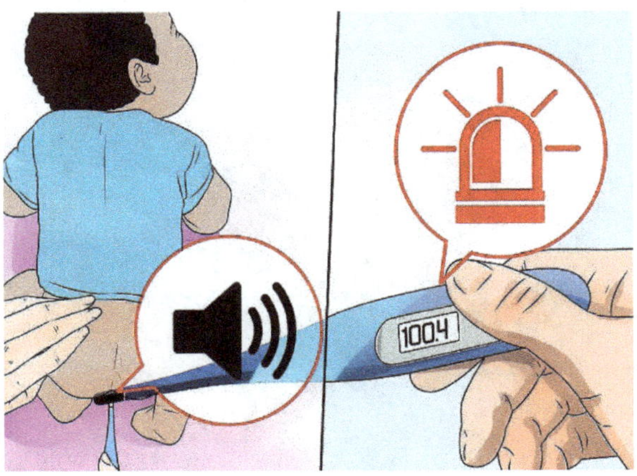

7. Once the beep sounds, carefully remove the thermometer. Read the thermometer to determine whether the child has a fever. A temperature of 100.4 °F (38.0 °C) or higher indicates a fever.

- If the child is under 5 months old, call the doctor for a fever 100.4 °F (38.0 °C) or higher.
- If the child is over 5 months old, call the doctor for a fever 101 °F (38 °C) or higher.
- If the person with the fever is an adult, call the doctor if it's 104 °F (40 °C) or higher.

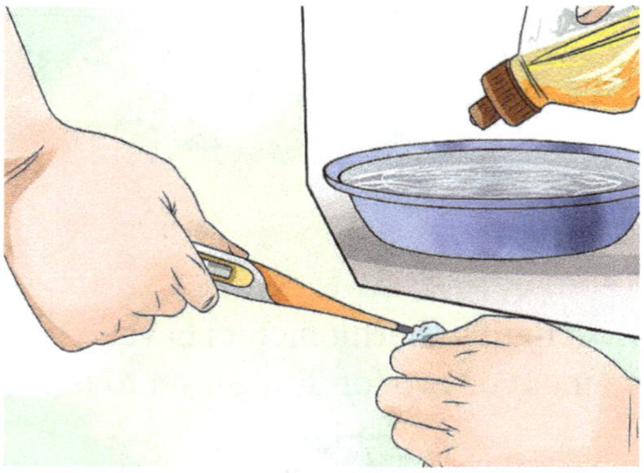

8. Wash the thermometer before putting it away. Use warm, soapy water as well as rubbing alcohol to cleanse the tip thoroughly.

How to use a Glucometer

One of the most valuable tools that a diabetic can have is an at-home blood sugar reader, otherwise known as a glucometer. This hand-held machine allows diabetics to monitor the amount of glucose in the blood, which helps in determining what food you can eat and how well any medication you are on is working, as well as how much insulin you may need to inject. Obtaining and properly using a glucometer at home can make diabetic care simpler and can help you to keep track of your blood sugars over time.

Method 1

Preparing for Daily Testing

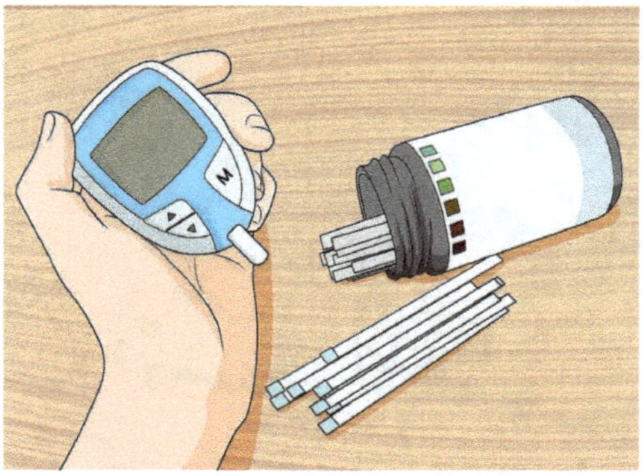

1. Obtain a glucometer and test strips. You can go to any drugstore and buy a blood sugar testing kit. Most kits contain lancets (testing needles), a lancing device, testing strips, and a meter to read the results.

- Many insurance companies will pay for your meter and test strips if you obtain a prescription from your doctor.

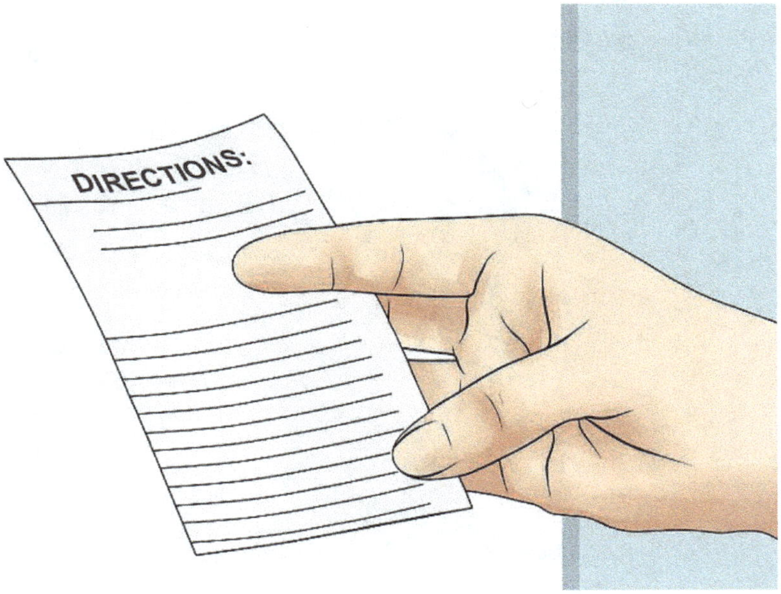

2. Read the materials and directions that come with your meter. Familiarize yourself with all the functions of your blood glucose meter, how much blood is required for testing, where you insert your test strip, and where the readout will be. Look at the pictures and read the instructions thoroughly, and if you have any questions or concerns then contact your doctor before trying to use the machine.

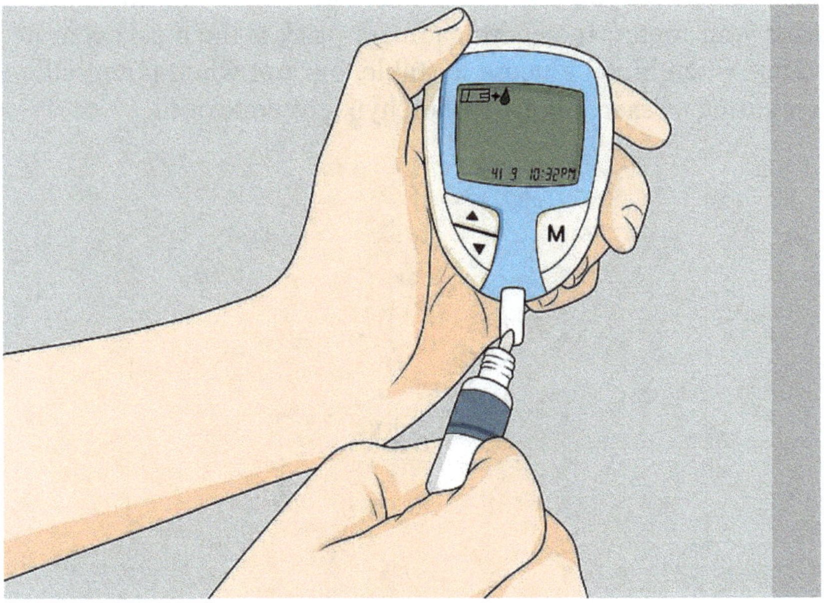

3. Test the glucometer before using it. Most glucometers include a way to test to make sure they are reading correctly. This could be in the form of a premade test strip or a liquid you place on a test strip. These are inserted into the machine and the reading should be within acceptable limits, which the instruction manual will provide.

Method 2

Testing Blood Sugar with a Glucometer

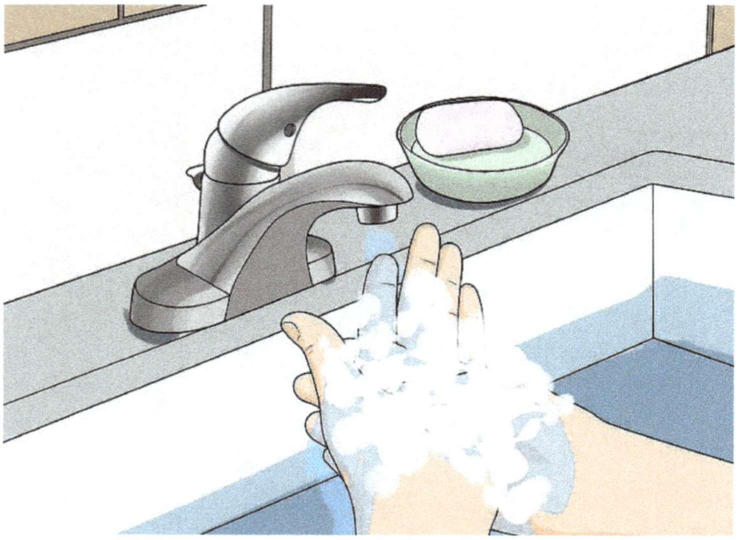

1. Clean your hands and sampling area. Use hot water and soap to wash your hands. Clean the finger you're going to prick with an alcohol swab, or with rubbing alcohol on a cotton ball. Alcohol evaporates rapidly so there's no need to dry the area; that will just recontaminate it. Let the alcohol air dry.

- Most glucometers instruct you to prick your finger for a sample, but some of the newer blood glucose meters let you use an area on your arm. Determine which of these areas is acceptable for your meter. In general, a finger prick is the most accurate. Alternative sites are okay to use when blood glucose is stable, but not when potentially changing rapidly, such as after eating or exercising, or when hypoglycemic or ill.

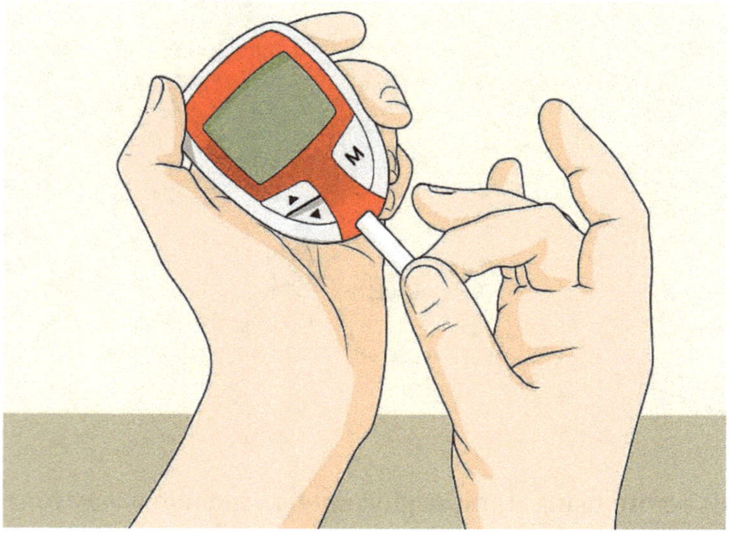

2. Assemble the device. Insert a test strip into the glucometer, ensuring your insert the proper end inward. Insert a lancet into the lancing device you use to prick your finger.

- Glucometers may differ in when you insert the test strip. Usually it is inserted in order to turn the machine on, but sometimes you have to put the blood on the strip and then insert it into the machine. Make sure you know which way your glucometer works before you prick your finger.

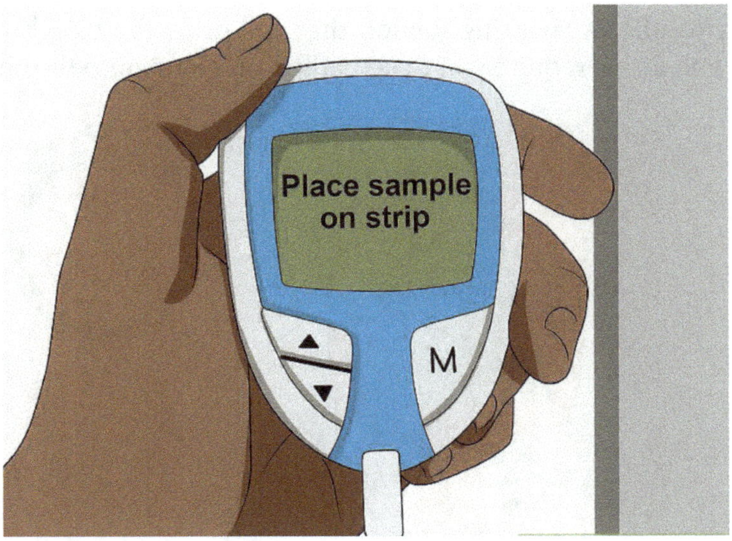

3. Wait for the glucometer to prompt you for a sample. A readout on the glucometer will tell you to put the drop of blood on the strip. The readout may actually say "place sample on strip," or it may give you a symbol, such as an icon that looks like a droplet of liquid.

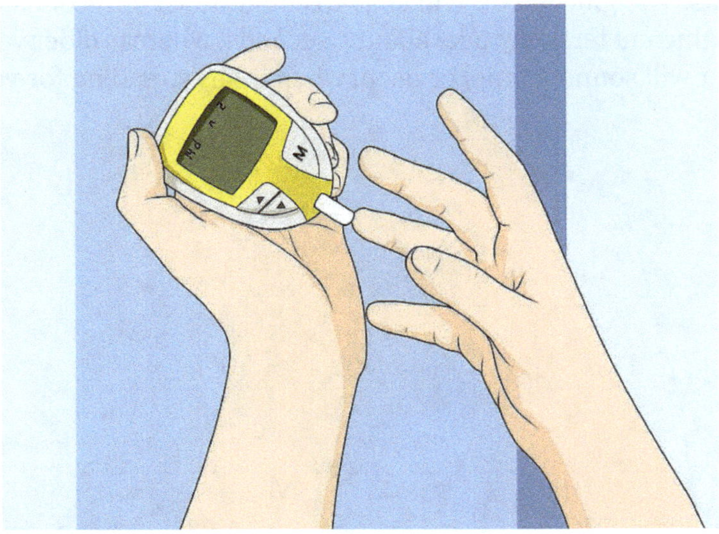

4. Test your blood sample. Prick your finger with the lancing device. This usually causes no, or very minimal, discomfort. You may need to squeeze or massage the finger you pricked on either side to squeeze out a drop of blood. Let the blood form a small bead on your finger. Hold the bead of blood to touch the tip of the strip at the right place, which should be indicated on the strip.

- Some people find it more comfortable to prick the side of the finger close to the fingernail, rather than the pad of the finger – there are fewer nerve endings on the side, making it a less sensitive area.

- If you find it difficult or painful to prick your finger, it may help to rinse your hand in warm water for a minute or two and then allow your hand to dangle at your side for another minute. This gets blood flowing to your fingers. Do this before you wash your hands with soapy water and use alcohol to clean the finger you're going to prick.
- The newer strips offer a "wicking" action that will draw the blood up into the test strip. Older meters and strips require you to actually drop blood onto the strip.

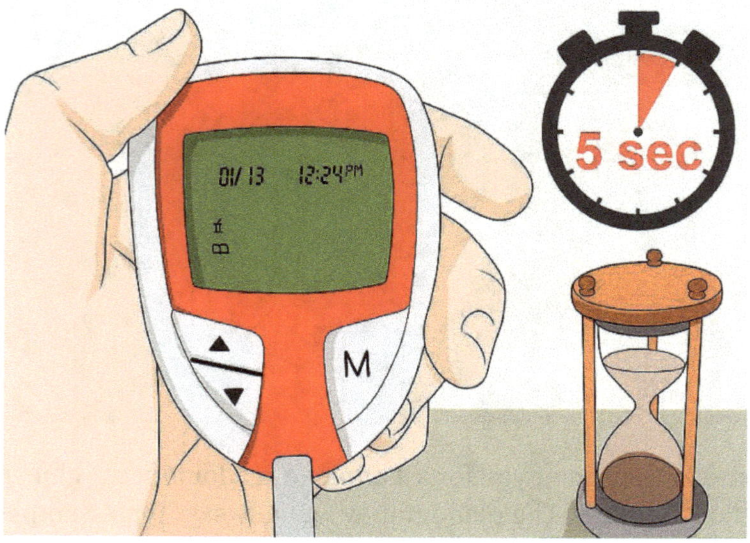

5. Wait for your results. The glucometer will start to count down in seconds until your results are ready to read. Newer glucometers only take about 5 seconds, whereas older versions may take10 to 30 seconds. The meter will sound a tone, or beep, when it has a reading for you.

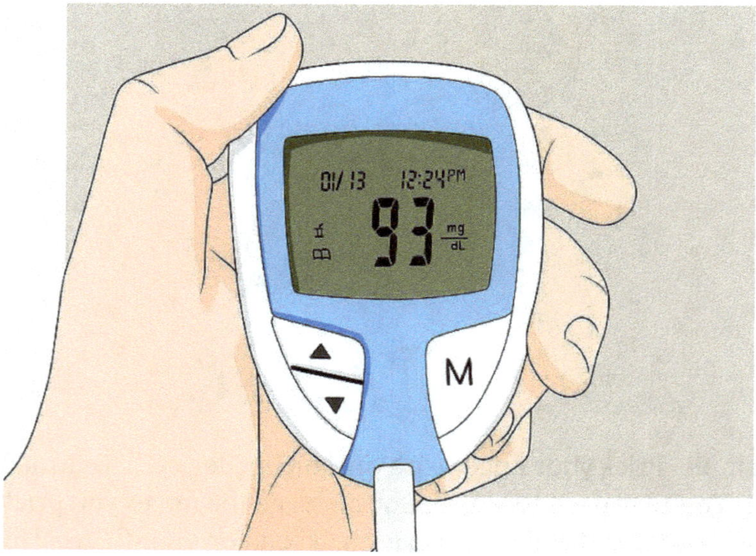

6. Read the results. The results will show up on the digital screen of your glucometer. Results will vary depending on what time of day it is, how recently you ate, and what you ate. There is no single good result for every person. You should discuss your diabetes with your healthcare provider and set goals for your blood sugar.

Method 3

Keeping Track of your Readings

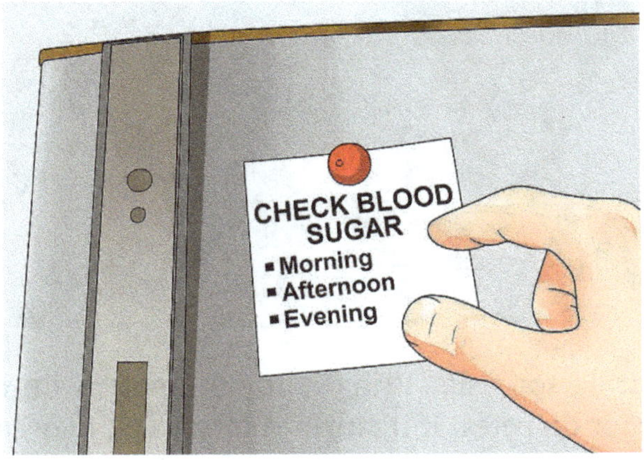

1. Create a system to help you remember to do your readings. You and your doctor will make a plan for how often and at what times you should use your glucometer to check your blood sugar. Sometimes this should be done three times every day. It might be hard to remember this, especially at first, but creating a system to help you remember can get you into the habit.

- Make a log that you have to check off for morning, afternoon, and evening. Put it on your refrigerator or bathroom mirror – somewhere that you look often throughout the day. Check off the boxes as you go.
- Be creative. Try keeping three small stones in your right pocket. As you do a reading, move a stone to your left pocket. By the end of the day you should have all stones in your left pocket. This can be a tangible reminder to do your readings. Come up with something that works for you.

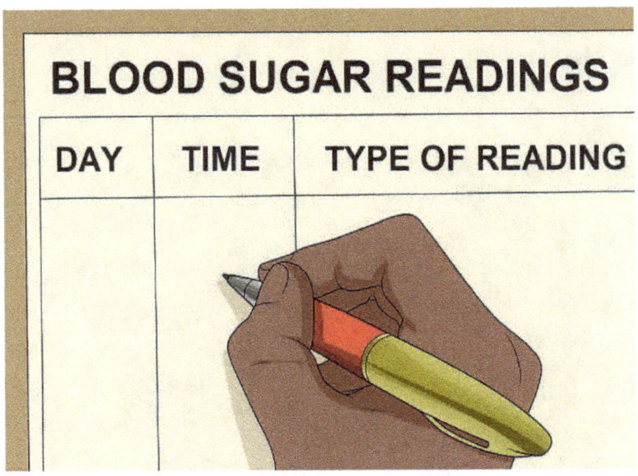

2. Keep a record of your results. Some diabetic glucose meters will store the readings for you in their on-board memory. With others, you will have to write your results down. Make sure you note the day, time and type of reading. For instance, was the reading taken first thing in the morning? This is known as a fasting reading. Was it taken 2 hours after a meal? This is known as a 2-hour postprandial reading.

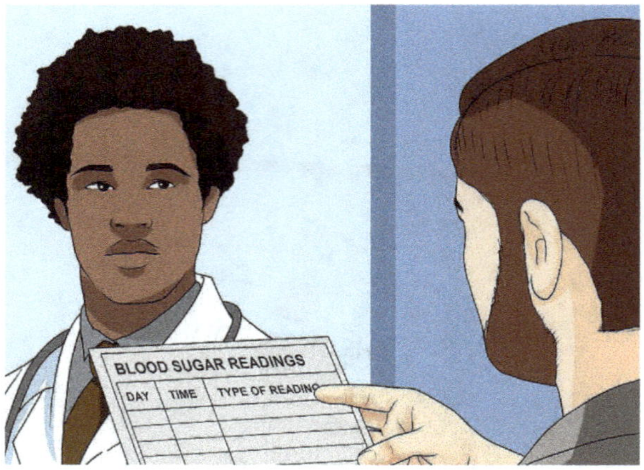

3. Bring your record to your doctor visits. Bring your glucometer with you every time you see the doctor who takes care of your diabetes. If it stores your results, they can access them directly. If your machine does not store your results, be sure to bring your written record with you. Bring your glucometer, as well, so your doctor can check to ensure it is working properly at every visit.

How to give a Sponge Bath

Sponge baths, or bed baths, are used to bathe people who are are bedridden or unable to bathe on their own due to health reasons. Giving a bed bath involves washing and rinsing the entire body one section at a time while the patient remains in bed. It is important to gather all the supplies needed before you begin so you do not have to leave the patient unattended. A good bed bath will leave the person feeling clean and comfortable.

Part 1

Preparing to Give the Bath

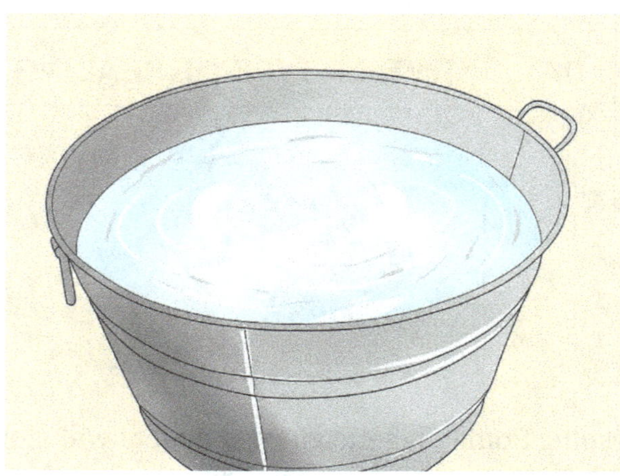

1. Fill two basins or washtubs with warm water. One is used for washing, and the other for rinsing. The water temperature should be 115 degrees F (46 degrees C) or less. You want it to be comfortable to the touch, but not too hot.

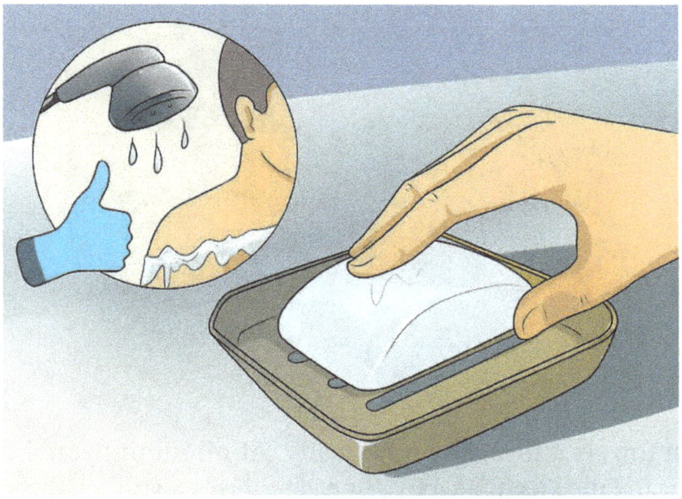

2. Choose soap that's easy to rinse away. Most bar soaps are fine to use. Body washes are also acceptable as long as they don't leave a residue. You may add soap to one of the basins to create a bowl of warm, soapy water for washing, or keep the soap separate and apply it directly to the patient's skin.

- Avoid using soap that has exfoliating beads or other substances that could end up staying on the patient's skin and causing irritation.
- No-rinse soaps are available at drug stores. This is a convenient solution for a quicker cleanse, but they leave a residue so you'll still need to rinse the patient's body from time to time.

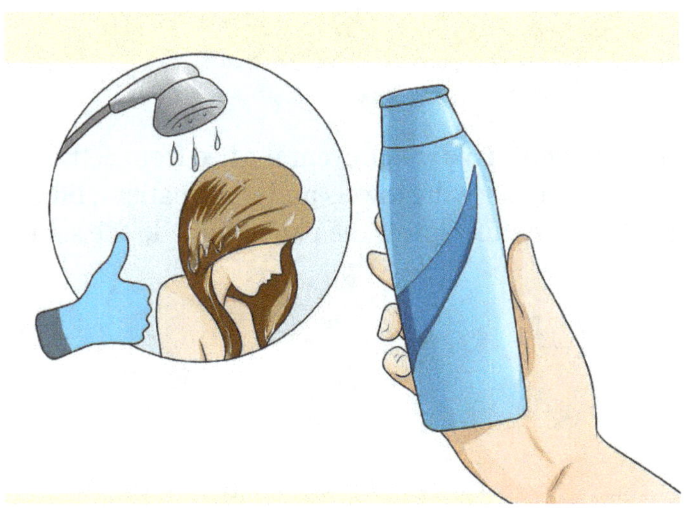

3. Get shampooing supplies ready. If you plan to shampoo the patient's hair, you'll need shampoo that's easy to rinse out (such as baby shampoo) and a special basin designed for washing hair in bed. You can find one at a medical supply store, and it's a big help when it comes to washing hair in bed without getting water everywhere.

- If you don't have a special basin, you can make do by placing an extra towel or two under the patient's head to protect the bed from getting too wet.

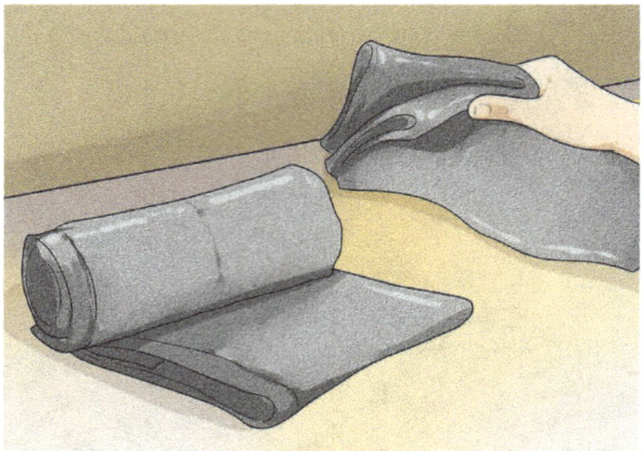

4. Have a stack of clean towels and washcloths ready. At minimum you'll need three large towels and two washcloths, but it's nice to have extra in case there's a spill or the supplies get soiled.

- It's convenient to stack towels, washcloth, the water basins and soap on a portable cart, such as a TV cart, so you can keep everything you need close to the bed.

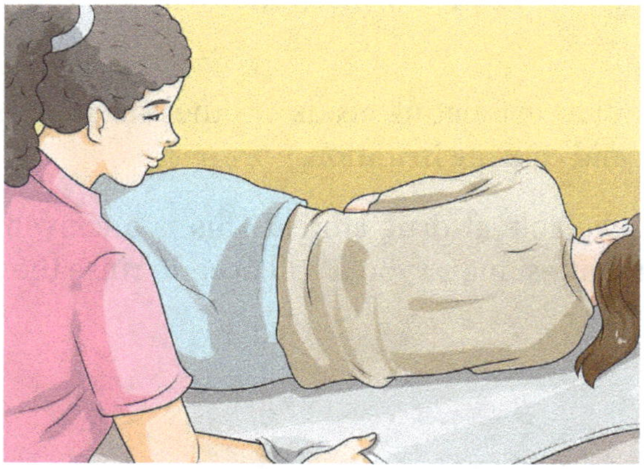

5. Place two towels under the patient. This will prevent the bed from getting wet and keep the patient comfortable during the process. To place the towels under the patient, lift the patient onto their side and scoot the towel under, then carefully lower the patient and do the same on the other side.

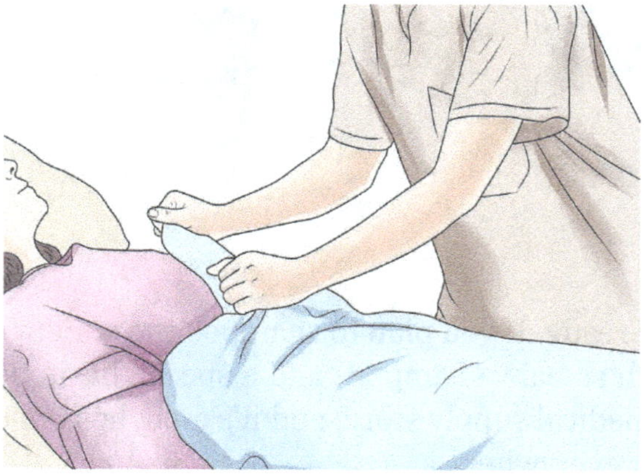

6. Cover the patient with a clean sheet or towel. This will ensure the patient stays warm during the bath as well as providing some privacy. The sheet or towel will stay on the patient's body the whole time.

- Be sure to adjust the temperature in the room if necessary, to prevent the patient from getting a chill.

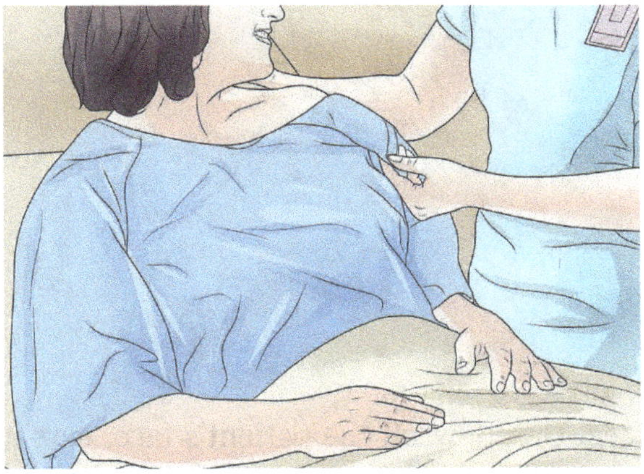

7. Remove the patient's clothes. Fold down the sheet or towel, uncovering the patient's top half, and remove their shirt. Replace the sheet over the top half of the patient. Fold the sheet back from the patient's legs and remove their pants and underwear. Recover the patient with the sheet.

- Try to keep as much of the patient covered as possible while you're removing the clothes.
- Keep in mind that this process can be embarrassing for some people, so try to work quickly and with a purposeful attitude.

Part 2

Bathing the Head, Chest and Legs

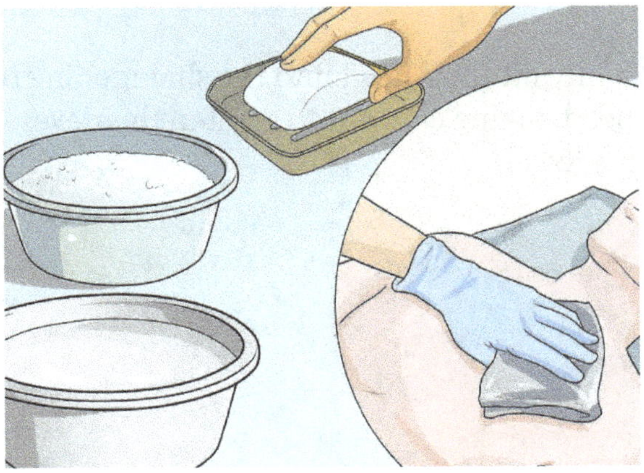

1. Use the same cleansing and rinsing method for the whole body. First apply soap or soapy water to the patient's skin. Scrub it gently with a washcloth to remove dirt and bacteria, then place the washcloth in the soapy basin. Dip a second washcloth into the rinsing basin and use it to rinse away the soap. Pat the area dry with a towel.

- Remember to rotate between the two washcloths: use one for soaping and one for rinsing. If the cloths become soiled, switch to clean ones.
- Replace the water in the basins as necessary.

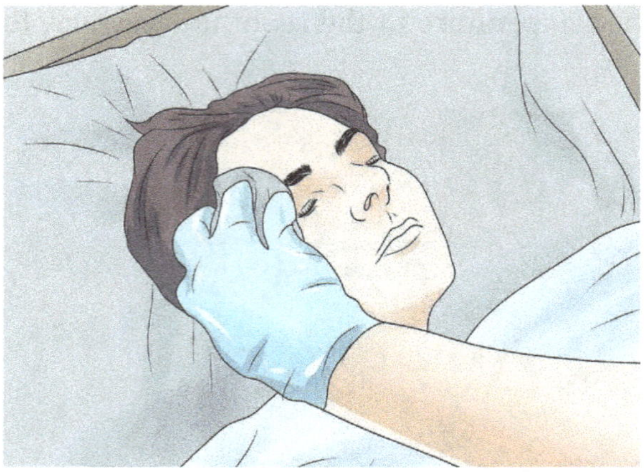

2. Start with the patient's face. Gently wash the patient's face, ears and neck with soapy water. Rinse away the soap with a separate washcloth. Dry the cleansed area with a towel.

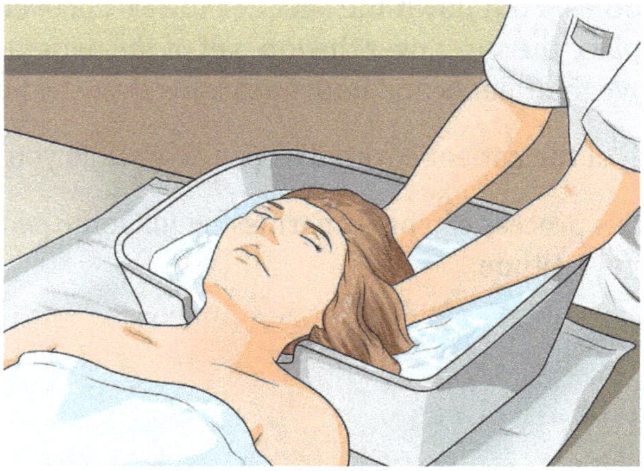

3. Wash the patient's hair. Gently lift their head into the shampooing basin. Wet the hair by pouring water over the patient's head, taking care not to get it in their eyes. Apply shampoo, then rinse it away. Pat the hair dry with a towel.

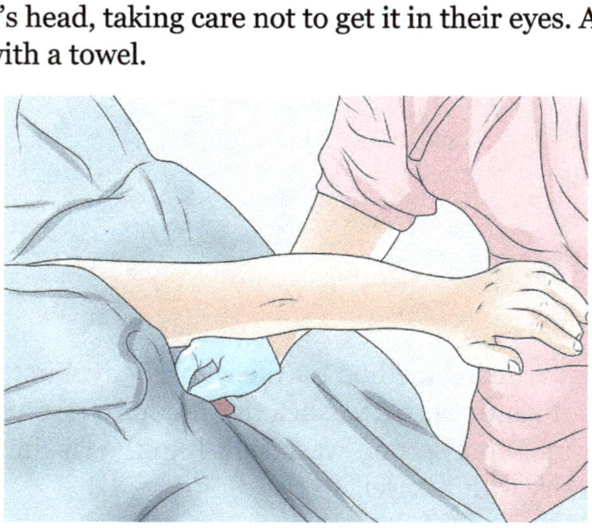

4. Wash the patient's left arm and shoulder. Fold over the sheet on the left side of the body down to the hip. Place a towel beneath the exposed arm. Wash and rinse the patient's shoulder, underarm, arm and hand. Dry the wet areas with a towel.

- Dry the washed areas thoroughly, especially the underarm, to prevent chafing and bacteria growth.
- Recover with the sheet to keep the patient warm.

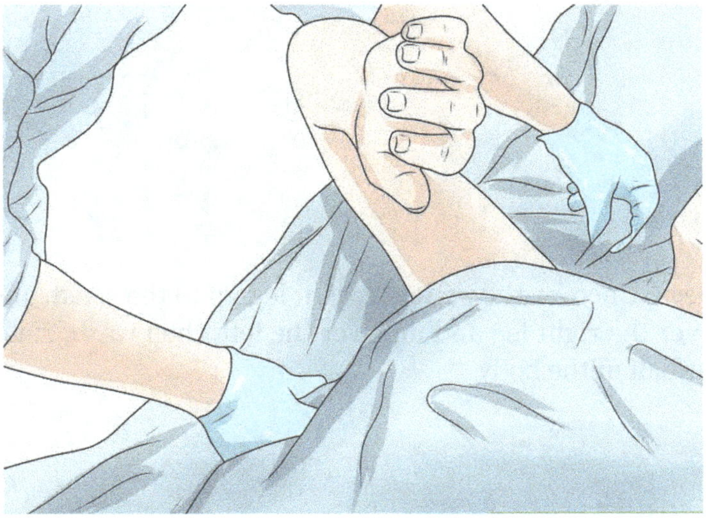

5. Wash the patient's right arm and shoulder. Fold over the sheet to expose the right side. Place the towel beneath the other arm and repeat, washing, rinsing and drying the right shoulder, underarm, arm and hand.

- Dry the washed areas thoroughly, especially the underarm, to prevent chafing and bacteria growth.
- Recover with the sheet to keep the patient warm.

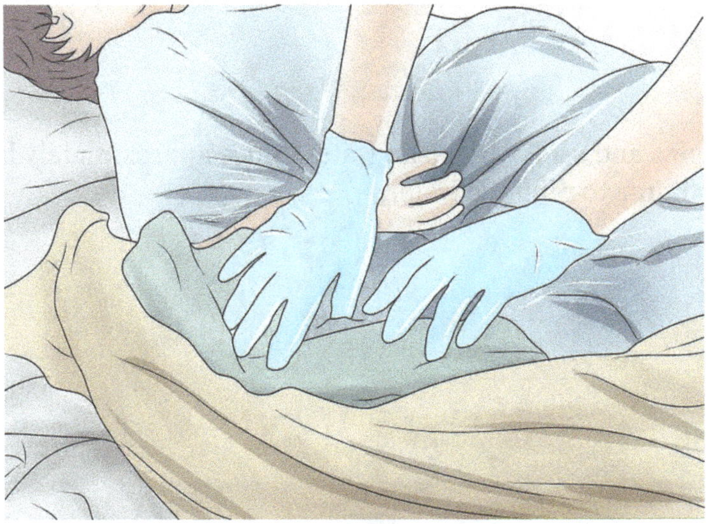

6. Wash the patient's torso. Fold the sheet down to the waist and gently wash and rinse the chest, stomach and sides. Be sure to wash carefully among any folds in the patient's skin, since bacteria tends to get trapped there. Dry the torso carefully, especially among the folds.

- Recover the patient with the sheet to keep the patient warm.

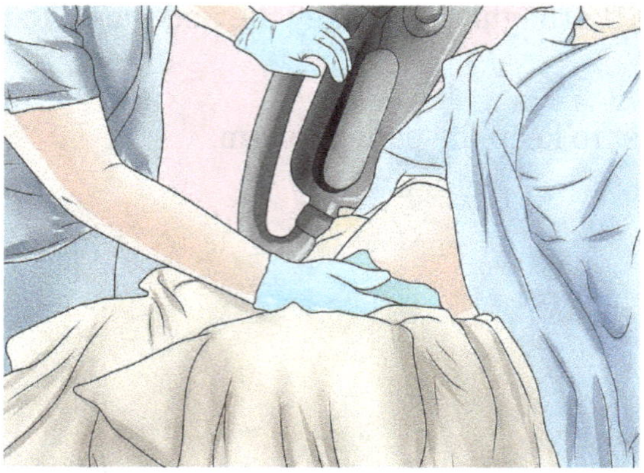

7. Wash the patient's legs. Uncover the patient's right leg up to the waist, and wash, rinse and dry the leg and foot. Recover the right leg and uncover the left, then wash, rinse and dry the leg and foot. Recover the lower half of the body.

Part 3

Bathing the Back and Private Area

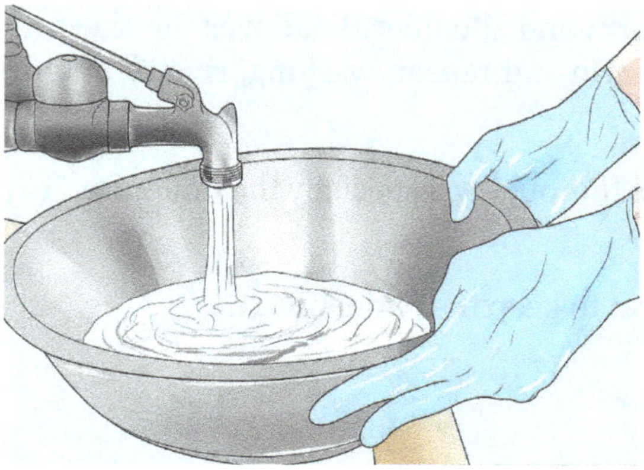

1. Empty the water basins and refill with clean water. Since approximately half the patient's body is now clean, it's a good time to refill the water.

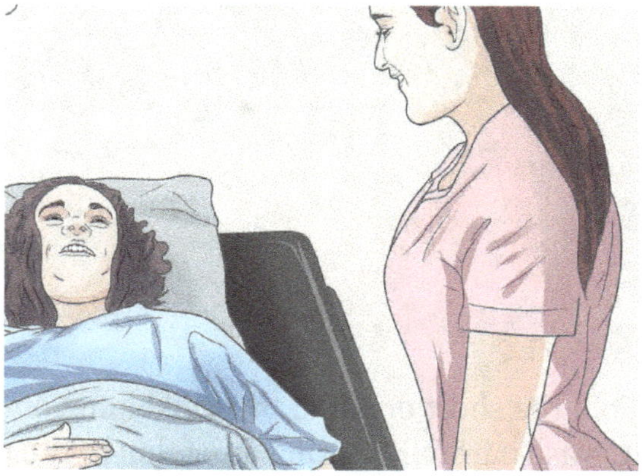

2. Ask the patient to roll on their side if they are able. You may have to assist the person. Make sure they are not too close to the edge of the bed.

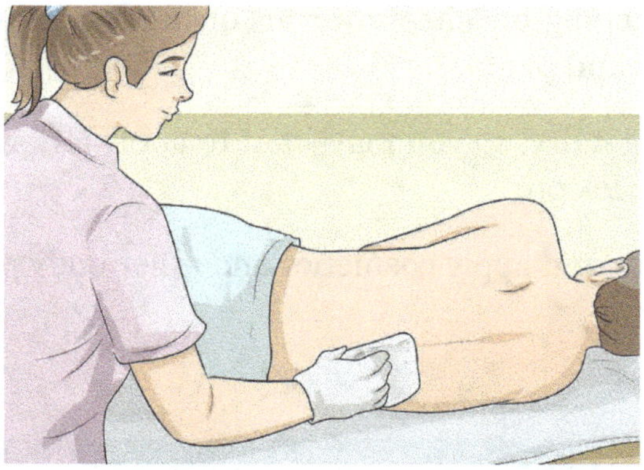

3. Wash the patient's back and buttocks. Fold the sheet over to expose the entire back side of the patient. Wash, rinse and dry the back of the patient's neck, back, buttocks and parts of the legs you may have missed.

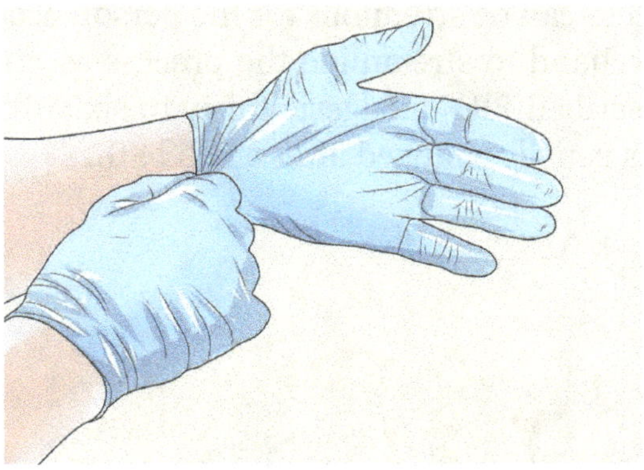

4. Wash the genital area and anus. Put on latex gloves if desired. Lift the person's leg and wash from front to back. Use a clean washcloth to rinse the area. Be sure to clean thoroughly between folds, and dry the area thoroughly as well.

- Males should be washed behind the testicles. Wash female's labia, but there's no need to clean the vagina.
- This part of the body should be washed every day, even when you're not giving a full-body bed bath.

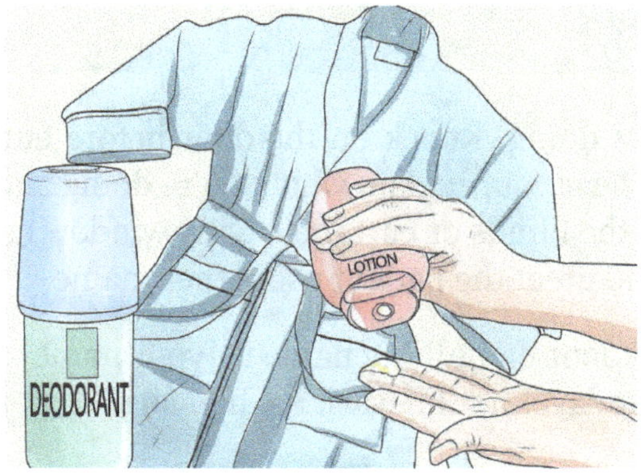

5. Redress the patient. When you're finished, dress the patient in clean clothes or a robe. First

replace the patient's shirt, keeping the sheet over his or her legs. Then remove the sheet and replace the person's underwear and pants.

- Elderly skin tends to get dry, so you may want to apply lotion to the arms and legs before putting their clothes back on.
- Comb the person's hair and apply cosmetics and other body products according to the patient's preferences.

How to Change Sheets in an Occupied Bed

Ideally, you should change bed sheets when a bed is empty. However, if a person is on bed rest and is either not supposed to or is unable to get out of bed, you'll need to change the sheets while the bed is occupied. This process can be strenuous for the person occupying the bed, so make sure your supplies are ready beforehand to streamline the process as much as possible. For patients experiencing pain, give a prescribed PRN analgesic thirty to sixty minutes before you change the bed linens. An occupied bed is usually changed after a bed bath.

Part 1

Setting up the Bedding

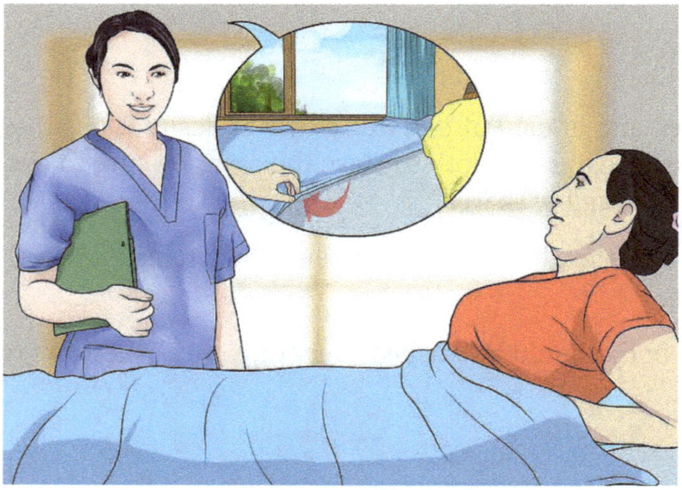

1. Tell the patient what you're doing. Knock on the door before entering the room. Whether or not you think the patient can hear you, explain what you're doing and make sure that you provide privacy for the patient. Close the blinds or curtains of any window as well as the patient's privacy curtain. Introduce yourself and greet the patient using their name.

- Try saying, "Hello, [patient name]! My name is [your name] and I'm the CNA who will be changing your sheets today. First I'll wash my hands, and prepare the supplies. I'll be right back, okay?"
- If the patient is sitting upright, ask if it is alright that you lay them down flat.

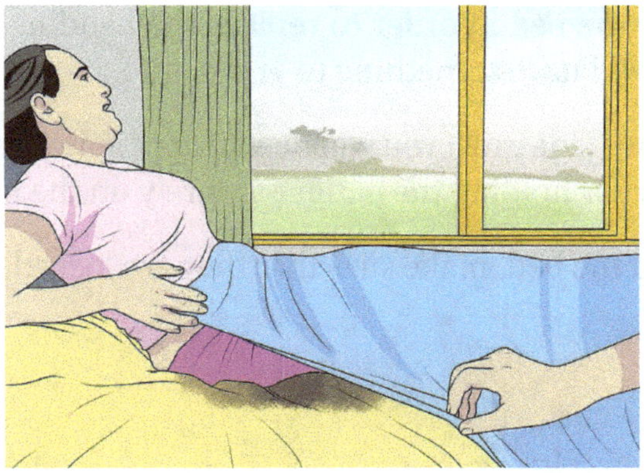

2. Check the state of the linens. You may not have to replace all the bedding every day. However, you may need to change the bottom and top sheets and the pillowcase regularly. The mattress pad, bedspread and blanket can remain if they are dry and unsoiled.

- Bedding that is at all dirty or wet from urine, stool, blood, emesis or perspiration should be changed.

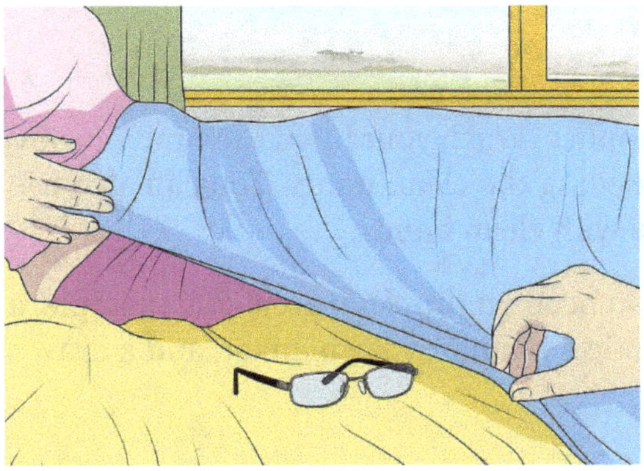

3. Check the bedding for items. Make sure there are no hearing aids, dentures, jewelry, glasses, tissues or other items in the bed before changing the linens. This way you will be able to remove soiled sheets without shaking them.

- Make sure no tubes are tangled in the bed sheets.

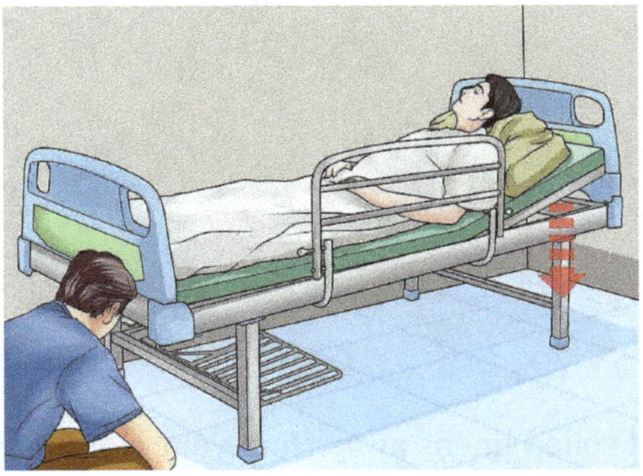

4. Adjust the bed. Put the bed at a comfortable height, and flat if possible. Ensure that you won't

have to stretch or bend over the bed in order to replace the bedding. Put the side rails up so the occupant won't roll out and will have something to grasp onto.

- If the bed does not have side rails, you will need two people for this process: one for making the bed and the other for holding the patient securely on the bed.
- If there are wheels on the bed, make sure that they are locked.

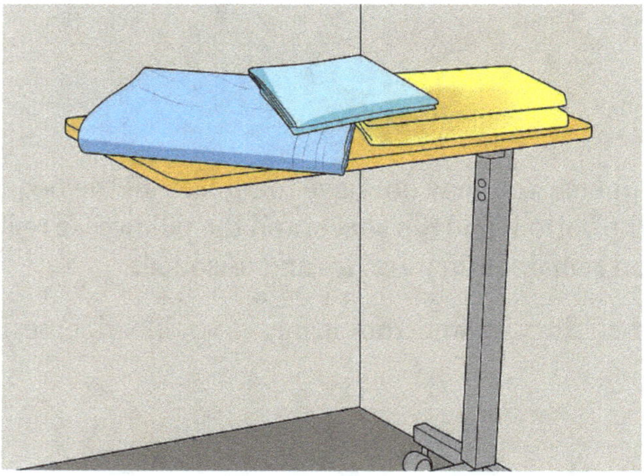

5. Create an area for clean supplies. Wash your hands and put on gloves. Have a clean surface such as a rolling table ready for holding the clean items. You can also use the overbed table as a work area. Only touch the supplies with clean hands.

- Put the clean items you need on the clean area. For example, a flat sheet, fitted sheet, and a pillow case. Also include a clean privacy blanket, and a draw sheet if desired.

Part 2

Changing the Sheets

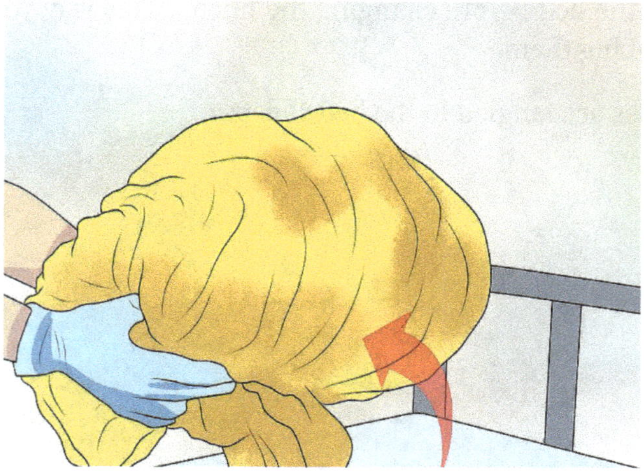

1. Remove soiled items. Hold soiled linens away from your clothing when transferring them to a hamper. Don't shake the linens, as this can introduce micro-organisms into the air. If the clean linens accidentally touch the floor, put them in the dirty hamper and get new clean sheets.

- Don't allow soiled linens to touch your face or uniform.
- If a hamper is not immediately available, place soiled sheets in a plastic bag or laundry basket. Never place them on the nightstand or floor, even temporarily.

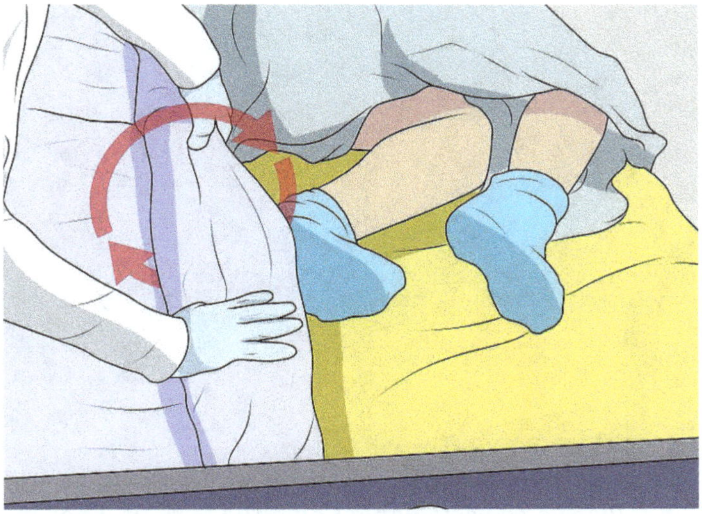

2. Change the fitted sheet. Gently roll the patient onto their side. Remove the fitted sheet by rolling it towards the patient. Put a pad where the patient's hips will lie. Then roll a clean linen towards you. Carefully roll the patient onto the clean linen.

- Tuck the corners and sides of the clean fitted sheet neatly under the mattress. Pull the clean linen tightly on the bed so that it's wrinkle-free.

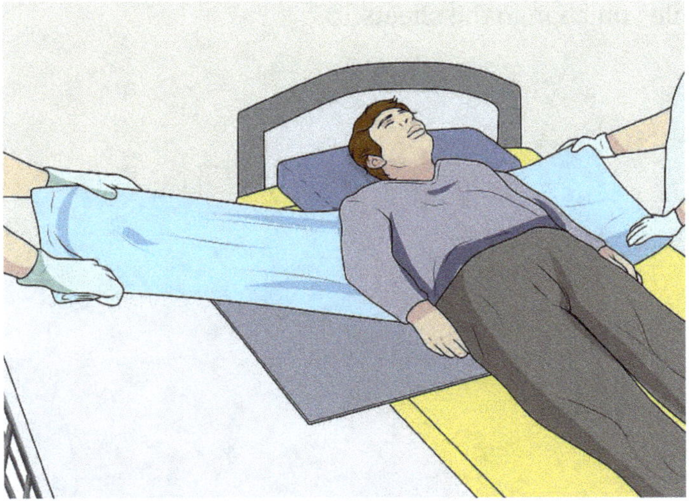

3. Use a draw sheet if you're working with a partner. This will allow you to move the patient from side to side during the process. Fold a sheet in half and stretch it across the middle of the bed to use for this purpose. Place the draw sheet on top of the bottom sheet, from the patient's shoulders to buttocks with at least six inches of sheet left on each side.

- Pulling the sheet on with a helper permits you to move even a large onto their side or higher up on the mattress. If you need a demonstration, ask an OT or PT.

Part 3

Changing the Remaining Linens

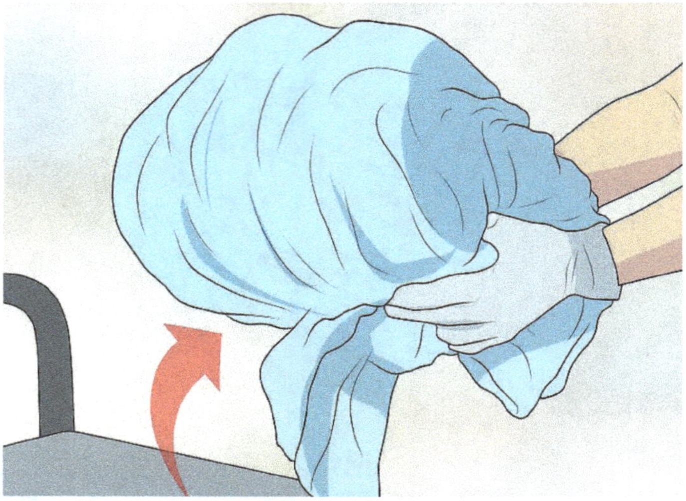

1. Remove the top bedding. Place a privacy blanket over the patient. Loosen the top bedding at the end of the bed. Fold the bedspread to the foot of the bed and take it away by holding it at the center. Repeat with the blanket.

- Only put the bedrail down on the side you're working on. Never step away from the bed at all when the side rail is down.
- If the blanket and bedspread are dirty, replace them with clean ones. Otherwise place them over a chair while you change the sheets.

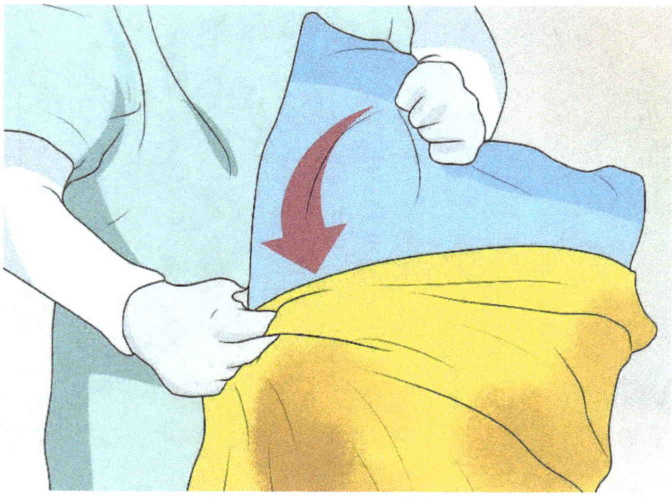

2. Remove the dirty pillowcase. Support the person's head and neck as you remove the pillow. Gently rest the patient's head back down on the bed. Remove the dirty pillowcase by unrolling it away from you. Put the pillowcase in the laundry hamper. Change your gloves to a clean pair.

- Try saying, "I'm going to use my hands to gently support your head and neck as I remove the pillow now, so that I can put on a fresh pillowcase for you."

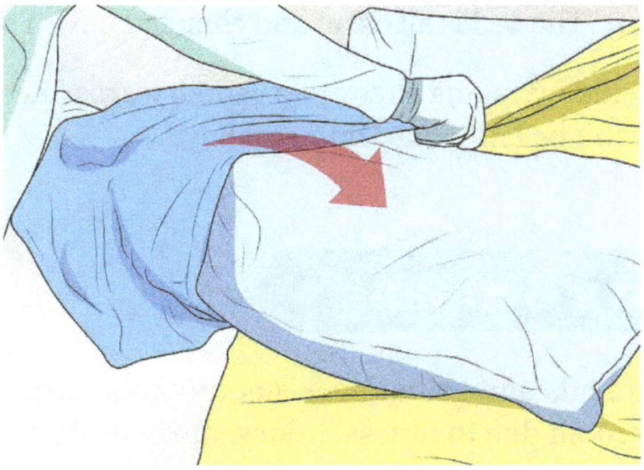

3. Put on a fresh pillowcase. Put the clean pillowcase over your hand and arm so that you can grasp the center of the pillow with your covered hand. Unroll the clean pillowcase onto the pillow. Carefully lift the patient's head and neck and put the pillow with the clean pillowcase on it under their head.

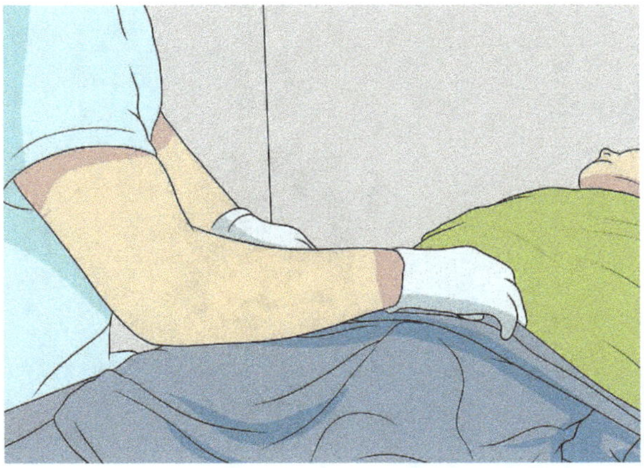

4. Cover the patient. Put a clean flat sheet and a blanket over the patient. Secure the lower corners of the sheet with mitered corners. Move the occupant into a comfortable resting position and adjust the bedding as needed.

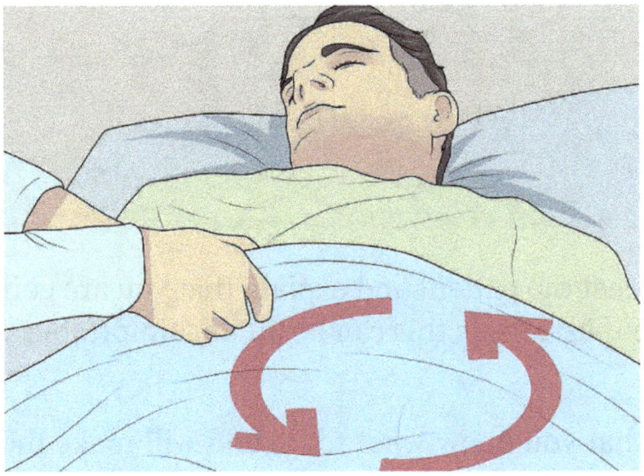

5. Replace the top blankets and finish up. If the bedspread and blanket were soiled, replace them with new, clean ones. If not, you can put the original ones back on. Dispose of your gloves and wash your hands.

- Try telling the patient, "The bed is all clean and changed now. Thank you for your patience!"
- Remove the dirty items by taking them to a laundry area. Keep them in a plastic bag or laundry bag if they can't be laundered immediately.

How to Position a Bedpan

Bedpans make bowel movements and urination easier and more hygienic for people who cannot easily go to and from a bathroom due to illness, injury, or infirmity. If you are assisting someone with using a bedpan, whether in a professional capacity or as a friend or family member, you need to be emotionally sensitive and physically gentle. Positioning a bedpan may seem intimidating, but as long as you follow proper procedures, you should be able to complete it without a problem.

Part 1

Preparing the Procedure

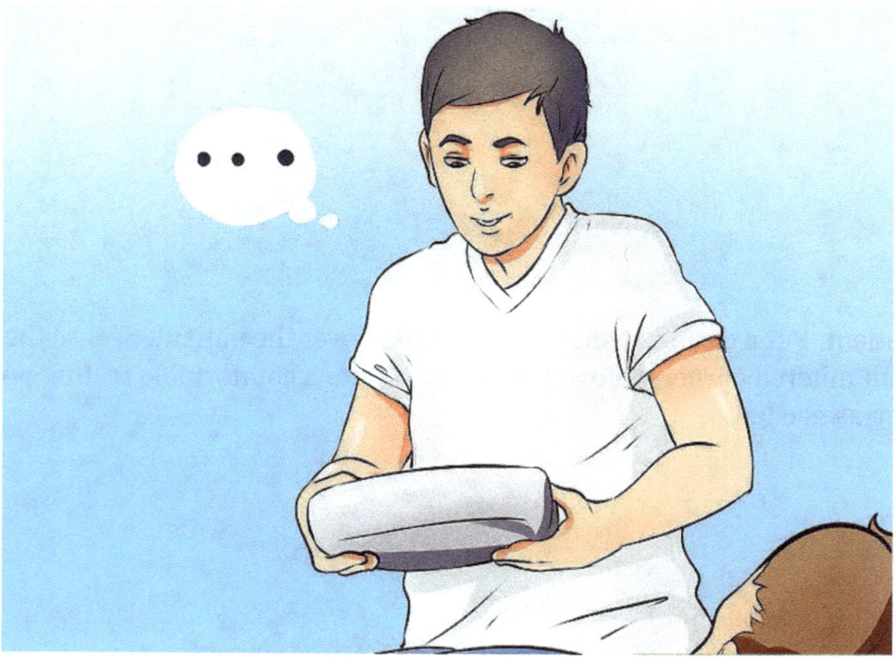

1. Explain the procedure. Greet the patient and explain that you are going to help him use the bedpan. Show patience and compassion, as this can be an uncomfortable and embarrassing situation for the patient.

- Assure the patient that you know what to do and will make the experience as pleasant as possible.
- Explaining this to the patient beforehand can help calm your patient and reduce his fear and uncertainty.

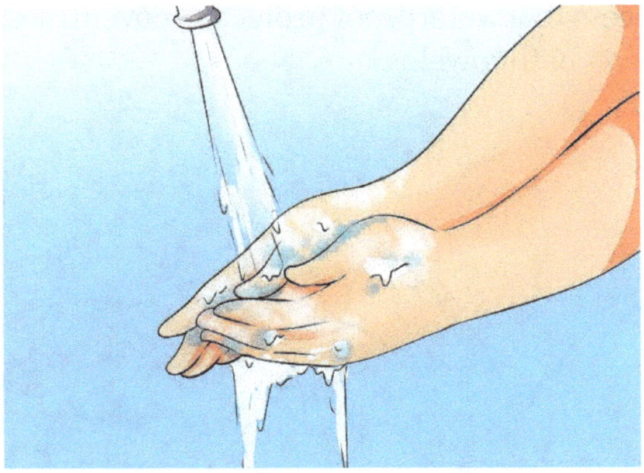

2. Wash your hands and put on gloves. Wash your hands thoroughly with hot water and soap. When finished, dry your hands and put on a pair of disposable gloves.

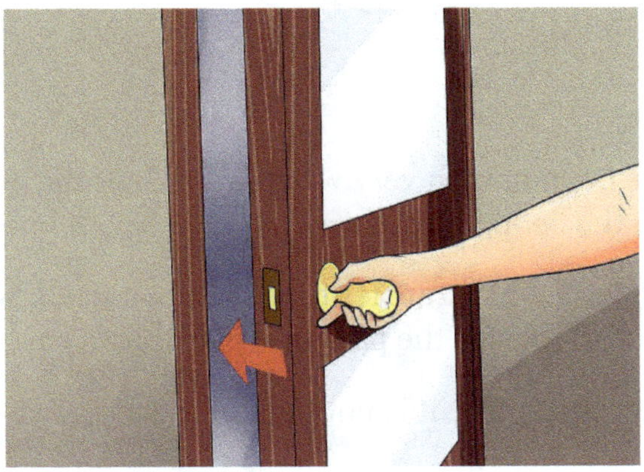

3. Provide privacy. Provide the patient with as much privacy as possible, now and throughout the entire procedure.

- Close the door and cover the windows with curtains.
- If the patient shares a room with someone else, draw the curtain separating the two beds.
- Keep the patient's legs covered with a blanket or sheet until you are ready to position the bedpan.

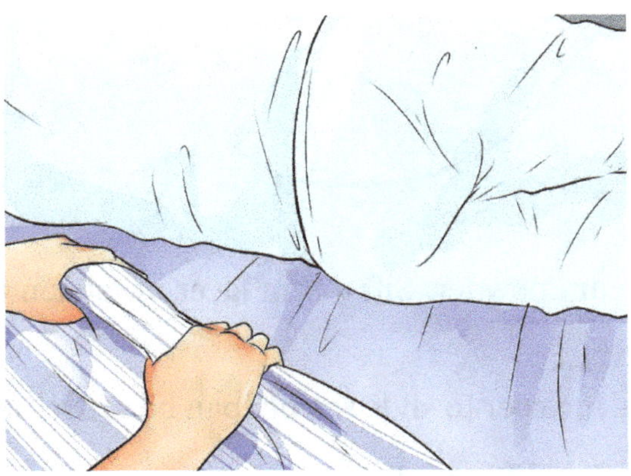

4. Protect the sheets. If possible, cover the sheets beneath the patient with a waterproof protector.

- If you do not have access to a waterproof protector, cover the sheets beneath patient's buttocks with a large, clean bath towel.

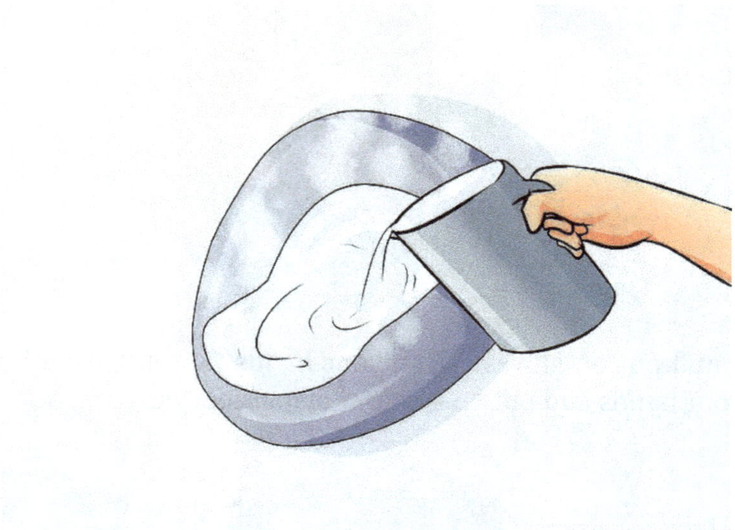

5. Warm the bedpan. Fill the bedpan with very warm water. Let the water sit for several minutes, then dump it out and dry off the bedpan.

- The heat from the water should transfer to the bedpan itself, warming it up. A warm bedpan will be more comfortable for the patient to use than a cold one.
- If it is a metal bedpan, make sure it is not too hot.

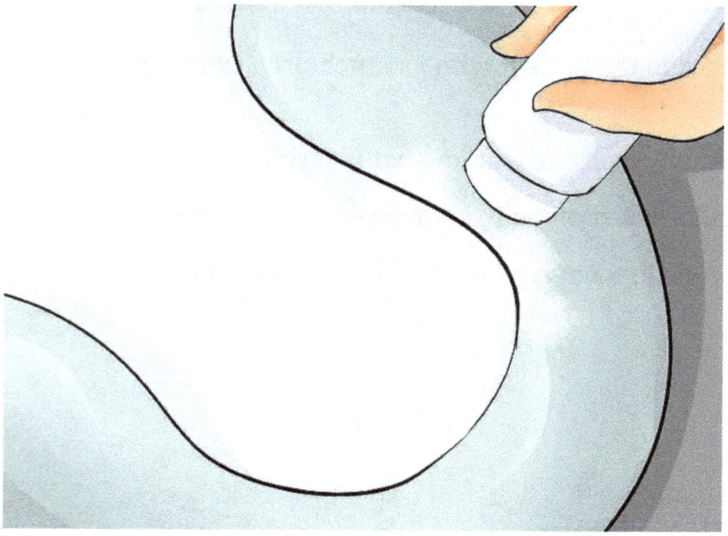

6. Sprinkle the edge with talcum powder. Sift a thin layer of talcum powder over the edge of the bedpan.

- The powder will make it easier to slide the bedpan beneath the patient.
- Only do this if the patient does not have any bedsores or cuts on her buttocks. Do not use talcum powder if the patient has any open wounds.

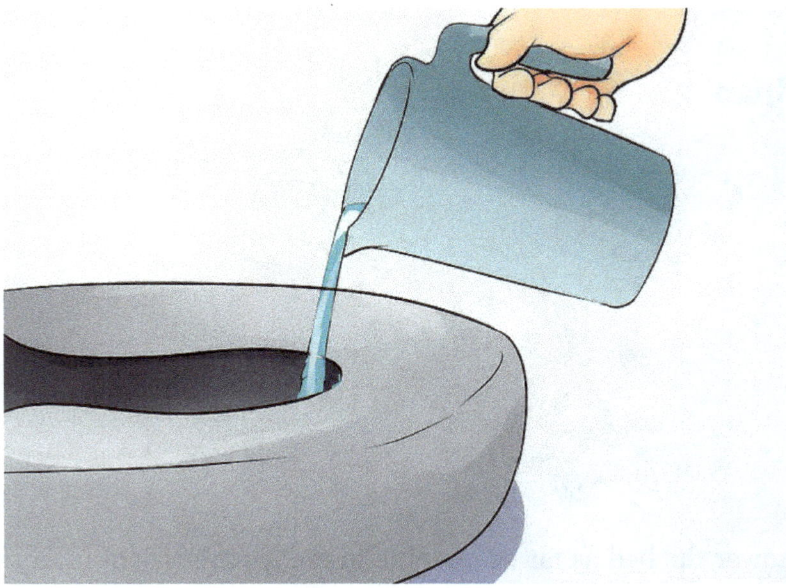

7. Fill the bedpan with just enough water to cover the bottom. Alternatively, you can place a few squares of toilet paper in the bottom of the bedpan or coat it with a little vegetable oil spray (if you are in a home setting).

- Any of these practices will make the cleanup process easier.

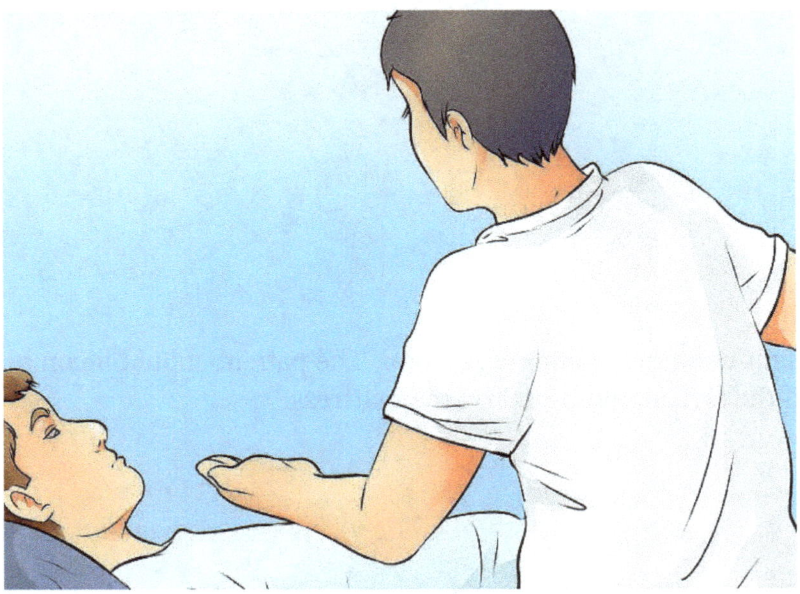

8. Ask the patient to remove his bottoms. Now that the supplies are ready, instruct the patient to remove clothing from the bottom half of his body.

- Assist the patient if he is unable to do this alone.
- If the patient is wearing a gown with an opening in the back, you can leave the gown on. If the gown has no opening, you will need to lift it above the patient's waist.
- You will also need to pull the top sheet or blanket back at this time.

Part 2

Placing the Bedpan

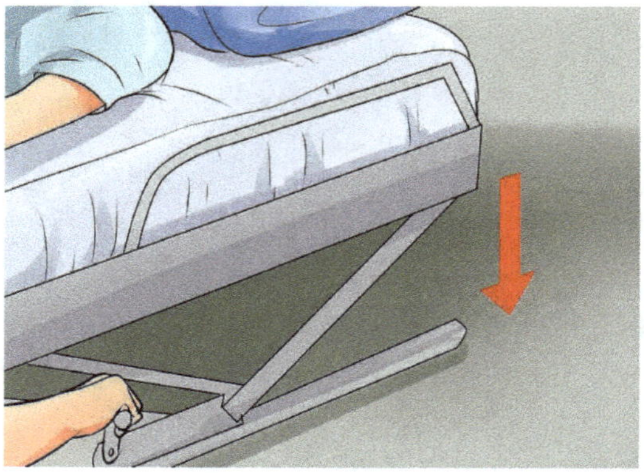

1. Lower the bed. Lower the bed as far as possible to reduce the risk of injury if the patient falls during the procedure.

- You should also lower the head of the bed at this time, since doing so may make it easier for the patient to lift or turn as needed.

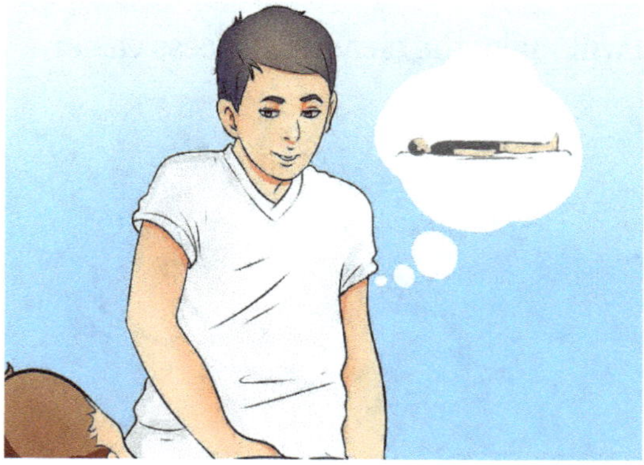

2. Instruct the patient to lie in the supine position. The patient should lie on her back. The knees should be bent and the feet should be flat on the mattress.

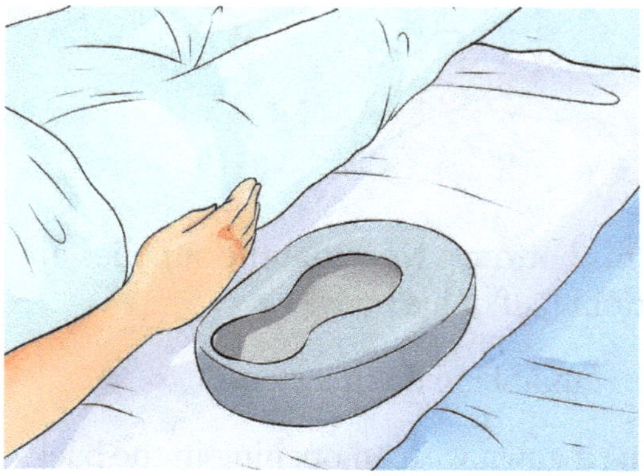

3. Place the bedpan next to the patient. Set the clean bedpan directly next to the patient's hips on the side of the bed.

- Positioning the bedpan as close as possible before moving the patient will cause less strain to the patient.

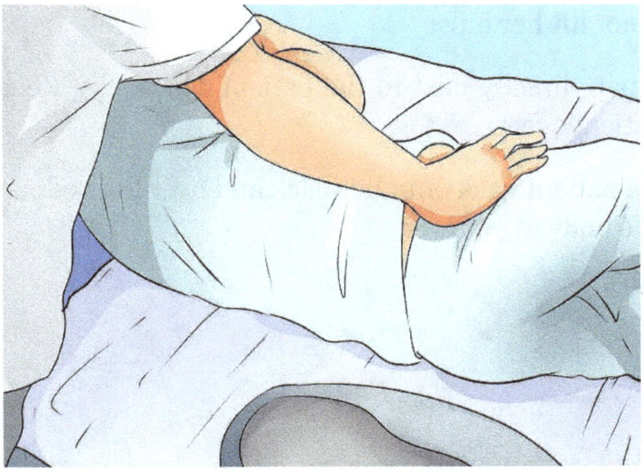

4. Help the patient shift away from the bed. The patient will need to raise his hips. If the patient does not have the strength to do so, you will need to turn the patient to his side instead.

- If the patient can lift his hips:
    - Instruct your patient to raise his hips on the count of three.
    - Support the patient by placing your hand beneath the lower back. Do not do any serious lifting with this hand. You should only provide light support.
- If the patient cannot lift his hips:
    - Gently turn the patient to the side facing away from you. Work carefully to prevent the patient from rolling onto his stomach or off the bed.

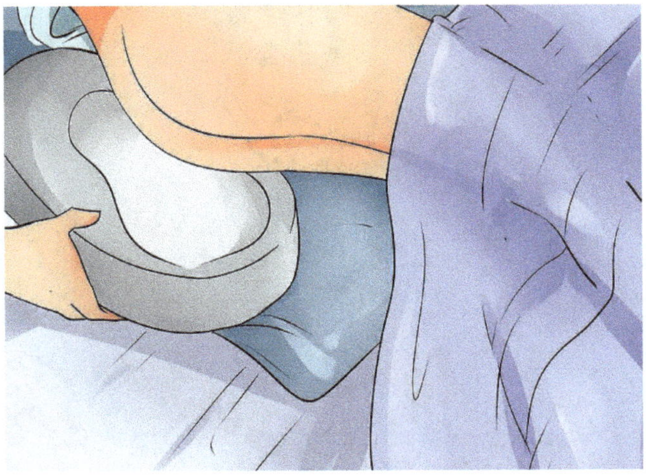

5. Place the bedpan under the patient's buttocks. Slide the bedpan beneath the patient's buttocks with the curved edge of the bedpan facing the back.

- If the patient can lift her hips:

    - Slide the bedpan underneath the buttocks and instruct the patient to ease down onto it, using your support hand to guide her.

- If the patient cannot lift her hips:

    - Slide the bedpan directly next to the patient's buttocks. Keep the open end pointing toward the patient's feet.

    - Gently roll the patient back onto her back and over the bedpan. Hold the bedpan close to the patient's body as you work.

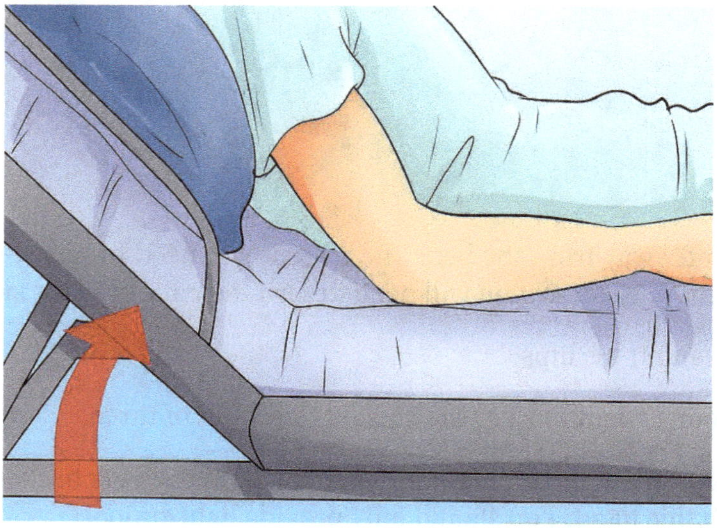

6. Raise the head of the bed. Carefully raise the head of the bed, bringing the patient's body up into a more natural toileting position.

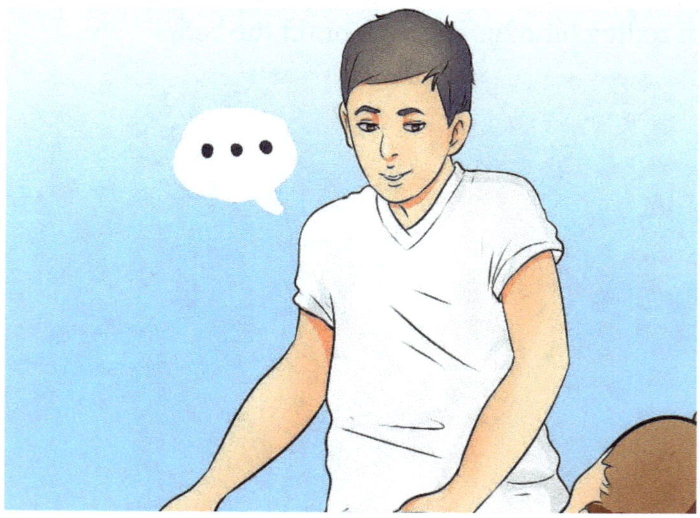

7. Verify the positioning. Ask the patient to spread his legs slightly so that you can verify proper bedpan placement.

- Essentially, you need to make sure that the bedpan is positioned securely beneath the entire area of the buttocks.

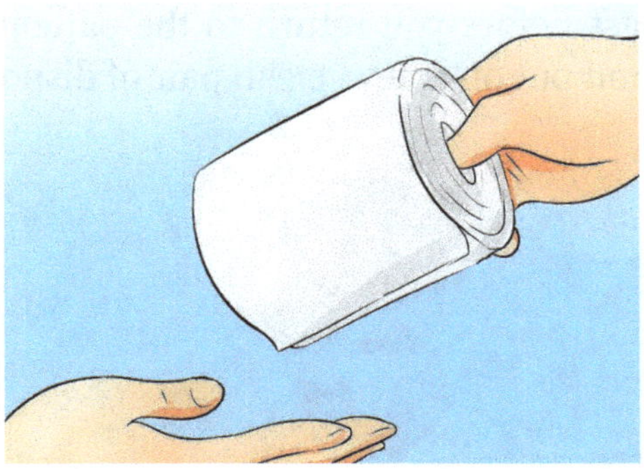

8. Provide toilet paper. Place toilet paper within the patient's reach. Let the patient know that it's there.

- You should also provide sanitary wipes for the patient's hands.
- Keep a signal cord, bell, or similar device near the patient, too. Instruct the patient to ring the signal when finished.

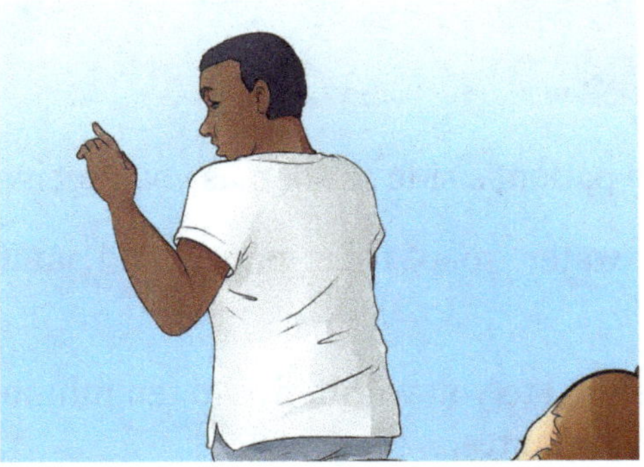

9. Step away. Give the patient privacy as she uses the bedpan. Let her know you will be back to check in a few minutes, but instruct the patient to ring for you if she finishes before then.

- Do *not* leave the patient if doing so would be unsafe.

Part 3

Removing the Bedpan

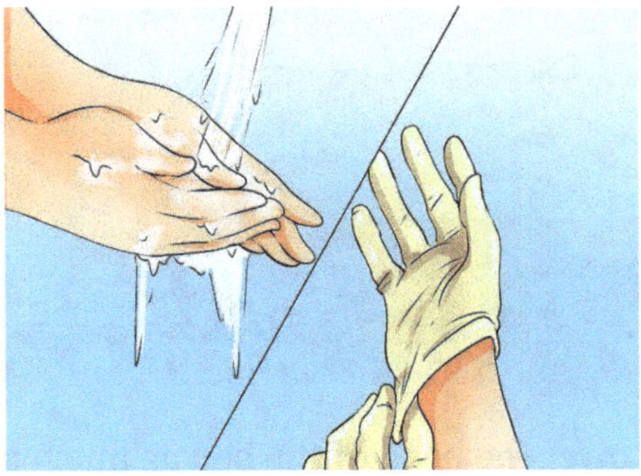

1. Wash your hands and put on new gloves. As soon as you leave the patient, you should remove your gloves and wash your hands.

- Several minutes may pass before you return to the patient again. Before doing so, wash your hands once more and put on a new, clean pair of disposable gloves.

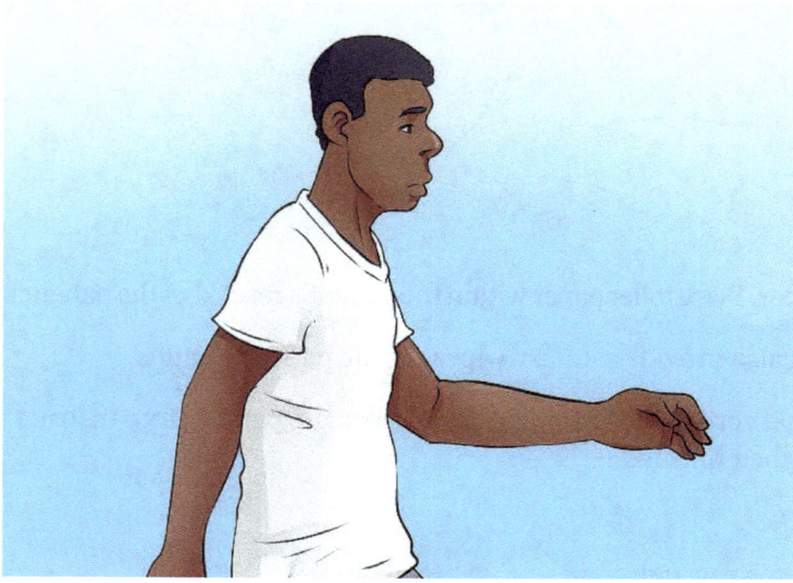

2. Return swiftly. Return to the patient's side as soon as you receive a signal from him.

- Bring a basin of warm water, soap, toilet paper, and sanitary cleansing cloths with you when you return.
- If the patient does not signal to you within five to ten minutes, check on his progress. Continue checking every few minutes.

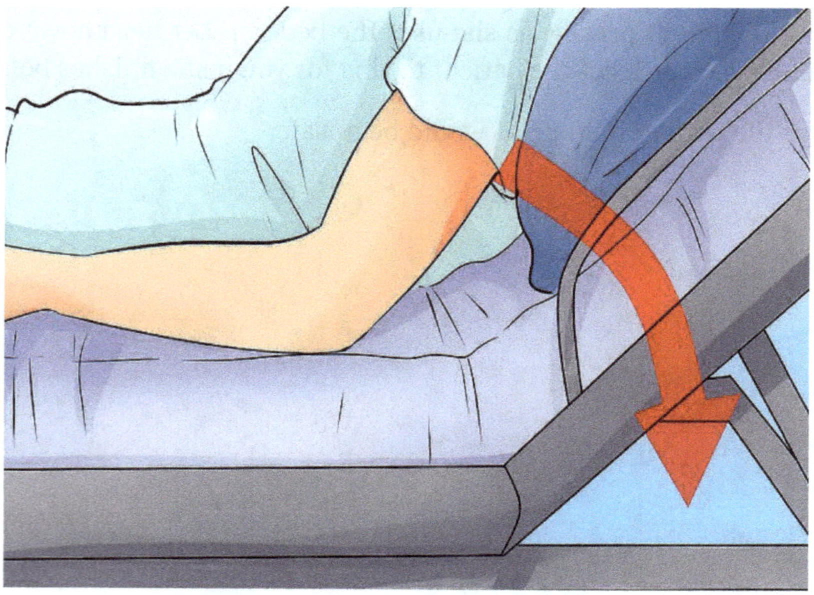

3. Lower the head of the bed. Lower the head of the bed as much as possible without making the patient uncomfortable.

- This position will make it easier for the patient to move off the bedpan.

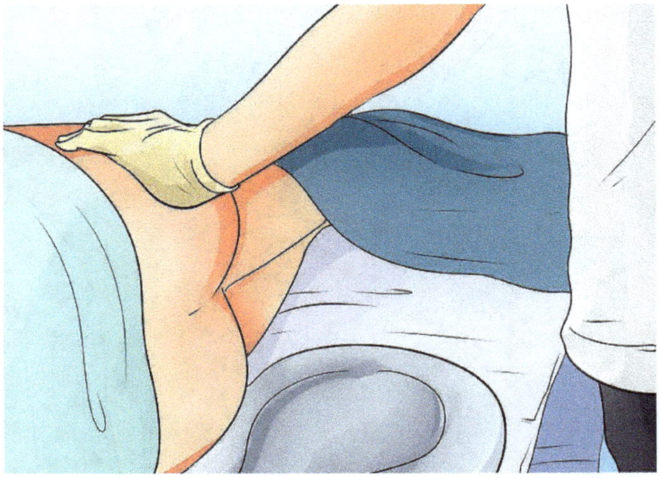

4. Assist the patient in moving away. If the patient lifted herself onto the bedpan, the patient should also lift herself off. If you need to turn the patient onto the bedpan, you will need to turn the patient off.

- If the patient can lift herself:
    - Ask the patient to bend her knees.
    - Instruct the patient to raise her lower half. Place your hand beneath the lower back to offer gentle support.
- If the patient cannot lift herself:
    - Hold the bedpan flat on the bed so that it does not spill.
    - Simultaneously roll the patient to the side facing away from you.

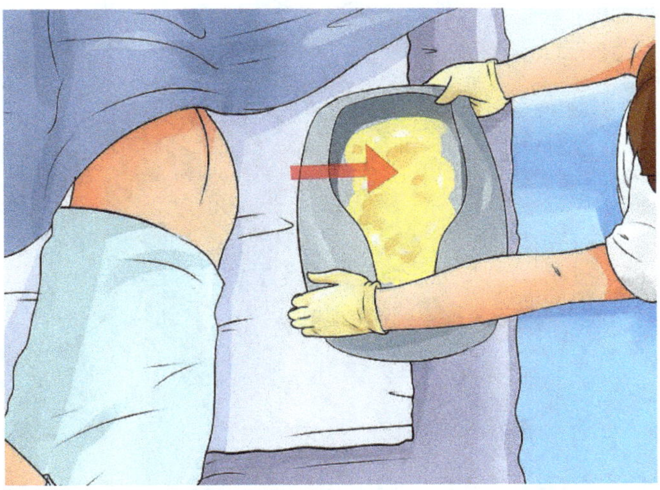

5. Slide the bedpan away. Slide the bedpan from its current position and allow the patient to rest.

- Work carefully and avoid sliding the bedpan against the patient's skin while removing it.
- Cover the bedpan with a towel and set it aside for the time being.

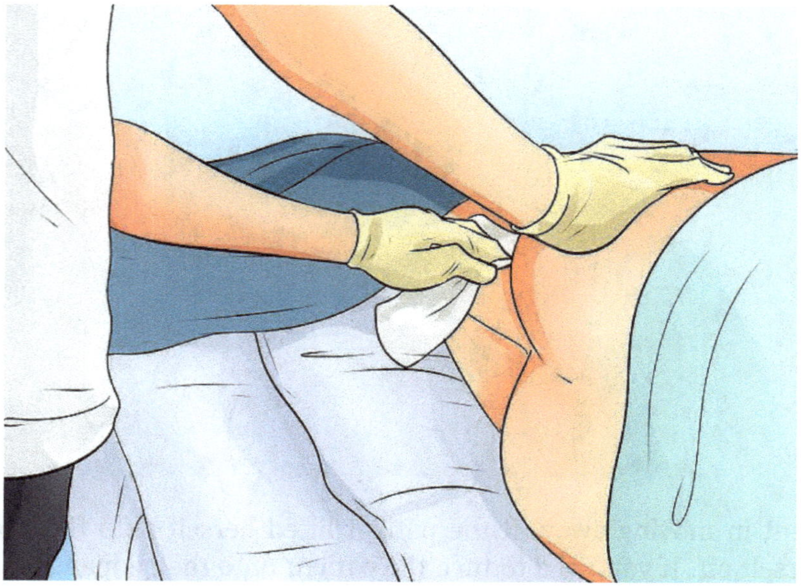

6. Clean the patient. Determine whether or not the patient was able to clean himself. If not, you will need to clean the patient.

- Clean the patient's hands with a wet, soapy washcloth or sanitary wipes.
- Clean the patient's bottom half with toilet paper. For female patients in particular, wipe from front to back to reduce the risk of contaminating the urinary tract with bacteria from the rectum.

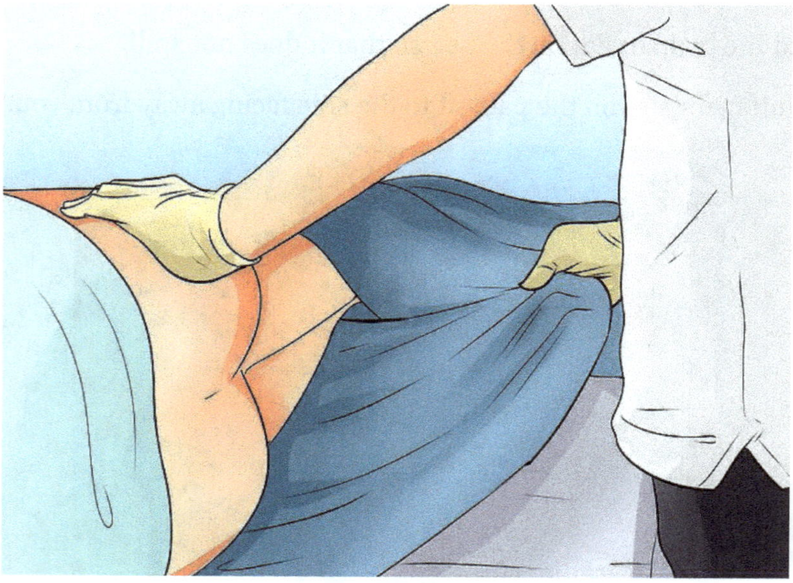

7. Clean the area. Once the patient is clean, remove the waterproof covering or towel.

- If a spill or other contamination occurs, you will need to change the bed linens and the patient's gown or clothing immediately.
- If there is an odor in the room, consider spraying an air freshener.

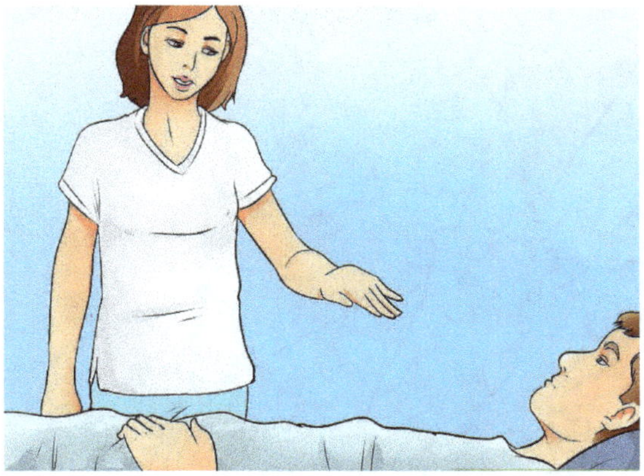

8. Return the patient to a comfortable position. Help the patient shift back into a comfortable resting position.

- If necessary, raise or lower the entire bed or the head of the bed to keep the patient more comfortable.

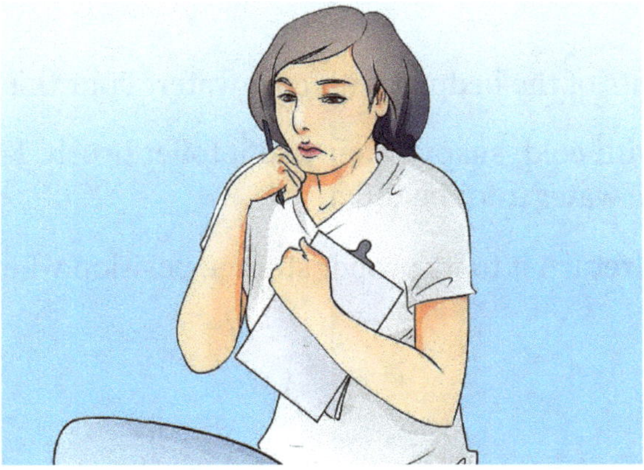

9. Observe or record the contents. Take the bedpan to the bathroom and check its contents.

- Look for anything unusual, like streaks of red, black, or green, as well as mucus or diarrhea.
- If necessary, measure and record the output.

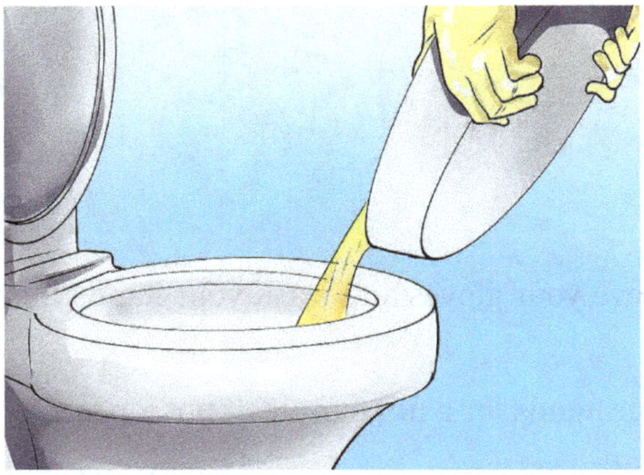

10. Dispose of the contents. Empty the contents of the bedpan into the toilet and flush them away.

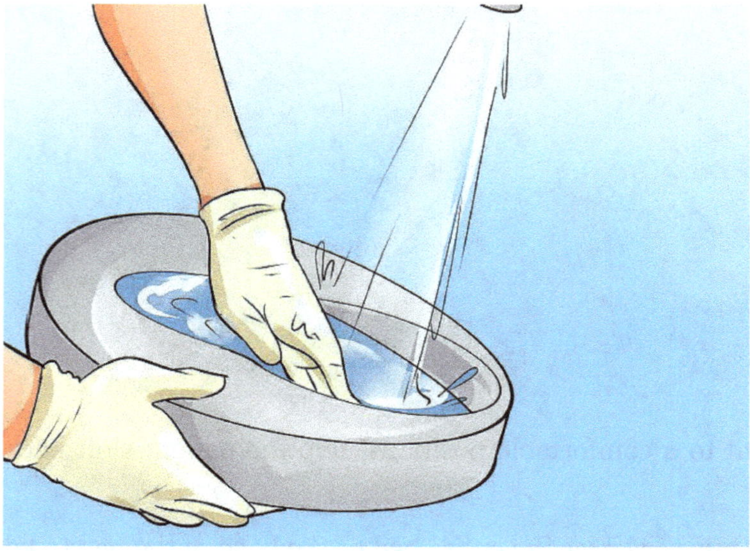

11. Clean or replace the bedpan. Unless the bedpan is disposable, you will need to clean it thoroughly before storing it.

- Flush out the contents of the bedpan with cold water. Pour this water into the toilet.
- Scrub the bedpan with cold, soapy water and a toilet brush. Rinse it with additional cold water, and dump the water into the toilet.
- Dry the bedpan and return it to its proper storage position when done.

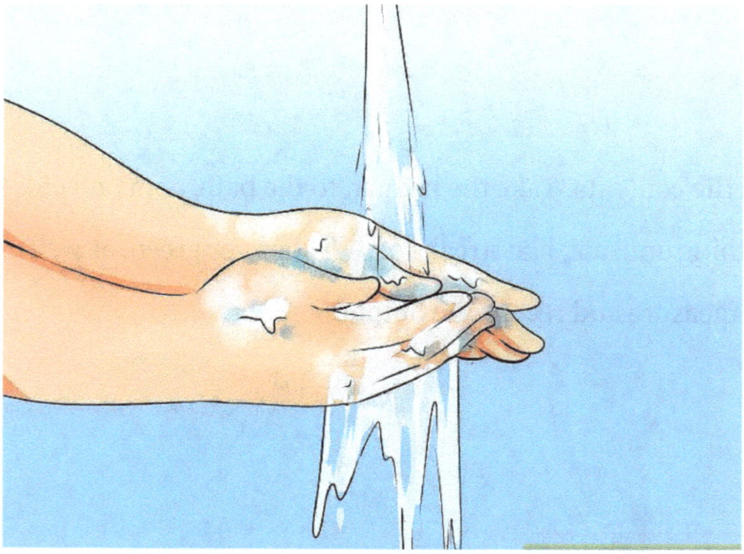

12. Wash your hands. Remove your gloves and wash your hands thoroughly with hot water and soap.

- You should wash your hands for a full minute, if not longer.
- Once everything is clean, you can return the room to its standard condition by opening curtains, windows, and doors that were closed for the procedure.

How to Perform a Full Physical Exam

This is the appropriate and thorough way to perform a physical exam on a patient.

Steps

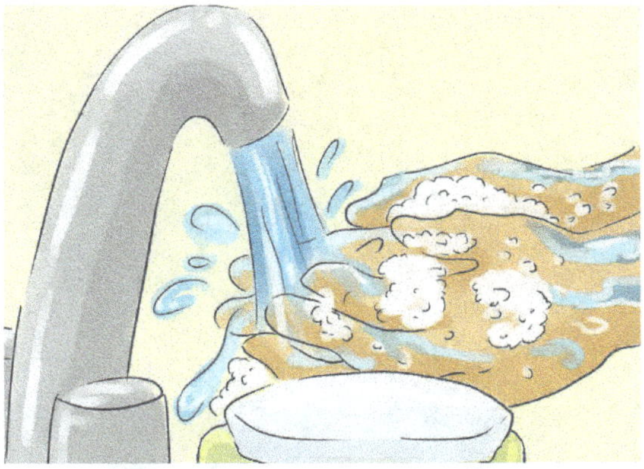

1. Wash your hands before the examination.

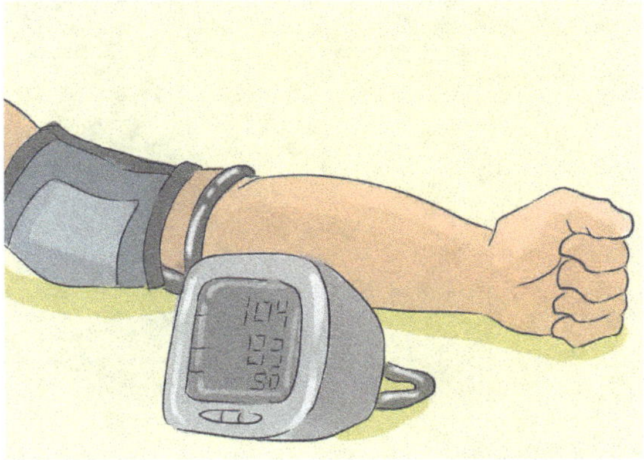

2. Take the patient's blood pressure.

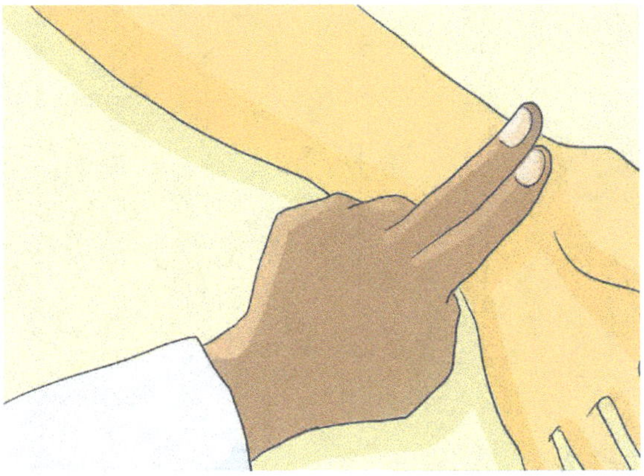

3. Take the radial pulse for 15 seconds if the pulse is normal. Take it for 30-60 seconds if the pulse is high or slow.

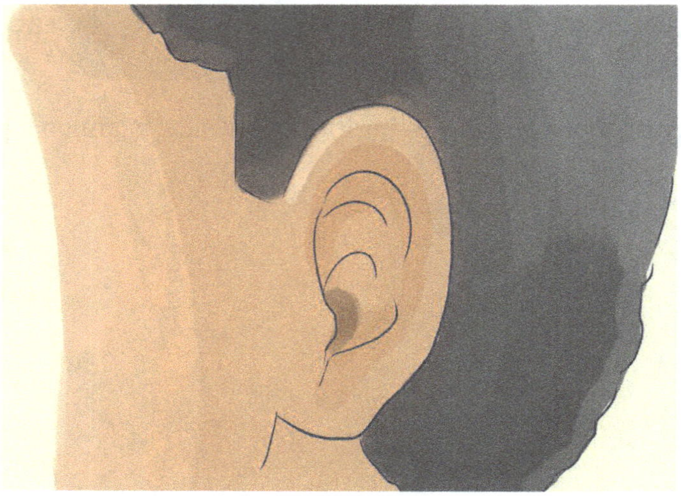

4. Check the patient's ears.

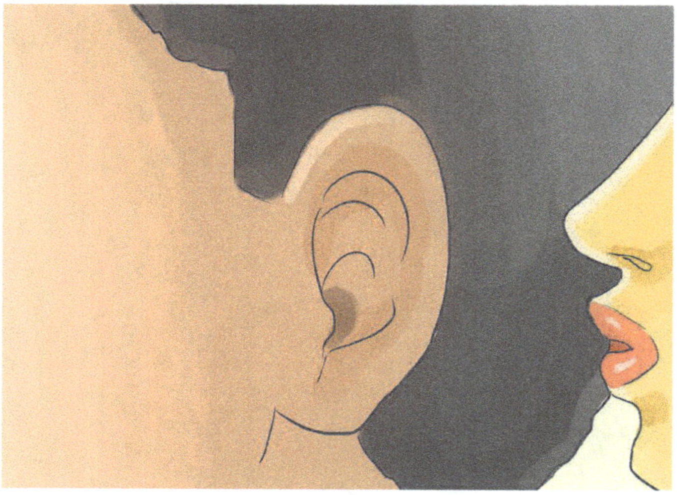

5. Do the hearing test. Use simple words and whisper them.

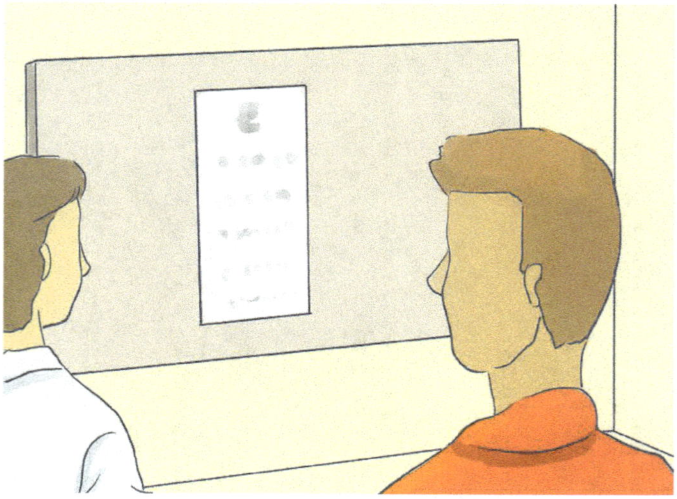

6. Give them the Snell test.

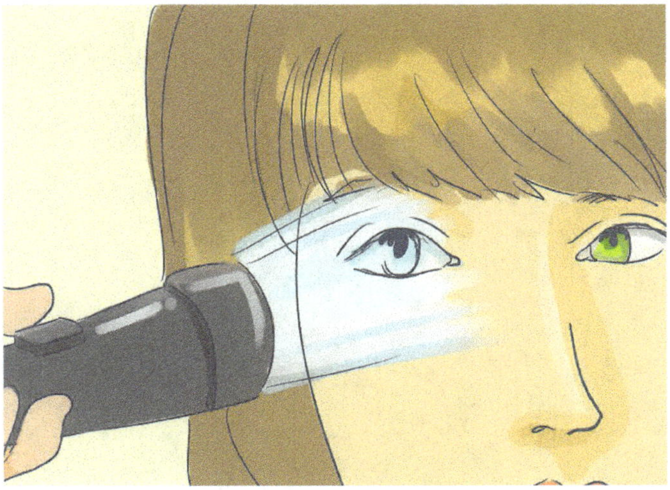

7. Test their eye reaction with a flashlight.

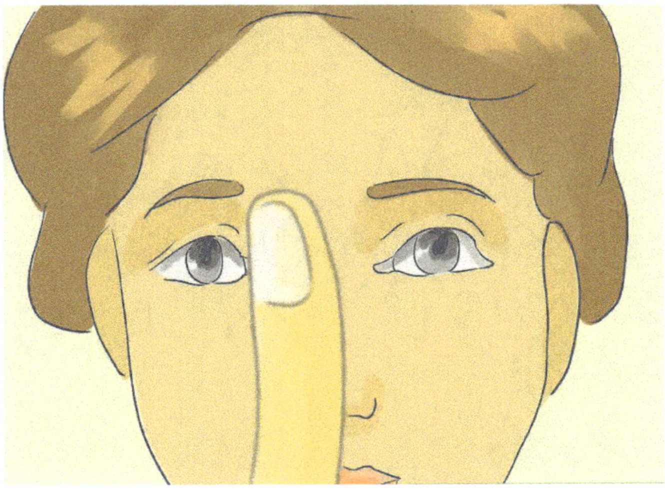

8. Get the patient to follow your fingers with their eyes.

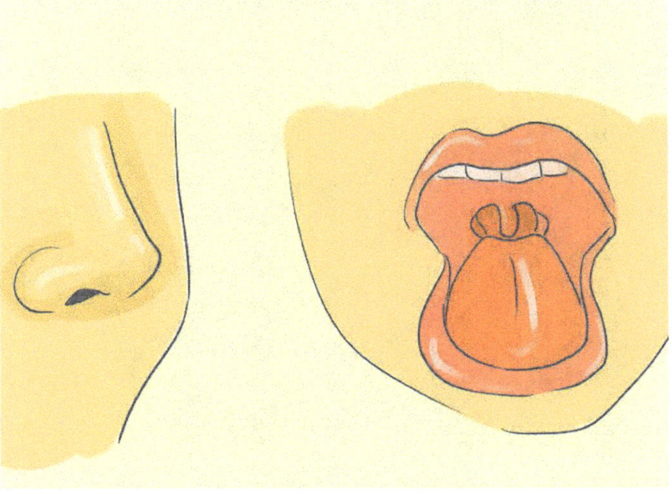

9. Check the nose and throat.

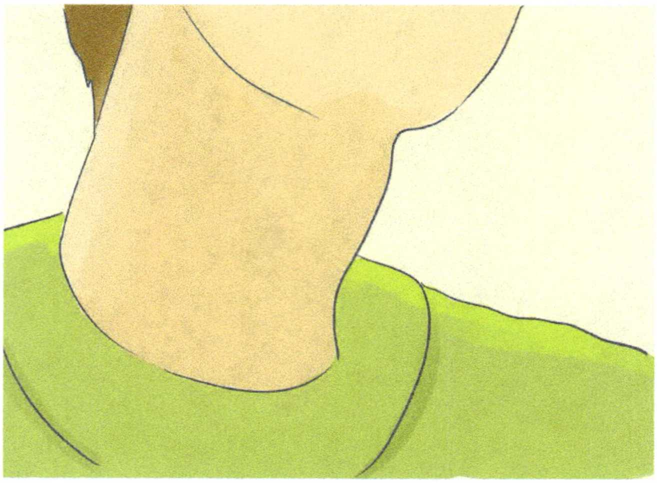

10. Check the neck. Get them to flex, extend, rotate, and bend the neck.

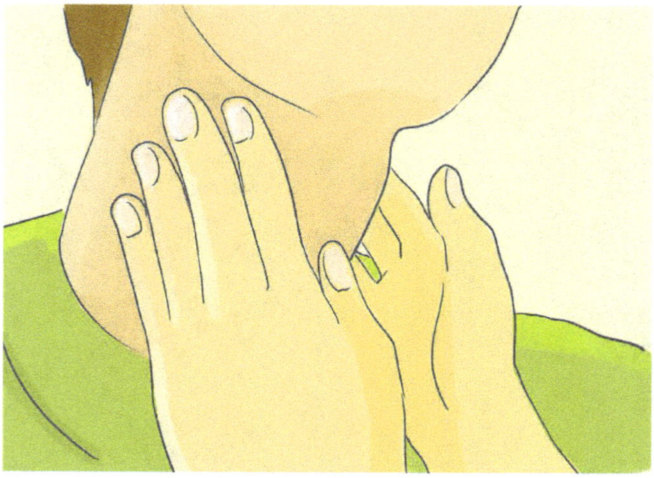

11. Check the thyroid gland.

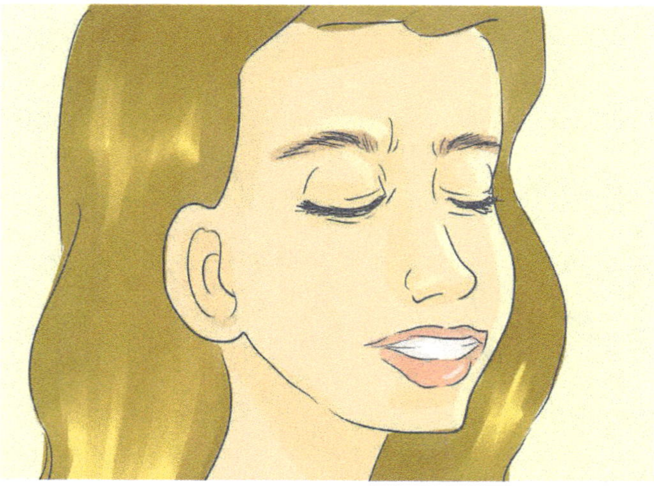

12. Check the cranial nerves. Ask them to raise their eyebrows, frown, close their eyes tightly, show their teeth, smile, and puff out their cheeks.

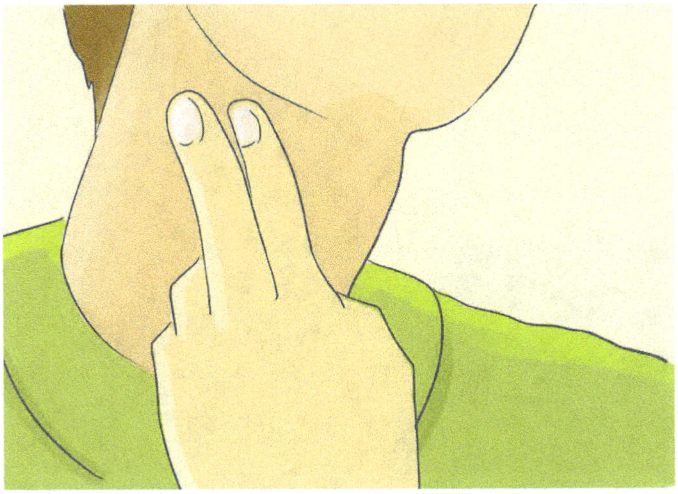

13. Check the lymph nodes.

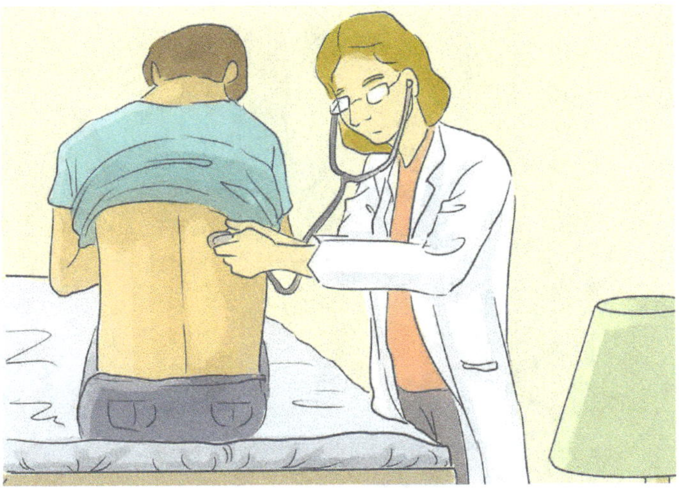

14. Do the lung exam. Do 3 spots on the back of each lung and 1 on the front of each lung.

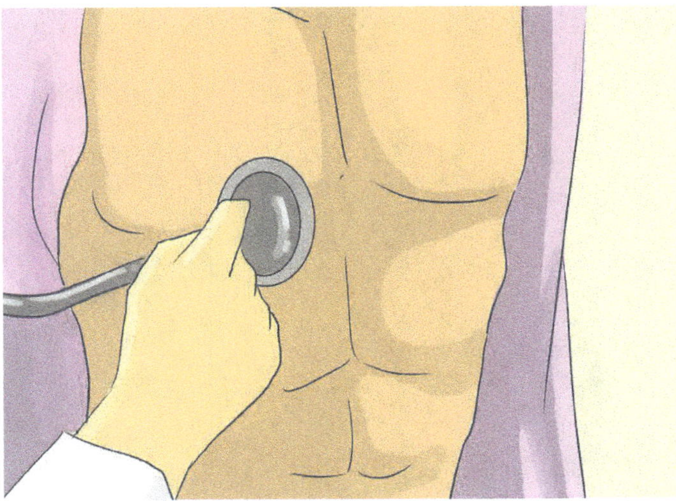

15. Now listen to the heart. After, move on to the carotids with the bell of the stethoscope.

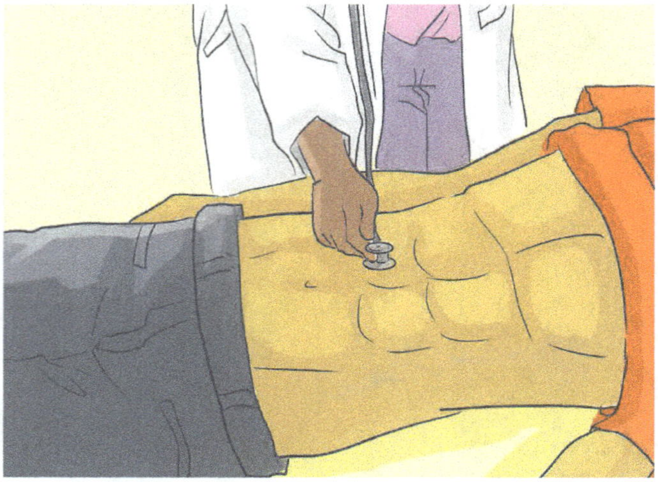

16. Proceed to the abdominal exam. Listen for bowel sounds in all 4 quadrants. Listen for an aortic bruit.

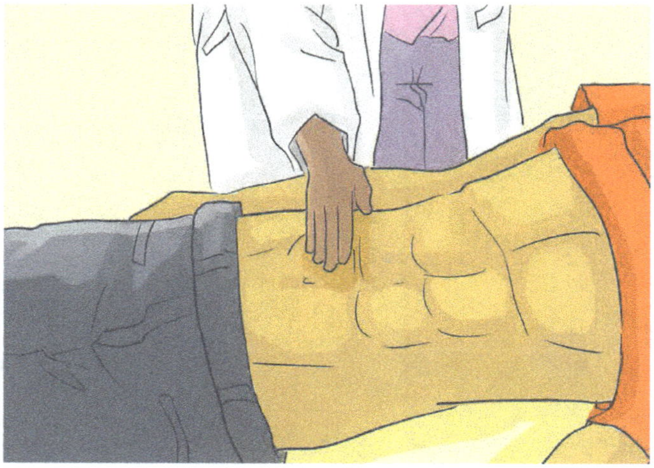

17. Palpate the four quadrants, liver, and spleen. Measure the vertical span of liver with a ruler.

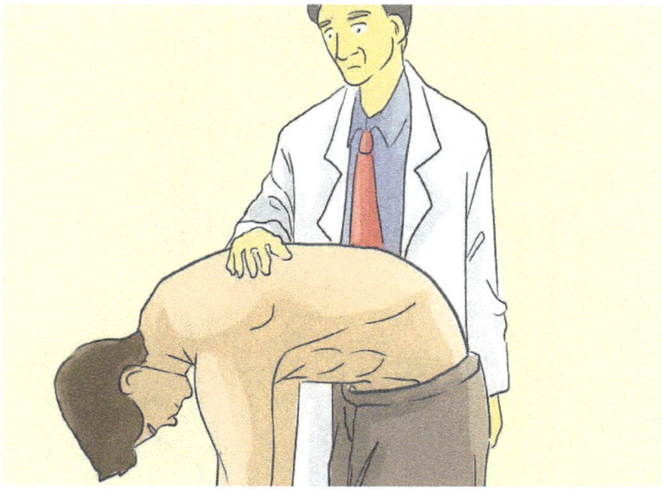

18. Look at the patient's spine. Get them to bend forward and touch the toes.

Chapter

5 Developing a Career in Nursing

Professional nursing has many specializations. These include maternity nurse, pediatric nurse, nurse anesthetist, psychiatric nurse, neonatal nurse, nursing consultant, etc. The topics discussed in the chapter are of great importance to broaden the existing knowledge on professional nursing.

How to become a Nurse Anesthetist

Nurse anesthetists perform a variety of duties including administering anesthesia, monitoring patients' vital signs, and overseeing patient recovery following surgery. They may serve as assists to physicians, dentists, anesthesiologists, and other medical professionals.

Steps

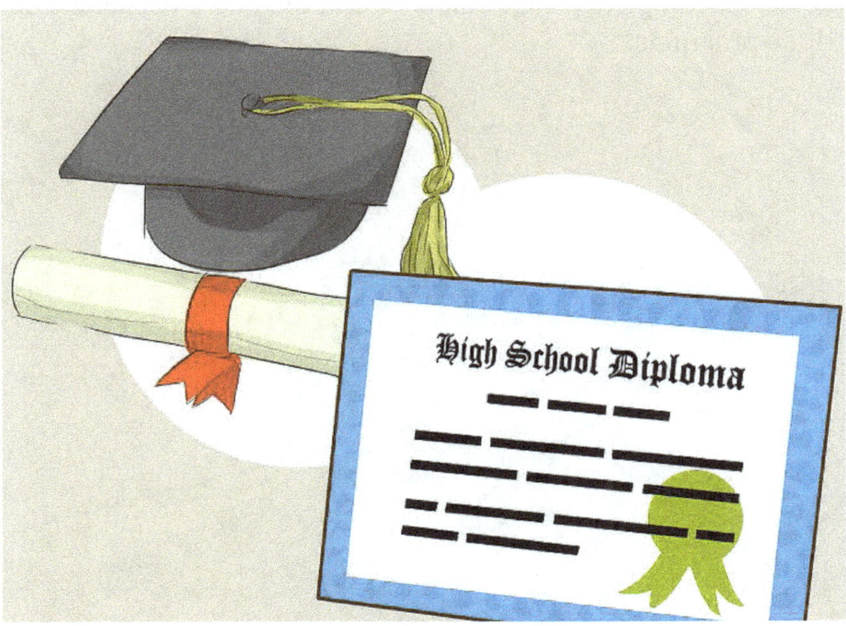

1. Graduate from high school or pass the General Education Development (GED) examination. This is the first step on the path to becoming a nurse anesthetist. Pay special attention to science courses like biology, physiology, and chemistry, as your performance in these types of courses early on will help you determine whether or not medicine is the right field for you.

- Take the SATs, the required standardized test for college admissions, your junior year and apply to more than one school to increase your likelihood of acceptance.

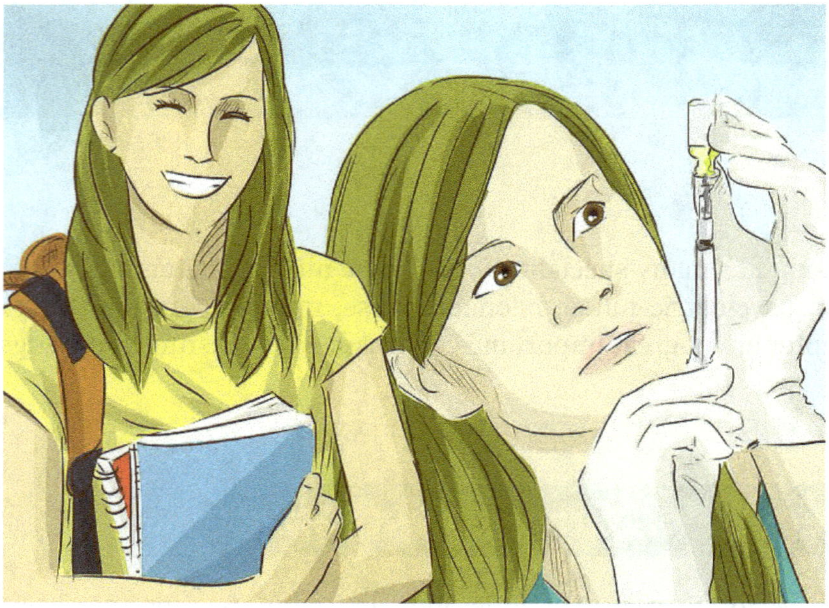

2. Get a Bachelor of Science in Nursing. While particular programs differ, coursework generally includes physiology, nursing theory, and biology.

- Though registered nurses don't necessarily need a bachelor's degree, nurse anesthetists do because they must complete postgraduate education, and a bachelor's degree is a prerequisite for these programs.

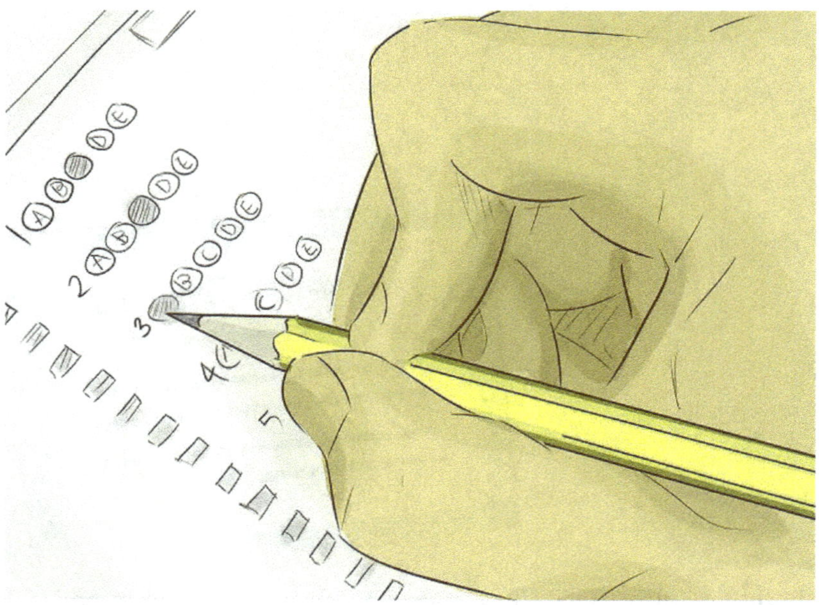

3. Become a registered nurse. You will need to take the National Council Licensure Examination for Registered Nurses and meet additional state requirements. You must become a registered nurse in the state in which you plan on practicing.

- Some states require that you complete a criminal background check and send your college transcripts in order to sign up for the national licensing exam.

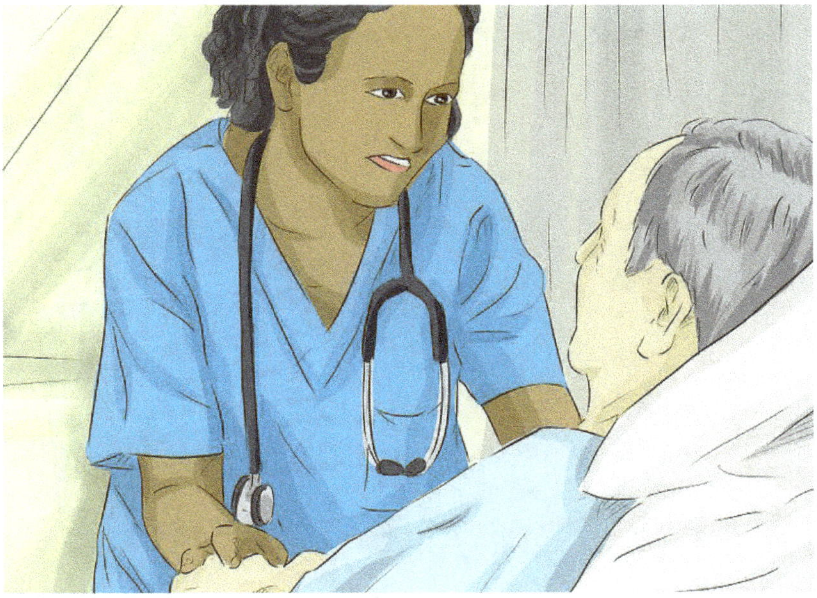

4. Complete at least one year of acute care experience. This includes working as a nurse in an ICU (Intensive Care Unit), ER (Emergency Room), or other acute care facility within a hospital.

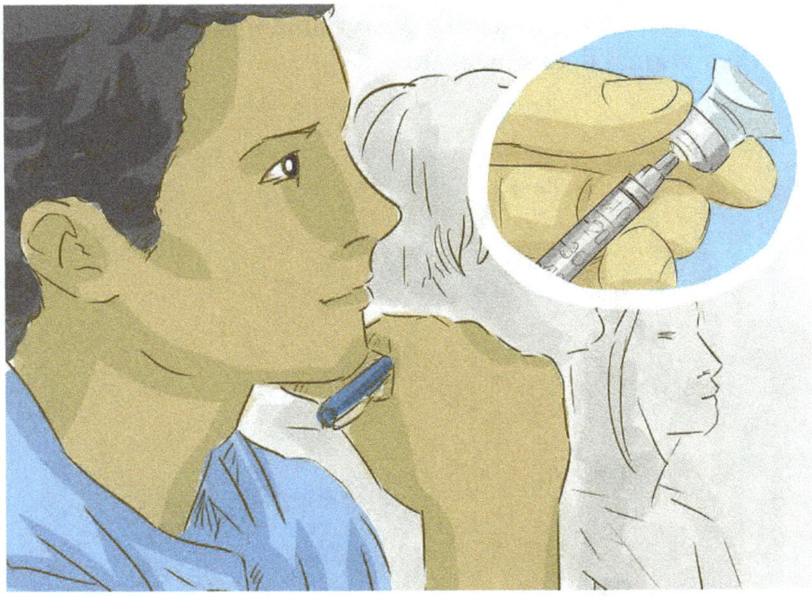

5. Complete an accredited graduate program in nurse anesthesia. These programs typically last between 2 to 3 years, and earn you a Master of Science in Nurse Anesthesia or other related Master of Science degree. Nurse anesthetist programs combine classroom instruction and hands-on clinical experience, focusing on subjects like anatomy, chemistry, physiology, and pharmacology. You will learn important skills like how to administer anesthesia for different types of surgeries.

- You will need to have a bachelor's degree, hold a nursing license, and show proof that you have completed one year of acute care in order to apply for a master's program in nurse anesthesia.

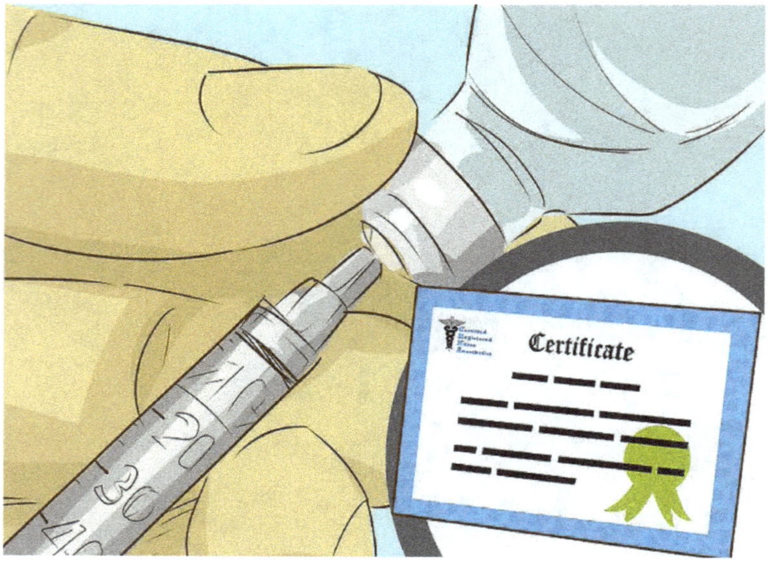

6. Take the national certification examination for CRNAs. This test is required in order to become a certified nurse anesthetist. Tests are administered several times a year, and there are a variety of programs designed to help you prepare for the exam.

- You must have successfully completed a postgraduate program in nurse anesthesiology to be eligible for the national licensing exam.

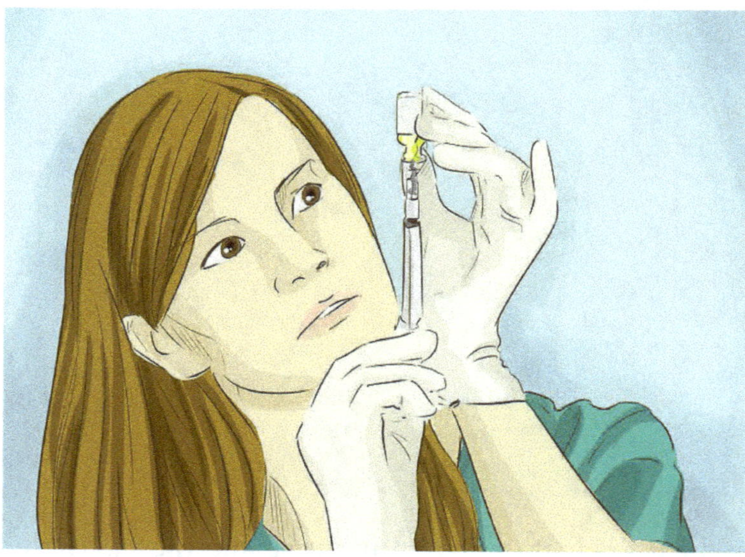

7. Find work as a nurse anesthetist. Certified nurse anesthetists can work in either the private or public sector, and typically work in hospitals, surgery centers, physicians' offices, dental offices, plastic surgeons' offices, podiatrist offices, and clinics.

- Nurse anesthetists earn one of the highest salaries within the nursing profession, with a median income of six figures.
- As populations continue to grow, there will continue to be an increased demand for nurse anesthetists and other medical professionals.

How to become a Maternity Nurse

With the exception of ICU nurses, labor and delivery or maternity nurses are considered to be among the most skilled nursing specialties. To be a labor and delivery nurse, you have to be able to take on multiple roles. Many labor and delivery nurses will help labor the patient, be the "baby nurse" for the newborn, be prepared to resuscitate the newborn, be able to work as a "scrub nurse", operating room circulator, and first assistant for the physician performing a cesarean. In addition to working in a variety of locations, maternity nurses can hold a variety of different licenses depending on their specialties and level of education. To become a maternity nurse you need to obtain the required education, experience, and training, and then seek employment in a healthcare setting.

Method 1

Training to be a Maternity Nurse

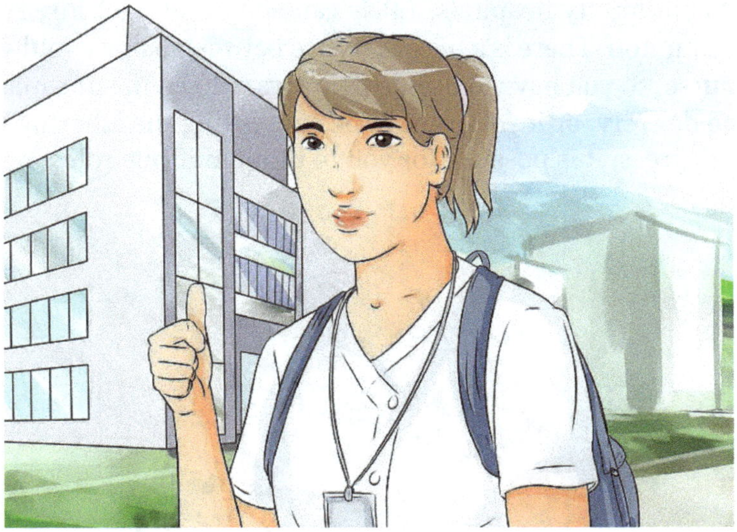

1. Decide what kind of nursing degree you would like to pursue. This will vary depending on what you would like to specialize in and how much time you want to spend in school. Options include:

- Licensed Practical Nurse (LPN) - A LPN program is 1½ years long. LPNs can become certified and licensed through community colleges or vocational schools. However, many LPNs are not used in a labor and delivery setting due to the specialty area that it is. Most LPNs are utilized in an office outside the hospital or medical surgical floor, rather than an ICU setting, Labor and Delivery, or pediatrics.
- Registered Nurse (RN) - The average registered nurse program is 2-4 years long, as it requires a bachelor's degree and 2 or 3 years of additional education. The RN's role as a labor and delivery nurse can range depending on the hospital setting you work in. They can specialize in a wide variety of roles, including labor and delivery, antepartum, and postpartum care.

- Clinical Nurse Specialist (CNS) - A CNS is a master's degree program. A CSN is an advanced practice nurse, a Master's degree program, that may prescribe medication and do other duties as a physician. Therefore, a CNS in labor and delivery may specialize in the management clinically of the woman during pregnancy and labor and delivery. The CNS is also a great resource for nurses on the division, specializing in education.
- Nurse Practitioner (NP) - A NP is a master's degree program. Nurse practitioners do specialize in neonatal care and are utilized in NICU and normal newborn nurseries. They usually help to triage patients and do not perform deliveries.
- Certified Nurse Midwife (CNW) - A CNW is a master's degree program. Midwives were the original nurse professionals in the labor and delivery world. Midwives are trained over a graduate level and are trained to support women in their pregnancy and labor and delivery. They are not able to do surgery on their patients, therefore, if a C-Section is needed or a vacuum or forceps assisted delivery, a physician will have to help them.
- Most major labor delivery centers are not using LPNs in labor and delivery and instead are using RNs. At community hospitals, LPNs can sometimes get hired in that role, but still RNs are more common. There is a big difference between being a midwife and being a labor and delivery nurse, so you have to decide if you want to be the one managing the labor and performing the delivery, or if you want to be supporting the laboring mom. Assuming you have the right degrees, it is possible for you to fulfill multiple roles.

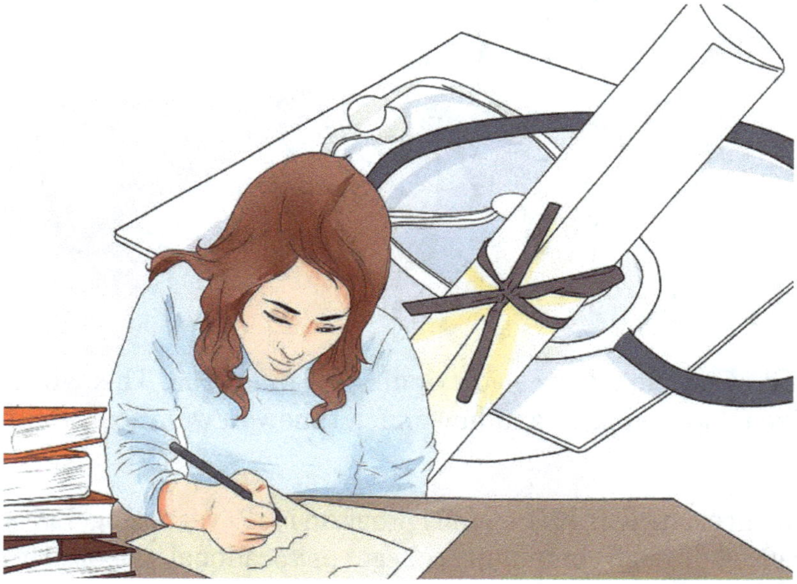

2. Train for general nursing during your degree program. Each nursing program has specific hours you will need to graduate, which are built into your nursing program. In addition to classroom learning, you will have to take hands-on courses, also known as clinicals. You will go through a short period of clinical experience in labor and delivery and postpartum care. This gives you a view into the world of a labor nurse to see if it is something you would be interested in pursuing.

- However, this experience will not give you thorough training like you will get once you are on the job.

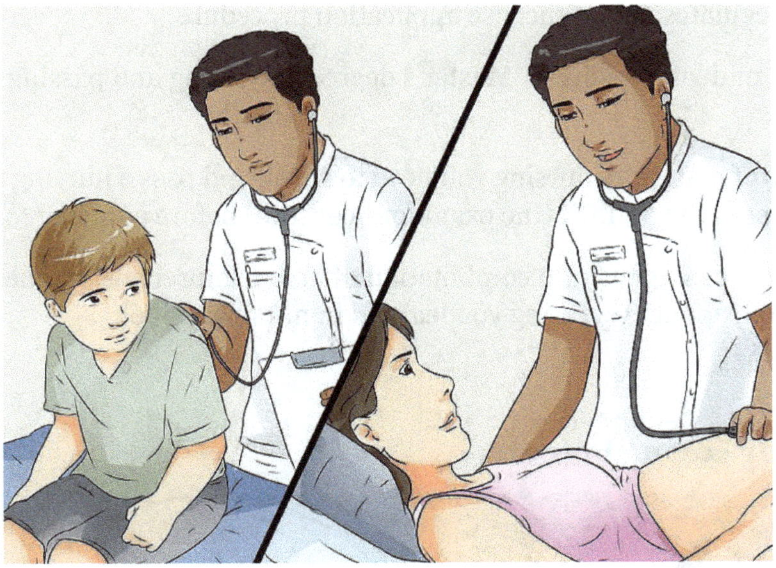

3. Learn the specifics of maternity nursing by working in a hospital maternity ward or obstetric practice, or by observing a practicing midwife. The variety of nursing jobs in the maternity ward vary from an antepartum nurse, triage nurse, labor nurse, delivery nurse, scrub nurse, circulating nurse (in the operating room), postpartum nurse, lactation nurse, and newborn nurse.

- Start by contacting your local hospital's volunteer program. The director can help guide you on a shadowing experience. This can be done during nursing school to see if it is a hospital you would like to work in.
- Maternity wards are not the same everywhere. Touring and volunteering your time can be a great way to see if you feel like you would fit in at that particular facility.

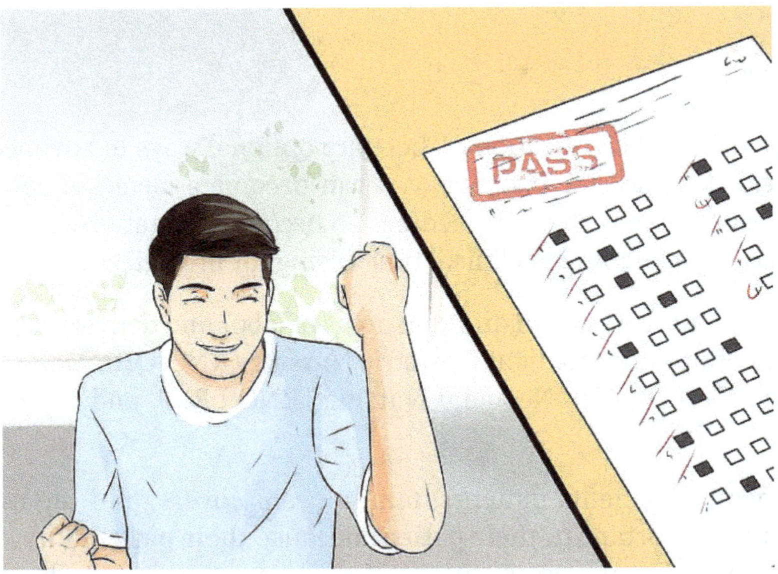

4. Get a nursing license in your state or region. You will need to visit the website of the state board of nursing in your specific state to see the qualifications for each test. Before you begin a specialty in maternity nursing, you must be a licensed nurse.

- Each state regulates its own license application procedure.
- Becoming a midwife requires a Master's degree in nursing and passing the midwifery certification.
- For all types of maternity nursing you need to enroll and pass a nursing program and apply to take and pass the NCLEX (the exam for licensure) before applying for a job.
- The nursing licensing test is a combination of high comprehension questions to make you critically think about everything you learned in nursing school.

Method 2

Maximizing your Hiring Potential

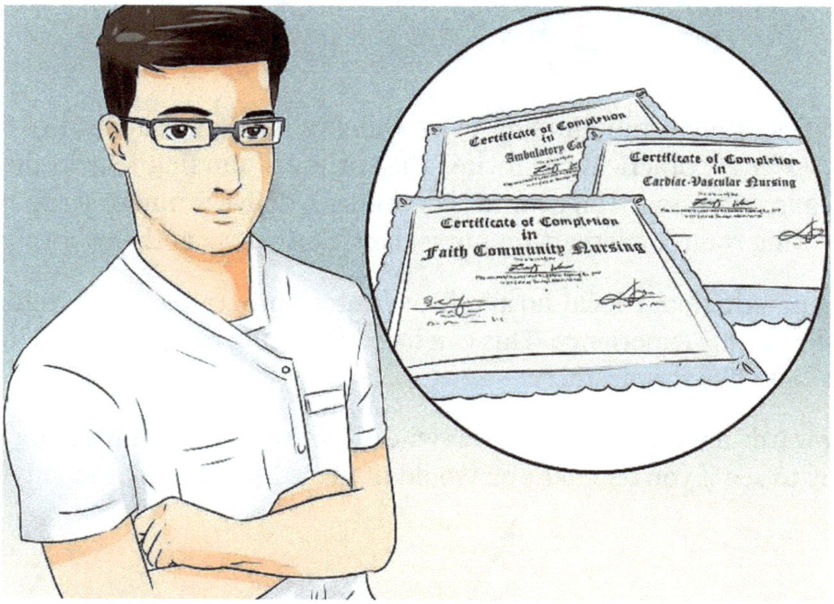

1. Consider getting additional certifications. There are optional ways to advance your degree even after you are a certified nurse. For instance, you can become a lactation consultant, which is a nurse who helps assist women with breastfeeding. To become a lactation consultant, you can take a specific exam and complete hours of clinical time caring for breastfeeding women.

- You can also become certified in different areas of labor and delivery. Options for maternity nurses certifications are Inpatient Obstetric Nursing (RNC-OB), Maternal Newborn Nursing (RNC-MNN), Low Risk Neonatal Nursing (RNC-LRN), and Neonatal Intensive Care Nursing (RNC-NIC).
- Nurse certification benefits patients, families, employers, and the nurse. The certified nurse becomes important to their patient because their patient knows they are experts in their specialty. Employers want certified nurses because it shows professionalism and retention. It shows the nurse loves what she or he does and wants to continue to learn. As for the nurse, it benefits him or her because of the sense of achievement in their career.

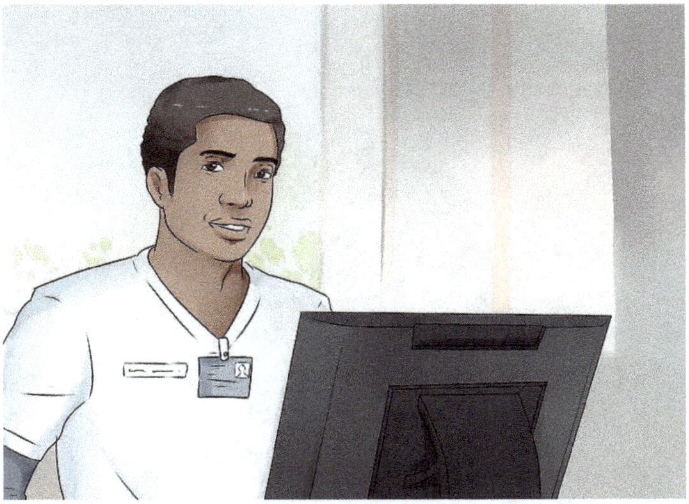

2. Get specific maternity experience anywhere you can. Work for doctors and midwives, or volunteer at the hospital. You can even try to become a nurse's aide in the area that interests you.

- Although you should try to get experience before you get the job, once you are hired you can expect on the job training that will prepare you for the actual work of maternity nursing.

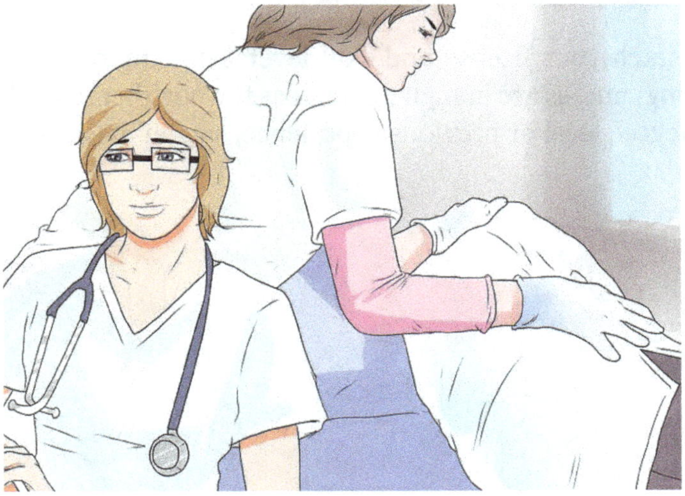

3. Work on the appropriate skills needed for maternity nursing. For example, you must be able to handle pressure and stay organized in stressful situations. In addition, communication and good interpersonal skills are essential.

- Learn to educate people. You will have to teach women how to nurse, partners how to encourage, and new parents how to care for their babies. Be sure you know exactly what you are teaching. Your patients will have questions and, as a specialized nurse, it is important to be able to answer those questions with accurate information.
- Work on staying physically and emotionally strong. Many new labor and delivery nurses are on night shift and that shift can exhaust anyone. Assisting doctors and women during childbirth can be exhausting, and you will need to be prepared for any possible outcome during the pregnancies of your patients.

Method 3

Finding Work as a Maternity Nurse

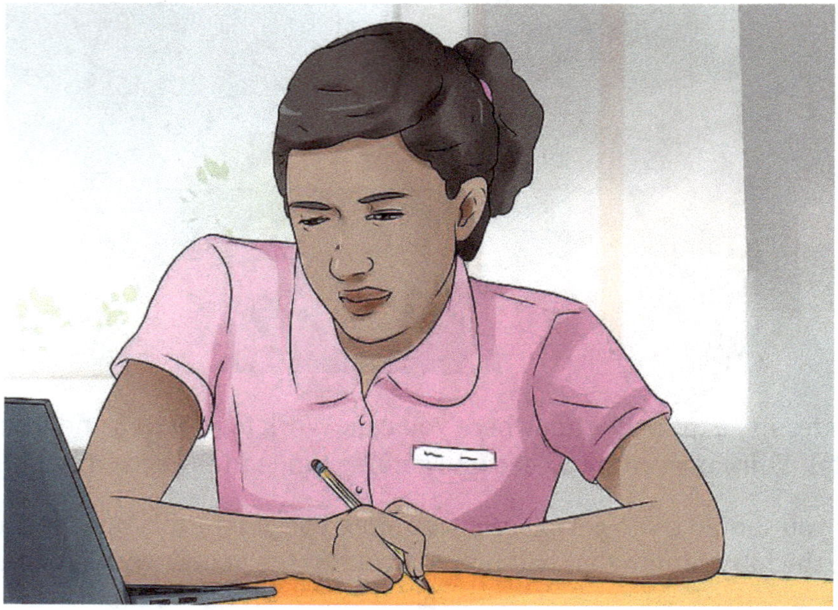

1. Look for jobs that match your license and skill level. The employment outlook for the entire nursing field is promising; nurses are in high demand as the healthcare field grows. Some positions will require a certain degree level or previous experience, so you may not qualify for all maternity nursing positions.

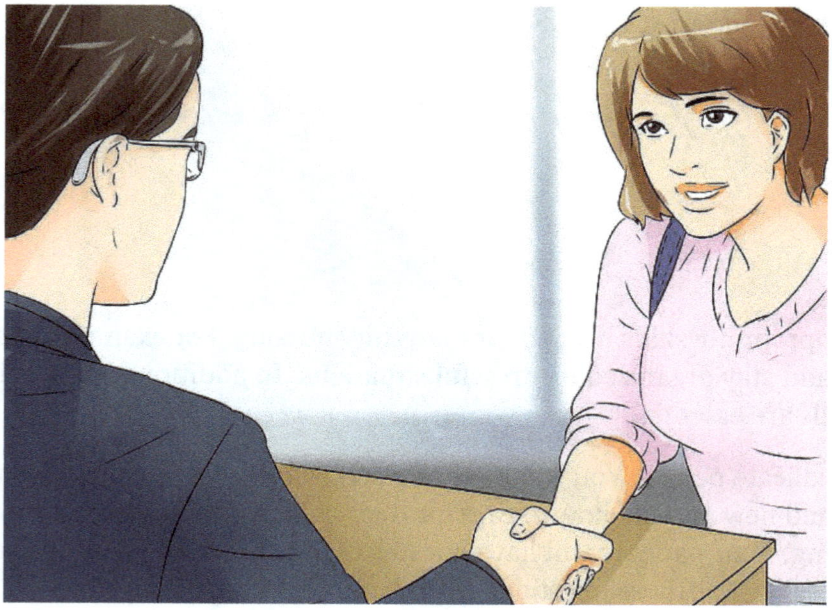

2. Begin your search before you leave nursing school. Take advantage of your program's job placement services to interview with different employers. Also be sure to make a good impression during your training and clinicals; you will often be supervised by working healthcare professionals who are looking for new talent.

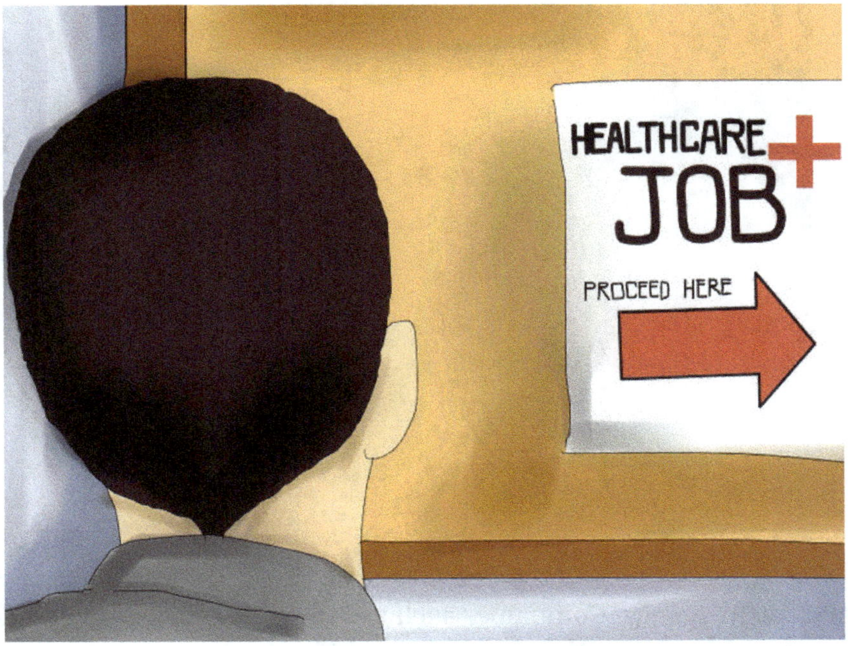

3. Attend healthcare job fairs. Talk to representatives about your interest in maternity nursing. Even if you do not find a job, your networking skills will improve and potentially lead you someone who can help you find the right job.

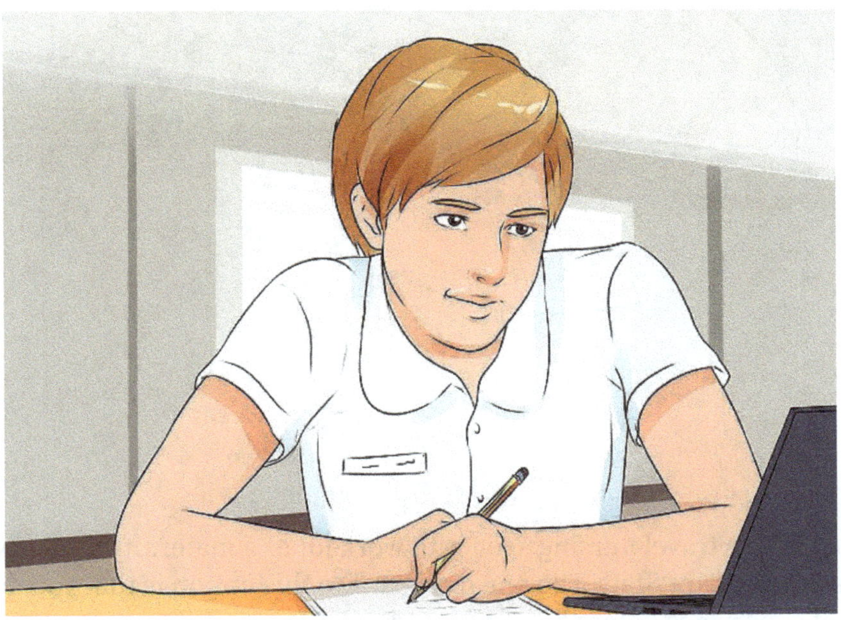

4. Check job listings. Many hospitals, physicians, and healthcare centers advertise for maternity nurses in the newspaper and online. Search general online employment sites, such as CareerBuilder, Indeed, and Simply Hired, but also look at nursing-specific sites as well. The most popular job sites for nurses of any specialty include nursingjobs.org and nurse.com. #Network with maternity nurses. Get to know the professionals in your field. They can become your friends and confidants but they can also share information with you when a job opening pops up.

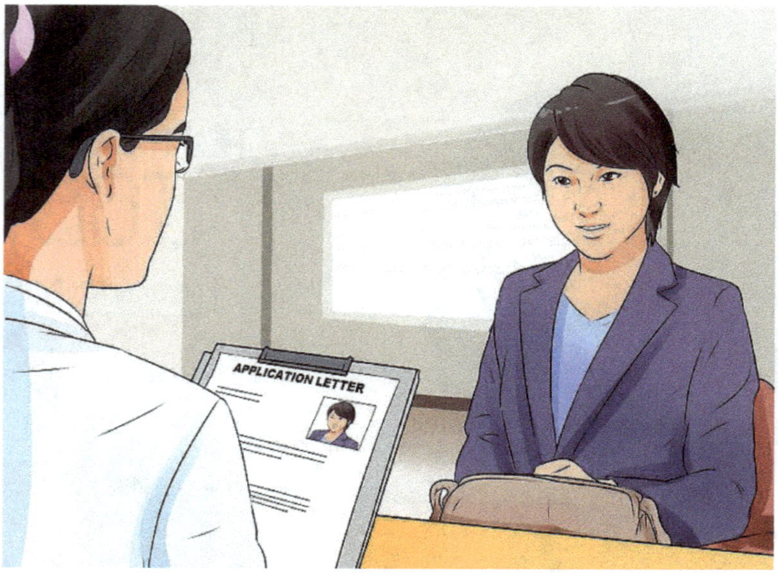

5. Enlist with a placement agency. Companies such as Maxim Staffing, NurseFinders and FlexRN specialize in placing nurses in jobs. Discuss your interest in maternity nursing with these agencies and see what they can find for you.

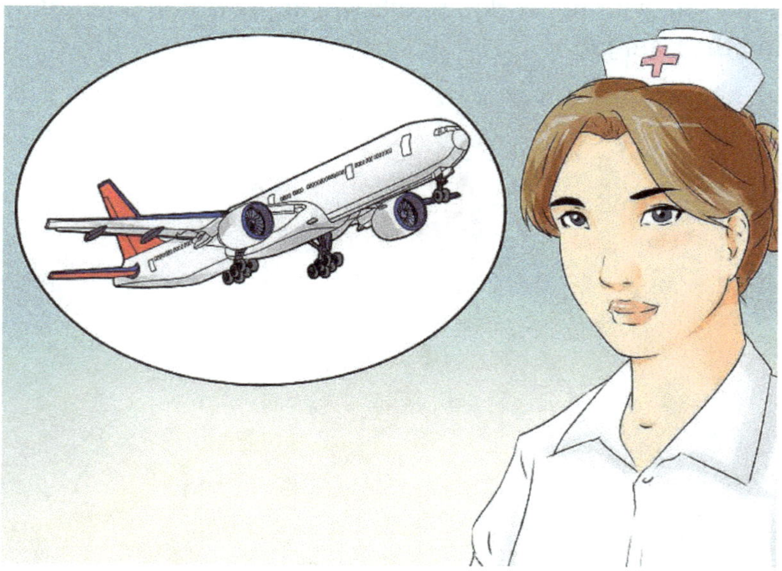

6. Be adventurous! Find a travel nursing agency to work for as a maternity nurse, with like Medical staffing solutions or Flex Care Staff. The one drawback to this option is that you do generally need at least one year of experience before becoming a travel nurse.

How to become a Pediatric Nurse

Pediatric nurses choose to face the unique challenges and rewards of working with children. They provide both preventative and acute care to their young patients, while helping to calm their fears (and those of their parents). They can work in settings ranging from hospitals to physician offices to schools, and are often the first line of medical care for their young patients. The path to becoming a pediatric nurse requires a general nursing degree, training and experience working with children, and often additional advanced certifications. The many benefits include a strong job outlook and the daily opportunity to make a positive impact on children's lives.

Part 1

Entering the Field

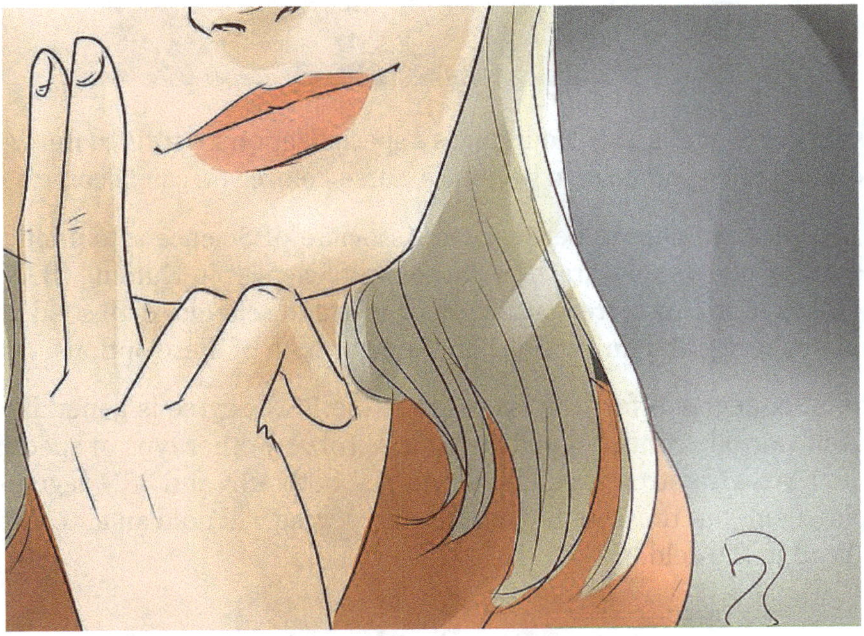

1. Consider your suitability for a pediatric specialty. Children are not just smaller adults, physiologically or psychologically. Their growing and changing bodies (and minds) require particular types of care and distinctive ways of providing it. Not all nurses, even exceptional ones, are cut out for pediatrics.

- First and foremost, you must embrace the challenges and rewards of working with children. You must also dedicate yourself to understanding their specific health needs.
- You must be patient, understanding, and ready to deal with the unexpected. You'll need excellent communication skills, including the ability to explain medical subjects to both small children and their parents.
- You need to be willing and able to be a major figure in office visits — you will often be the "first line" of medical care. You need to be able to provide vaccinations to crying infants, exams to tantrum-throwing eight year olds, and sound advice to know-it-all teenagers.
- Patient education and preventative medicine are of particular importance for pediatric nurses. It helps to have an interest in going out into the community — visiting schools, working at health fairs, etc. — to provide advice and care.

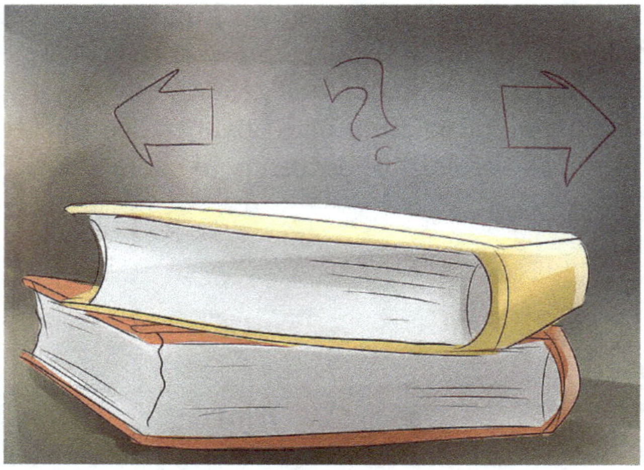

2. Choose a nursing program. Pediatric nursing is a specialization for trained nurses, not a separate career path. In other words, you have to become a nurse before you can become a pediatric nurse.

- In the U.S., you can choose between an Associate of Science in Nursing (ASN) degree, which normally takes two years, or a Bachelor of Sciences in Nursing (BSN) degree, which typically takes four. An increasing number of trade schools, dedicated nursing schools, community colleges, and universities offer one or both of these options.
- While the ASN degree offers the faster path, the BSN degree is generally considered the better path toward becoming a pediatric nurse (or any other type of specialized nurse, for that matter). With the strong demand for nurses, both ASN and BSN degree-holders should find employment, but those with the advanced degree will hold an automatic advantage in getting ahead in the field.

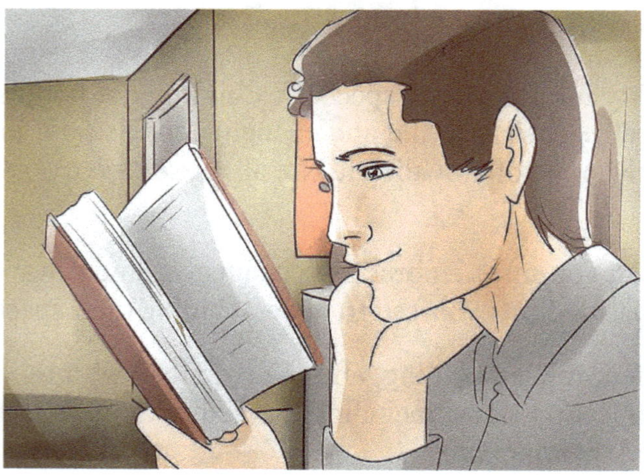

3. Take courses related to pediatrics. Most nursing schools do not have a specific track for pediatric specialties, but they usually do offer courses with a pediatric emphasis. If you are serious about a career as a pediatric nurse, take as many of these classes as possible while in nursing school.

- For instance, courses in child health and child psychology should be particularly useful. If you are in a nursing program at a college or university, you can probably find an array of elective courses that deal with childhood development.

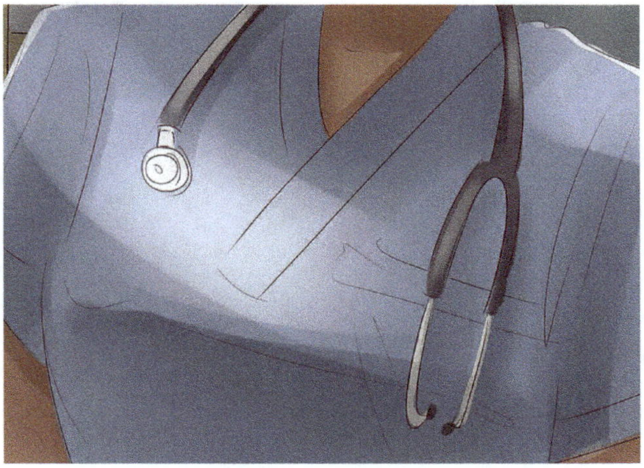

4. Become a Registered Nurse (RN). By doing so, you will achieve official status as a nurse, and can then begin directing your career toward a pediatric specialty. To become an RN in the U.S., you must complete an ASN or BSN degree program and pass the NCLEX exam.

- The National Council Licensure Exam for RNs is offered by the National Council of State Boards of Nursing (NCSBN). The exam takes approximately six hours to complete, and is offered regularly in numerous locations.

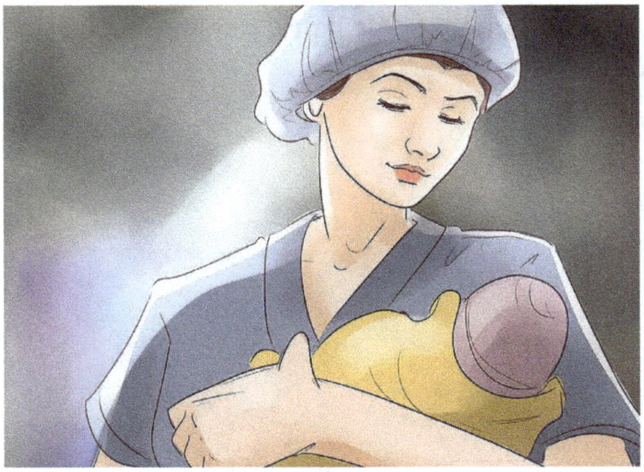

5. Gain experience working with children. Start while you are a nursing student, using your time to learn all you can about the pediatric nursing field. Read books, look at websites, talk to your teachers, and talk to current pediatric nurses.

- The Society of Pediatric Nurses website offers information on the field, and the organization produces the Journal of Pediatric Nursing.
- Volunteer in the pediatric wing of your local hospital, or a clinic, or anywhere else that provides care to children.
- Apply for intern programs that offer new nurses training specifically for pediatrics.
- Apply to work at sites that provide care to children, such as a pediatrician's office or pediatric after-hour care facility.

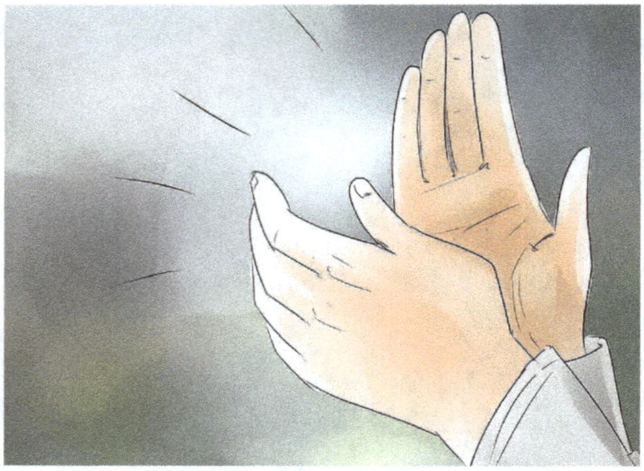

6. Seek recognition as an Advanced Practice Nurse (APN) by your state board of nursing. Research the nursing requirements that are set up in the state you plan to practice in.

- Consider earning APN status as a step toward additional advanced certifications and licensures that are also either required or highly recommended for pediatric nurses.
- You may also want to look into extending your education to earn a Master of Science in Nursing degree (MSN), which normally requires an additional two years of coursework. As discussed in the following Part of this topic, the MSN is a stepping stone to several advanced degrees and certifications in pediatric nursing, such as becoming a Certified Pediatric Nurse or Pediatric Nurse Practitioner.

Part 2

Advancing your Career

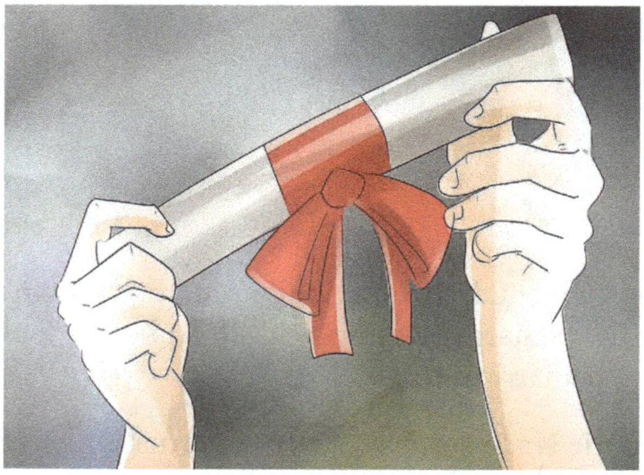

1. Become a Certified Pediatric Nurse (CPN). In some states, CPN status is required for pediatric nurses, but it is recommended for everyone in the field. It demonstrates that you are certified to give specialized care to pediatric patients, and to educate them and their families on health topics.

- To become a CPN, you need to already be an RN and have at least 1,800 hours of documented experience in pediatrics during the previous two years. This experience can include work, training, or coursework in an MSN program, among other options.

- You also need to pass an exam to become a CPN. The Pediatric Nursing Certification Board (PNCB) oversees the exam, and can offer valuable information on locating exam sites, fees for the exam, and procedures for registering for and taking the exam.

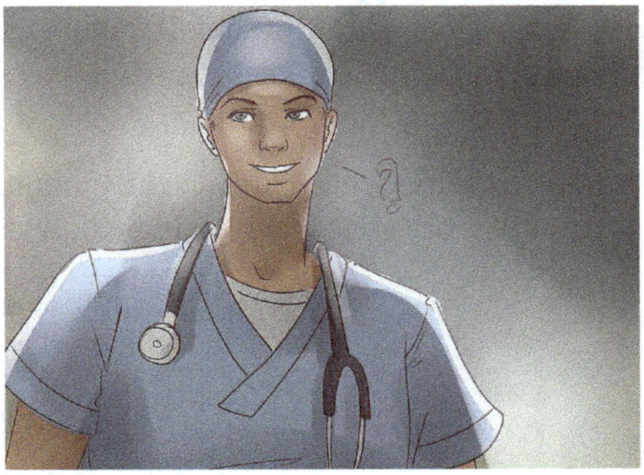

2. Determine your preferred work setting once you become a pediatric nurse. Just as the roles and requirements for pediatric nurses are different than those for other nurses, the setting in which you practice will make a significant difference in the type of work you do.

- You'll always face the unexpected as a pediatric nurse, but if you prefer providing primary care services like vaccinations, checkups, and dealing with bumps, bruises, and stuffy noses in a somewhat more regimented environment, you may want to work in a pediatrician's office or become a school nurse.
- If you want to care for acute, chronically ill, or critically ill children, you'll want to concentrate on acute care and specialty services, such as the PICU (Pediatric Intensive Care Unit). You can seek out advanced certifications in such fields from organizations like the PNCB.
- Consider your temperament, your ability to deal with children in varying stages of illness or injury, your ability to handle stress, and more practical matters like job availability and pay rates as you determine your preferred setting.

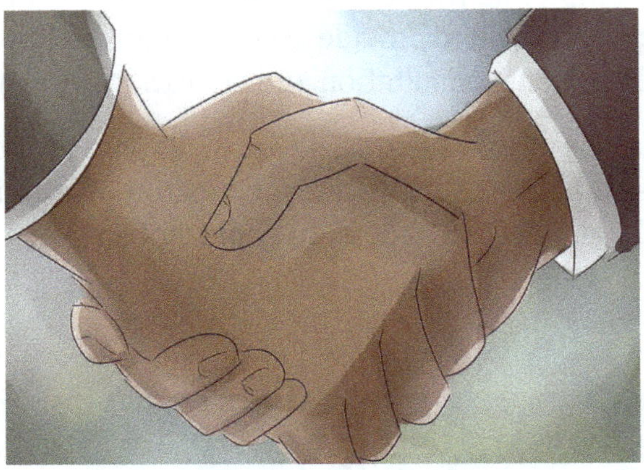

3. Find a pediatric nursing job that suits you. Employers may not necessarily be falling at your feet offering you great nursing jobs, but the demand for nurses (pediatric and otherwise) is exceptionally high in the U.S. Additionally, the future outlook indicates continued growth in demand and job openings.

- Utilize the placement office at your nursing school, as well as connections you've made through coursework, internships, and so forth.
- The demand for pediatric nurses is typically greatest in hospital settings, so that may be the easiest place to secure your first job in the field. If that is not your preferred setting, you may want to gain experience in the hospital setting while keeping an eye out for a job at a pediatrician's office, school, clinic, government agency, etc.
- In addition to real-world work experience, advanced training and certifications will most likely make it easier for you to score your ideal job in pediatric nursing.

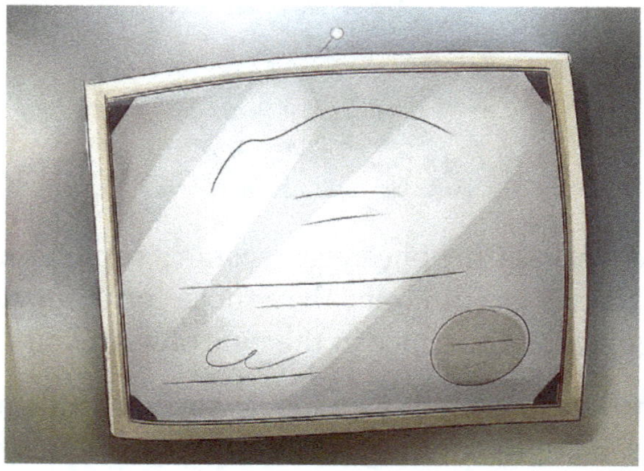

4. Look into additional licenses and certifications. As with any job in the healthcare field, a pediatric nurse's training is never truly done. As you settle into your career, it makes sense to always consider your next steps, including additional training and certifications that can enhance your work (and potentially earn you a bigger paycheck).

- There are numerous specialized certifications available for pediatric nurses, and they usually entail some sort of coursework and passing an examination.
- Pediatric nurses with a Masters in nursing (MSN) can choose to become a Clinical Nurse Specialist (CNS) by completing the requirements, which include a nationally-administered exam. CNSs are specially trained to provide a family-centered approach to care and to provide enhanced expertise in patient consultation and education, among other distinctive aspects.
- The MSN degree also permits you to seek certification as a Pediatric Nurse Practitioner (PNP). PNPs possess advanced diagnostic and treatment training, and have the power to prescribe medicine in all fifty U.S. states. In some states, PNPs are also permitted to practice independently.

How to become a Psychiatric Nurse

Psychiatric nurses, also called psychiatric-mental health nurses, help patients who are mentally ill. Patients suffering from conditions like schizophrenia or psychosis, or who are suffering from mental distress caused by traumatic events such as the death of a spouse or a cancer diagnosis, often find themselves under the care of a psychiatric nurse. Psychiatric nurses may work in hospitals or in the community, determining their patients' mental health status and helping meet those needs. To become a psychiatric nurse, you must first earn a nursing degree.

Part 1

Becoming a Registered Nurse

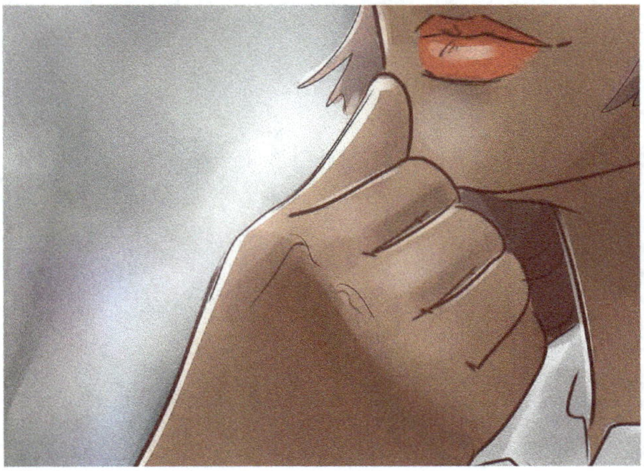

1. Choose a nursing program to complete. You can choose an Associate Degree in Nursing (ADN) program or a Bachelor of Science in Nursing (BSN) program. The ADN is a two-year program, where the BSN is a four-year program.

- You will need a high school diploma or GED to enroll in an ADN or BSN program.
- Second baccalaureate and entry-level master's of science in nursing programs are available for people who already have bachelor's degrees in fields other than nursing.
- BSN graduates may be preferred by employers over other degree types.
- Consider earning a master's degree in psychiatric-mental health nursing. The degree will enable you to diagnose and treat some mental health problems yourself. In some states you can also prescribe medication.

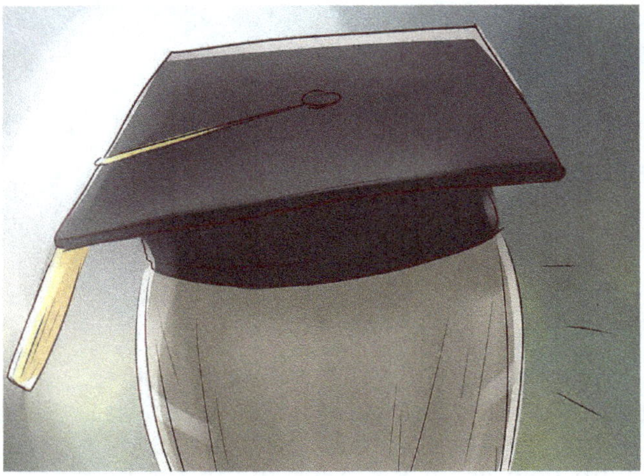

2. Complete the nursing program you have chosen. Programs accredited by the Commission on

Collegiate Nursing Education (CCNE) or Accreditation Commission for Education in Nursing (ACEN) ensure a path to RN licensure. Complete all requirements to graduate from the program you have chosen with your degree.

- Meet with your advisor to make sure you are completing the program requirements.

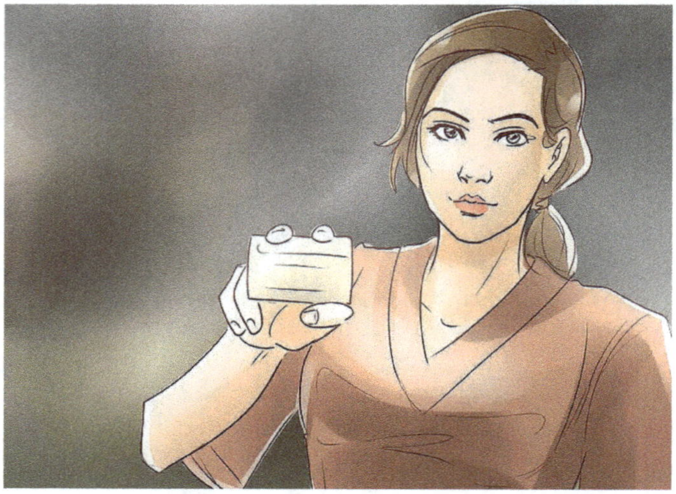

3. Get licensed as an RN. To get licensed as an RN, you must pass the National Council Licensure Examination (NCLEX-RN). This examination is given by the National Council of State Boards of Nursing. The license you receive after passing the exam must be periodically renewed, so you will have to take some continuing education courses.

- Requirements for licensure vary by state, so check with yours to see what requirements you may have to meet.

Part 2

Gaining the Necessary Experience

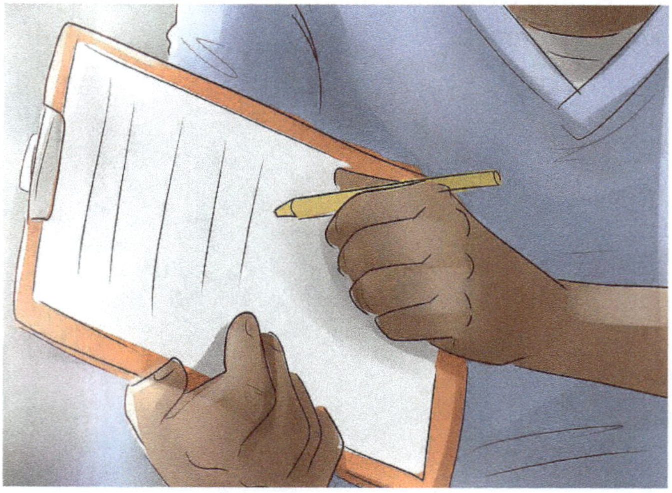

1. Work in the mental health field as an RN. Working in the psychiatric-mental health field as an RN translates to clinical practice, of which you will need 2000 hours should you desire to get

certified as a psychiatric-mental health nurse. Look for jobs in this field to secure a position and get the experience you need. You can ask for a psychiatric rotation at a hospital if that's where you work, volunteer in a community program, or work as a psychiatric aide.

- Many employers will provide tuition reimbursement or assistance if you pursue an ADN, BSN, MSN, or DNP. Check with your employer to find out if this is something they offer.

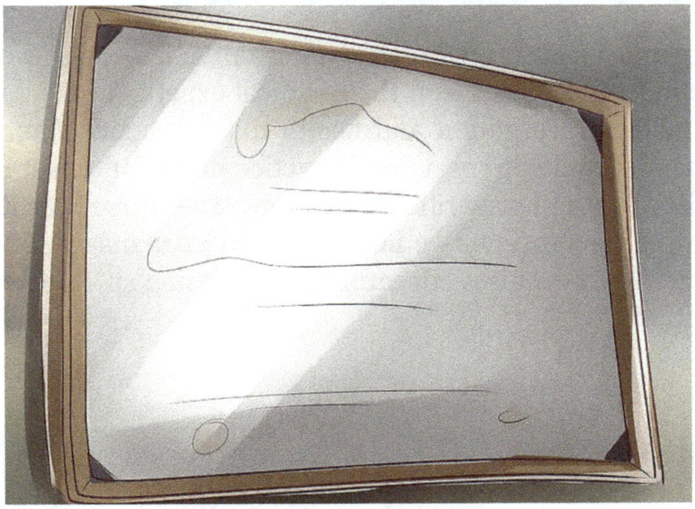

2. Get board-certified as a psychiatric-mental health nurse. Certification is not required to work in the psychiatric-mental health field, but it can be useful for finding a job and could mean higher salaries. You'll need an RN license, two years' experience working as an RN, 2000 hours of clinical practice in the psychiatric-mental health field within three years, and 30 hours of continuing education in the psychiatric-mental health field within three years.

- Certification is administered by American Nurses Credentialing Center (ANCC).

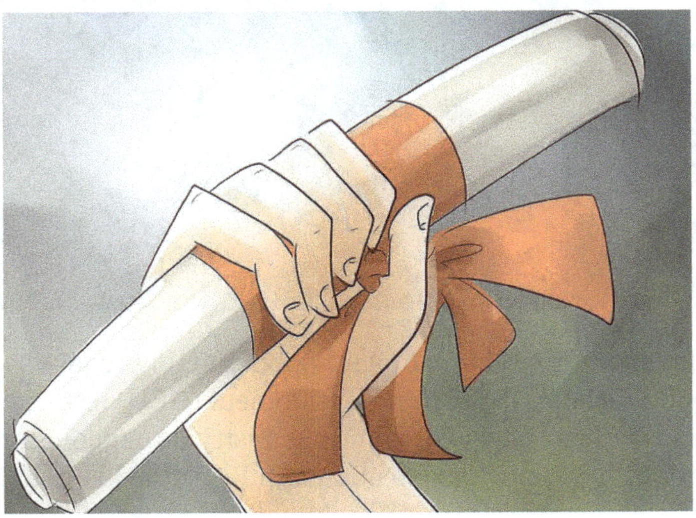

3. Maintain your certification. Board-certified psychiatric-mental health nurses must be recertified every five years. The American Nurses Credentialing Center (ANCC) requires professional development plus either 1000 hours of practice as a psychiatric-mental health nurse or passage of the certification exam.

- Professional development includes continuing education, academic credits, presentations or publication/research, professional service, or teaching hours (preceptorship).

How to become a Nurse Practitioner

Nurse Practitioners are one of several types of advanced practice nurses who are important partners in the healthcare industry. They blend their clinical expertise in diagnostics and treatment with an emphasis on disease prevention and health management. Often a Nurse Practitioner works alongside a general, family or specialized practice physician to set up and analyze health screenings, diagnose illnesses, and prescribe medications. The Nurse Practitioner also grants doctor referrals and arranges for preventative health as well as manages follow-up appointments. Becoming a Nurse Practitioner requires education and licensing as a Registered Nurse, graduate education and certification.

Part 1

Becoming a Registered Nurse

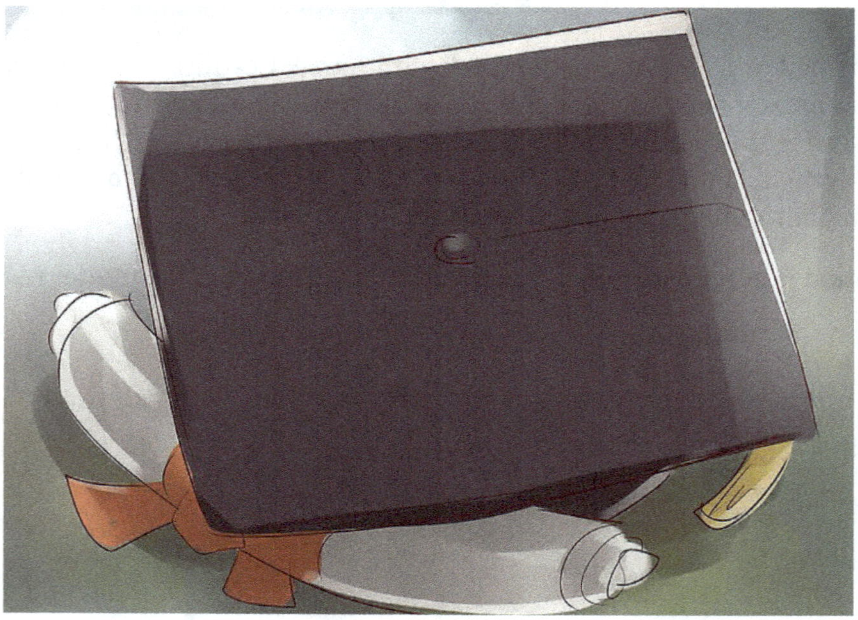

1. Get a high school diploma. Admission into a school of nursing requires a high school diploma or, alternately, passing the General Education Development (GED) test. If you want to be a nurse, pay attention courses like biology, physiology, and chemistry throughout high school. This knowledge will be very important in gaining qualification as a Registered Nurse (RN) and then a Nurse Practitioner (NP).

- The foundation of nursing is science. If you don't like science but find yourself interested in nursing throughout high school, speak with your school counselor about arranging a day or two to shadow a nurse.

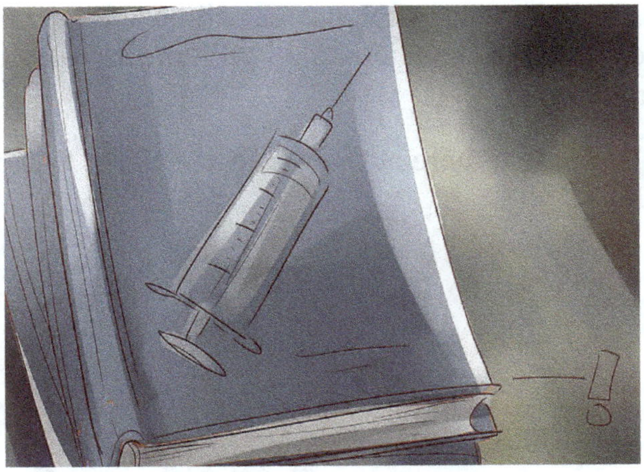

2. Undertake post-secondary education in nursing. There are three ways to become a registered nurse. In all cases, coursework includes physiology, biology, chemistry, nutrition, and anatomy.

- *Bachelor's degree in nursing (BSN).* This level of education is awarded by a college or university and usually takes four years to complete. Class offerings more diverse than other settings and include community health, pharmacology, health assessment, microbiology, human development and clinical practice. A BSN qualifies you for a higher pay grade and a wider variety of certifications and promotions on the job.
- *Associate's degree in nursing (ADN).* This is the most common way to obtain a registered nursing license and involves a two-year program at a community or junior college. Many students transition to BSN programs after having completed an ASN and holding an entry-level nursing position.
- *Diploma from an accredited nursing program.* You can also be eligible for licensure by completing a vocational nursing program. These accredited programs are often associated with a hospital and vary in length, though they are typically up to three years long. This education path is on the decline since the National Advisory Council on Nursing Education and Practice recommends that at least 66% of the workforce hold a BSN in nursing or higher.

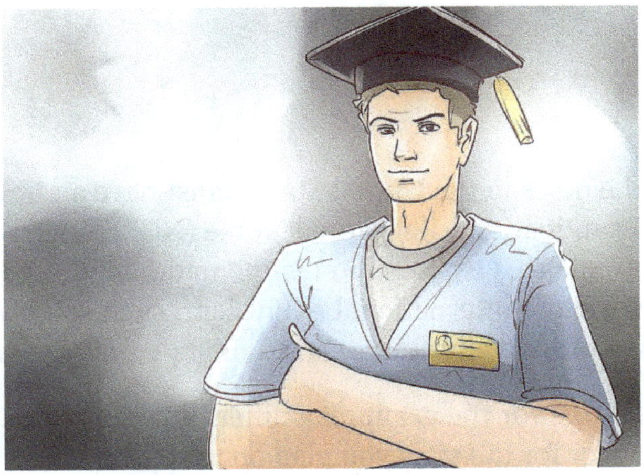

3. Note that you need a BSN to become a Nurse Practitioner. It is necessary to first become a Registered Nurse with a BSN before you can start a Master's of Science in Nursing (MSN) to become

a nurse practitioner. With a diploma or ADN, nurses will be able to move on to their bachelor's degree through accelerated programs and potentially with the assistance of their employers via a tuition reimbursement program.

- You may also wish to earn a more advanced degree called Doctorate of Nursing Practice instead of the MSN.

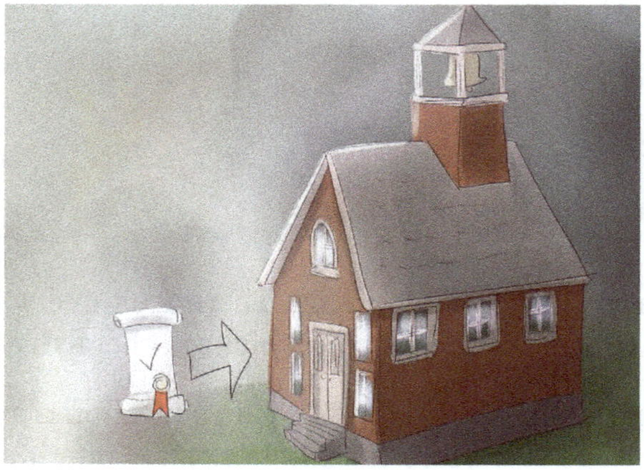

4. Make sure your school is accredited. The national accreditation agency for nursing schools is the Commission on Collegiate Nursing Education. This agency ensures the quality and integrity of bachelor, graduate, and residency programs in nursing. Accreditation is voluntary but ensures that colleges and schools providing nursing education are operating at the same professional level and educating future nurses in a manner which ensures that they can provide effective and standardized care.

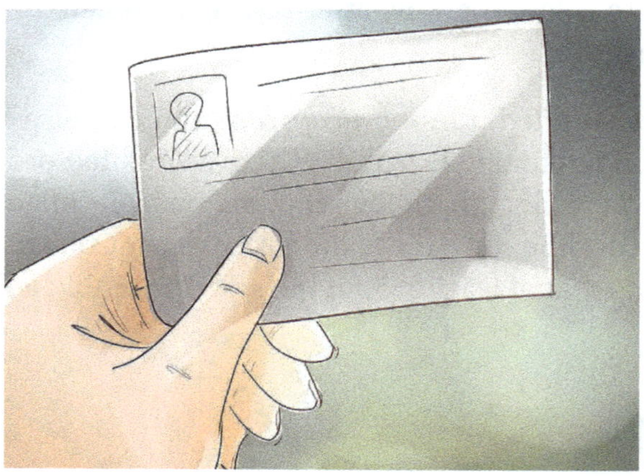

5. Get licensed. Registered Nurses in the United States must have a nursing license. Take the National Council Licensure Examination - Registered Nurse (NCLEX-RN) once you have graduated from your accredited program. This examination is the nationally recognized licensing exam for registered nurses. Prepare for the international equivalent, such as CGFNS International, if you plan to work overseas or if you are an international student planning to work in the United States.

- Prerequisites to and fees for the exam may differ between states. Check with the requirements for your state, or for the state you plan on practicing in.
- Be aware as well that each state has their own scope of practice for nursing. It is important to know scope of practice so you know what you can or can not do as a nurse in your state.

- Most states have reciprocal agreements, meaning that if you pass your exam in one state, you'll be able to apply for and receive a license in any other state without retaking the test as long as your license if free from any encumbrances (such as a felony conviction).

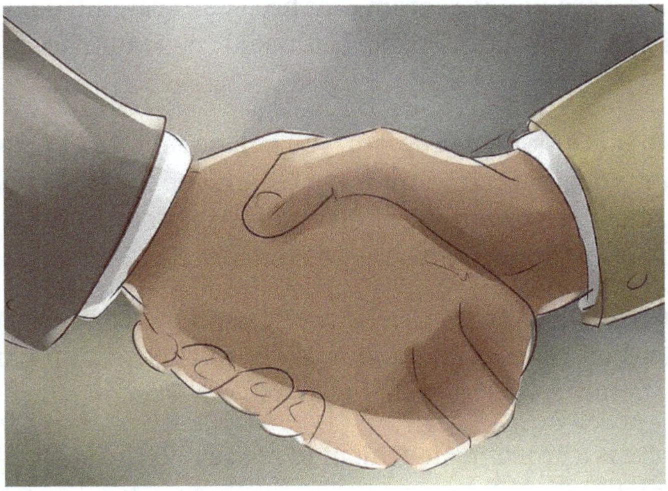

6. Find a job as an RN. Build some experience on the road to becoming a nurse practitioner by seeking entry-level work in a clinic or a hospital setting to get registered nursing experience. There are more than 2 million nurses in the United States, making the profession the largest in the health-care field. There are a variety of settings in which a nurse can work, including hospitals, physician's offices, elderly care homes, prisons, college campuses and schools.

- Entry-level work as an RN usually serves as a stepping-stone to a higher-level career as an advanced practice nurse, like a Nurse Practitioner. You can also work as an RN as you pursue the further education required to become a Nurse Practitioner. There is great flexibility in being able to work as RN while obtaining advanced degree.

Part 2

Becoming a Nurse Practitioner

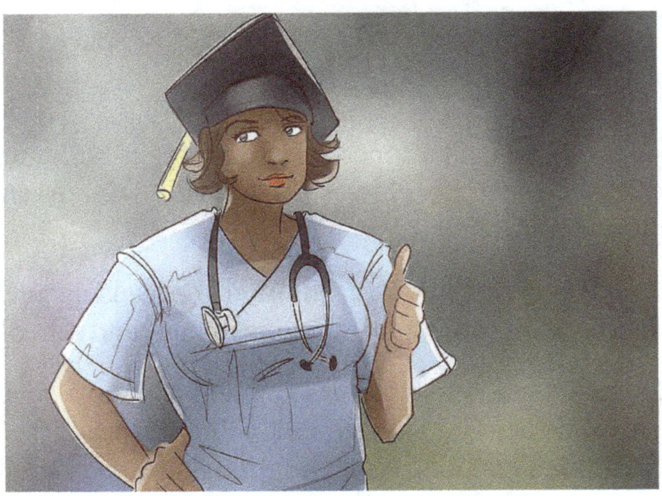

1. Get graduate education in nursing. Most Nurse Practitioners have obtained a Master's Degree of

Science in Nursing (MSN). Master's programs are often designed around the needs of a working professional and frequently offer night and weekend classes. A MSN may take between two and seven years to complete, depending upon if the applicant is pursuing the degree full-time or part-time. Make sure to choose a graduate program that has been accredited by either the Commission on Collegiate Nursing Education (CCNE) or the National League for Nursing Accrediting Commission (NLNAC).

- To be admitted to this graduate program, you will be required to have a Registered Nurse's license, a bachelor's degree, and a minimum GPA in the bachelor's degree as determined by the prospective school. Applications often require a statement of purpose, personal history or professional history. Applications may also require an interview.
- A MSN degree, particularly one with a Nurse Practitioner concentration, prepares students for careers beyond entry-level and allows them to choose a specialty such as pediatrics, women's health, family care or geriatrics, among other fields.
- Be aware that there is a growing movement to require all Nurse Practitioners to have a Doctor of Nursing Practice (D.N.P.) degree, or basically a doctoral degree. This degree requires three to four years of further education after a bachelor's degree in nursing.

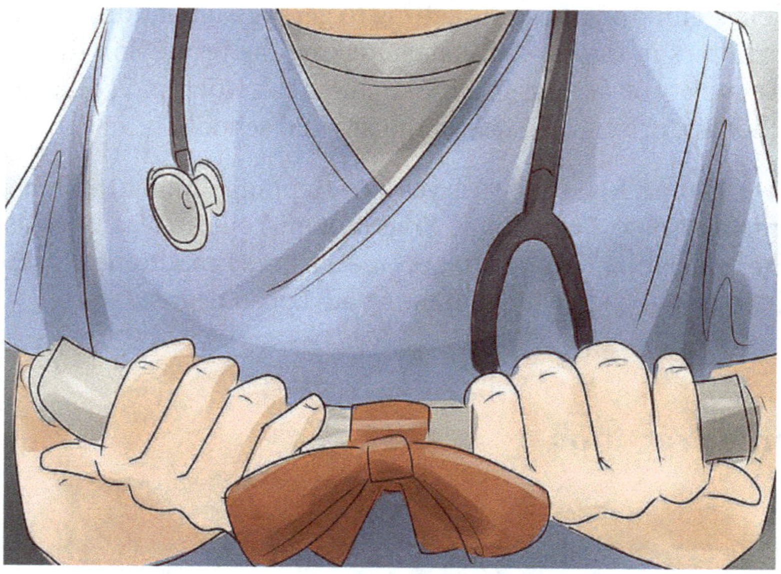

2. Get certified to work as a nurse practitioner. After earning a MSN, take the certification examination administered by the American Nurses Credentialing Center (ANCC) or the American Academy of Nurse Practitioners (AANP).

- Specialties that require certification in addition to licensing include pediatrics, family health, mental health, acute care, diabetes management and school nursing.
- Once certified, Nurse Practitioners can also choose to take a specialty examination that certifies they have additional knowledge and ability to practice. These specialty certifications include pain management, rehabilitation, cardiac rehabilitation, college health nursing, forensic nursing, diabetes management, nurse executive, pediatrics, and school nursing.

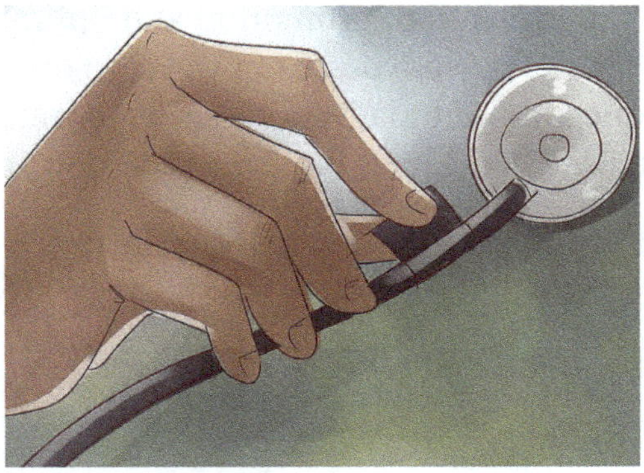

3. Get a job as a Nurse Practitioner. Nurse practitioners are valued members of the healthcare team, providing cost effective care in the diagnosis, treatment and management of many acute and chronic illnesses. This variety in practice and ability to specialize offers practitioners many options in the work place. Jobs are available in hospitals, private practices, nursing homes, clinics, health departments, urgent care settings, healthcare technology companies, and Health Maintenance Organizations (HMOs), among many other institutions. Different ways of getting a job include consulting online job websites, contacting headhunters in nursing, consulting local hospital job postings, and networking with physicians, nursing managers and community clinics, among other methods.

- The average salary of a NP is is $90,583 and the job outlook for NPs is considered excellent at present. This is because the numbers of primary care physicians is decreasing as the demand for healthcare services is rising thanks to the aging baby boomer generation.
- Other professional opportunities include teaching in schools and universities and working for governmental and military agencies.
- Note as well that about 15% of all Nurse Practitioners have their own private practices. There are also a growing number of nurse-run healthcare centers in the United States in which all healthcare is provided by nurse practitioners and other professionals. Keep in mind that not every state allows this – independent practitioners can only do this if it is within their state's scope of practice.

Part 3

Understanding Nursing

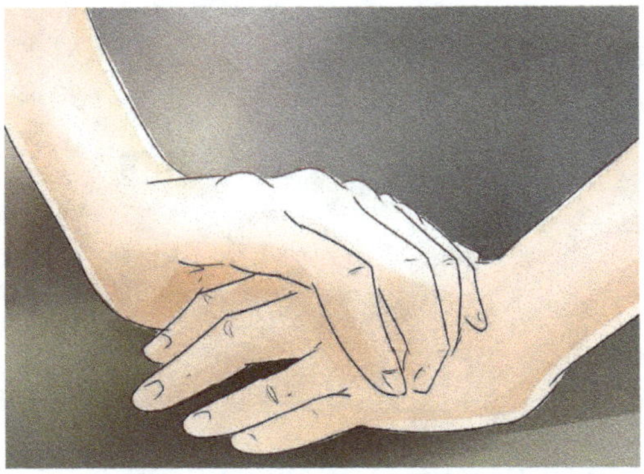

1. Understand the nursing profession in general. According to the American Nurses Association,

nursing today is designed for the protection, promotion and optimization of health and the prevention of illness and injury. Nurses are advocates in the care of individuals, families and communities. The standardized education of today's nurses, in contrast to the past, reflects the high expectations communities and physicians have on the men and women who fill these roles.

- The nursing profession is not just for women; there are over a hundred thousand registered male nurses working in the US.

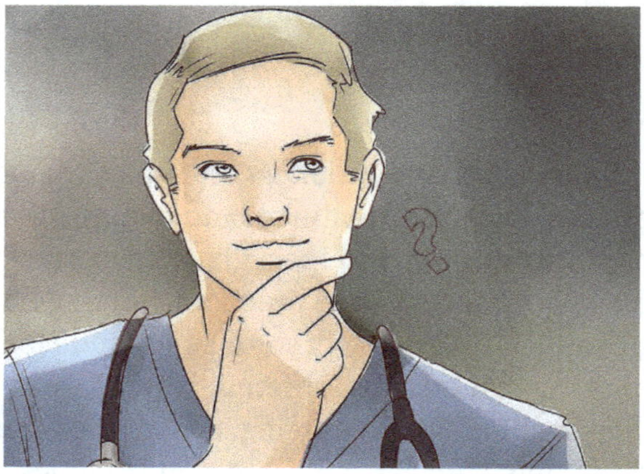

2. Determine if the general responsibilities of nursing interest you. The foundation of all nursing practice is based in human anatomy and physiology. The chief mission of the nursing field is to protect, promote and optimize health. Key responsibilities for nurses include:

- Performing physical examinations and taking medical and family histories.
- Providing counseling and education about health promotion and injury protection.
- Administering medication and providing wound care.
- Coordinating care and collaborating with other professionals including doctors, therapists and dietitians.
- Directing and supervising care and providing education to patients and family, which enable patients to be discharged sooner.

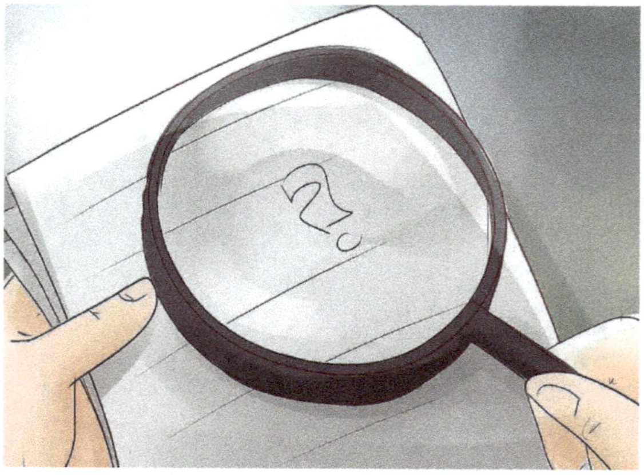

3. Consider the specific job of a Nurse Practitioner. Nurse Practitioners are advanced practice nurses who have obtained graduate education which in turn increases their professional responsibilities.

Nurse practitioners can serve in multiple roles, including providing direct care to patients, research in healthcare, consulting and education. Some of their duties can include:

- Undertaking physical examinations of patients
- Providing immunizations
- Diagnosing and treating common illnesses and injuries
- Managing chronic health problems (e.g., diabetes, high blood pressure, etc.)
- Ordering and interpret diagnostic tests (e.g., X-rays, EKGs, etc.)
- Prescribing medications and/or therapies
- Counseling patients on lifestyle and healthcare decisions

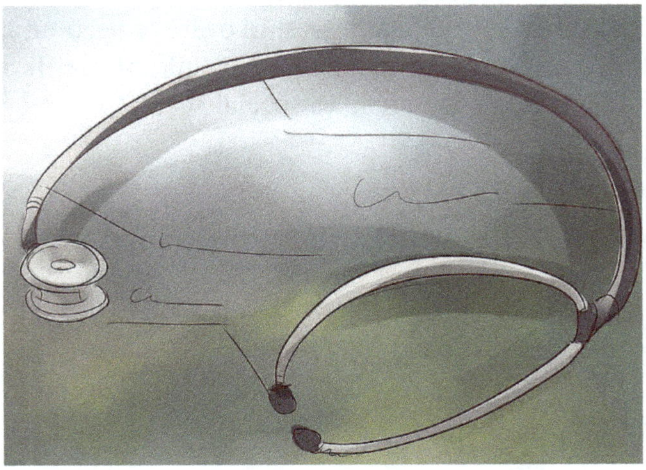

4. Know the skills and qualities required of Nurse Practitioners. Beyond having a breadth of knowledge in medicine (and being someone who does not get squeamish easily!), a Nurse Practitioner must also be skilled in other areas. In this sense, nursing is like any other profession in that there are specific individual qualities that make the job easier and a more natural fit for some people. It's important to determine whether your personality and abilities can accommodate the various responsibilities and tasks that come with being a NP. Key qualities include:

- *Critical thinking*: Nurse Practitioners must be able to assess changes in the health status of their patients from a variety of sources (what the patient says, diagnostic tests, clinical examinations, etc.) and make a quick and evidence-based recommendations.
- *Interpersonal and communication skills*: Being an NP requires working with people everyday—doctors, other nurses, technicians, patients, caregivers, and others. To communicate information and do their jobs effectively and clearly, nurses need strong interpersonal skills, patience, and the ability to break down complex information into something that is accessible for ordinary people (i.e., non-specialists).
- *Compassion*: Caring and empathy are valuable when taking care of individuals who are in sick or injured. Remember that patients may be scared or in pain and need to be comforted, reassured, and motivated to fight through their illnesses.

- *Detail-oriented and organized*: NPs often work with multiple patients and healthcare professional at a time and so they need to be able to keep track of what has been done and what needs to be done. In addition, attention to detail is key; one small mistake can have a big impact on a patient's condition and life.
- *Effective coping with stress*: Nurse Practitioners should be able to cope with stress in effective and healthy ways because they often work in urgent, emergency and/or other sensitive situations and face continual workplace pressures and stressors.

How to become a Nursing Consultant

Nursing consultants play an important role during legal cases by using their expertise and professional knowledge to advise attorneys and businesses. In order to become a nursing consultant, you must have the proper education, obtain a Legal Nurse Consultant Certificate, and master the skills necessary to the job before deciding which field to specialize in.

Part 1

Obtaining the Necessary Education and Training

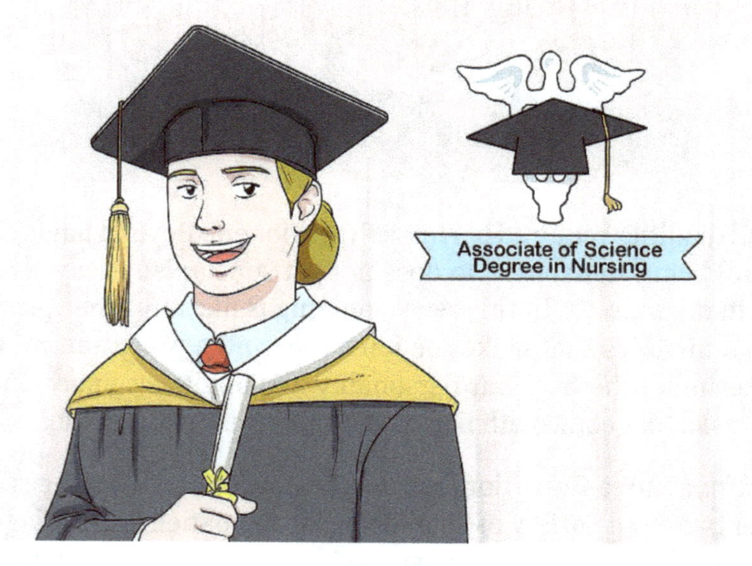

1. Obtain an Associate of Science Degree in Nursing. Before becoming a nursing consultant it is necessary to have a specialized educational background. Nursing consultants are required to at least have an Associate of Science Degree in Nursing, which is a two year program. This means a high school education, or a GED, is necessary as well.

- An Associate of Science Degree in Nursing is a good route to take if you are trying to expedite the education process, as it is a shorter program than other diplomas.
- You can receive your nursing diploma through a hospital or the military to expedite the process even further.

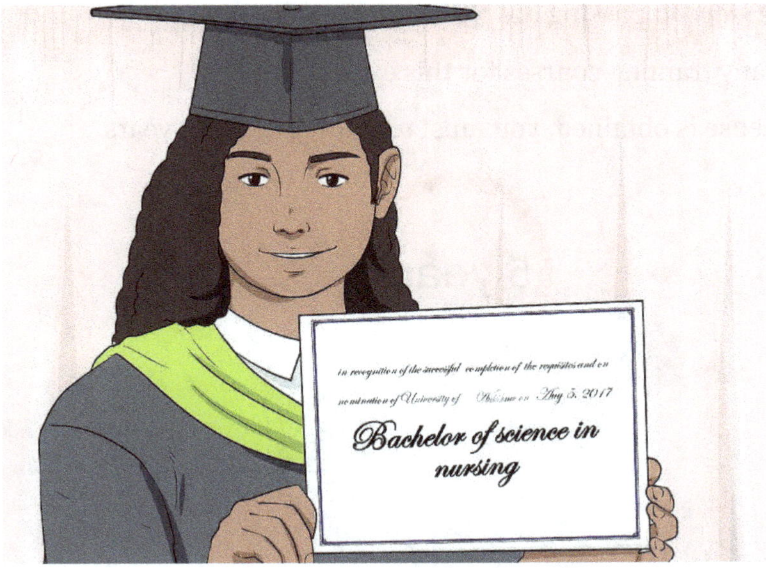

2. Receive a Bachelor of Science Nursing degree if you have more time. A Bachelor of Science Nursing diploma will take four years to receive and will provide you with more knowledge, as you will spend two more years becoming educated. Although this degree is not mandatory, it will better prepare you for your career as a nursing consultant in the long run.

- Applying for financial aid is a great way to get through this education process without retaining too much debt.
- Many nursing consultants are specialists and receive their Master of Science Nursing degree after their undergraduate degree.

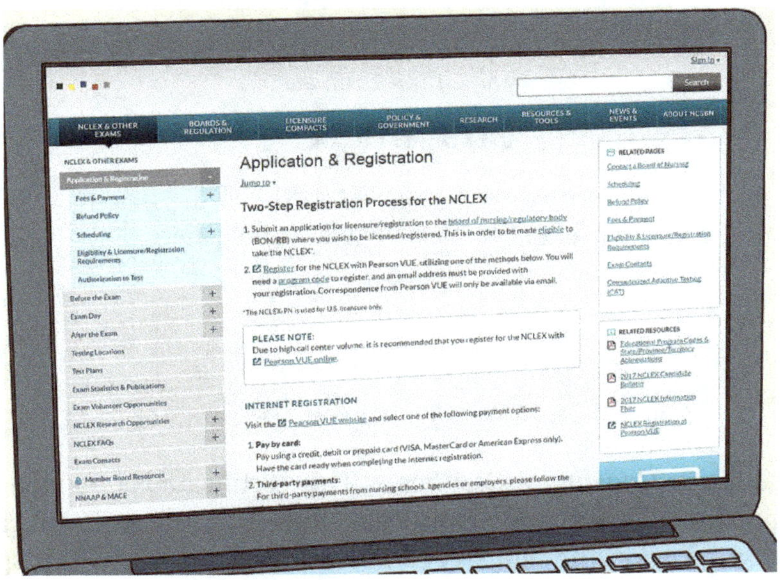

3. Become licensed as a registered nurse. In order to become a practicing nurse, and a nurse consultant later on, you must pass the National Council Licensure Examination for Registered Nurses (NCLEX RN). Because licensed nurses are the only competent professionals able to address nursing practices, becoming registered as a nurse is an essential step.

- Follow these steps to passing the NCLEX RN exam.
- There are many training courses for this exam.
- Once this license is obtained, you must renew it every five years.

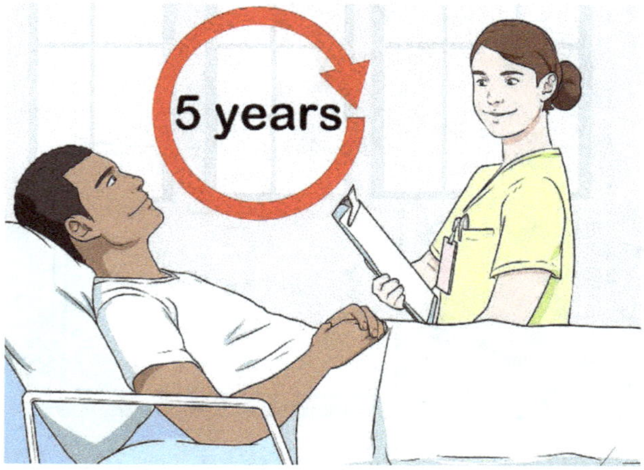

4. Practice as a nurse for a minimum of five years. As a nursing consultant, you must be an expert in the field, ready to use your knowledge in legal matters, so having clinical experience as a registered nurse is essential. Spend five years in the field to obtain the necessary amount of experience and expertise before beginning your career as a consultant.

- Because many legal cases take place in the critical care field, it is recommended to have a broad background in the medical-surgical or critical care/trauma fields. This will provide you an expertise that will allow you to critically analyze a wide variety of medical legal cases.

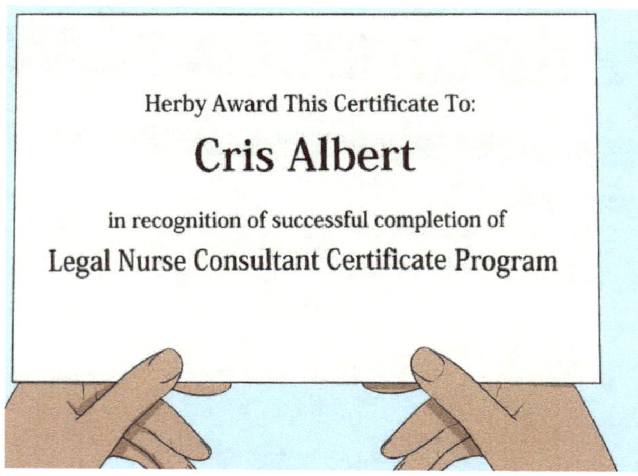
Herby Award This Certificate To:
Cris Albert
in recognition of successful completion of
Legal Nurse Consultant Certificate Program

5. Obtain your Legal Nurse Consultant Certificate. This certificate is obtained through an examination that is administered by the American Legal Nurse Consultant Certification Board and is considered the gold standard in the industry of nurse consulting. There are specific criteria that you must have before taking the exam and you have to meet the same rigorous standards as clinical nursing certification programs.

- In order to take the exam, you must have a full and unrestricted nursing license at the time of your application.

- You must have five years of experience as a registered nurse by the time you apply.
- You also have to have evidence of 2,000 hours of legal nurse consulting experience within three years of your application.

Part 2

Developing the Necessary Skills

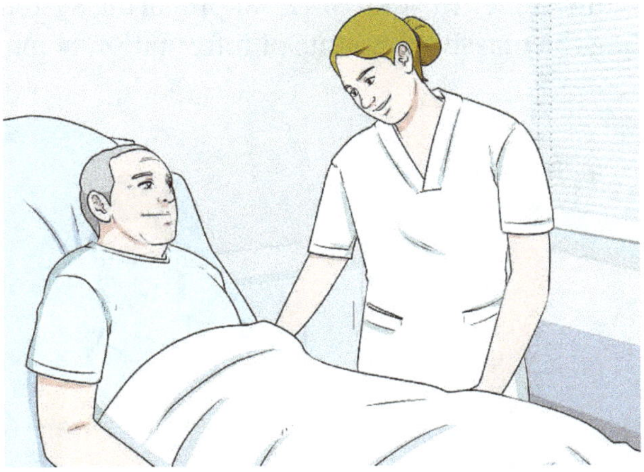

1. Become an articulate communicator. As a registered nurse, you will develop strong interpersonal and communication skills. However, once you begin a career as a nursing consultant, these skills will have to be sharpened. As you will be consulting attorneys or businesses on legal manners, you must strengthen your skills and become extremely good at communicating your opinions efficiently and effectively.

- During your clinical training, observe how other nursing consultants communicate and adapt the techniques you find most effective.
- If you plan to practice independently, you must also be able to communicate your business to the public and be a skilled marketer.

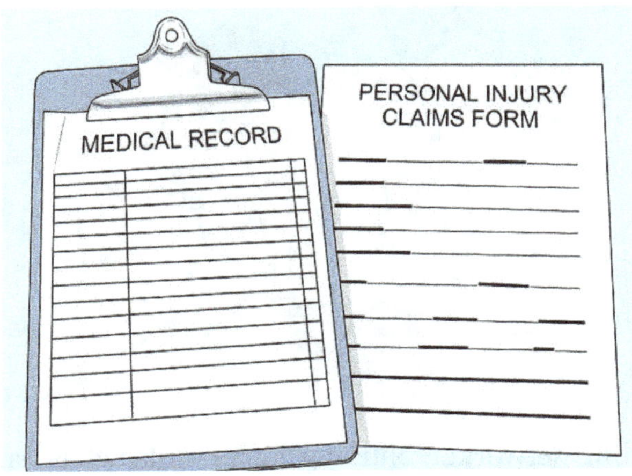

2. Master the art of organizing and analyzing information. While working on a case, whether it be malpractice or personal injury, a nursing consultant must be able to organize and analyze massive

amounts of information, including medical records and litigation materials. Being detail-oriented and being able to consolidate information allows nursing consultants to make objective, fact-based consultations.

- You will need to prepare some research on your own as a nursing consultant, including preparing chronologies of healthcare events and comparing them to the allegations relevant to a case, conducting client interviews, and conducting literature searches and summaries.
- Clients will expect consistency in your work, so preparing systems of organization will be necessary in handling the massive amounts of information being processed in each case.

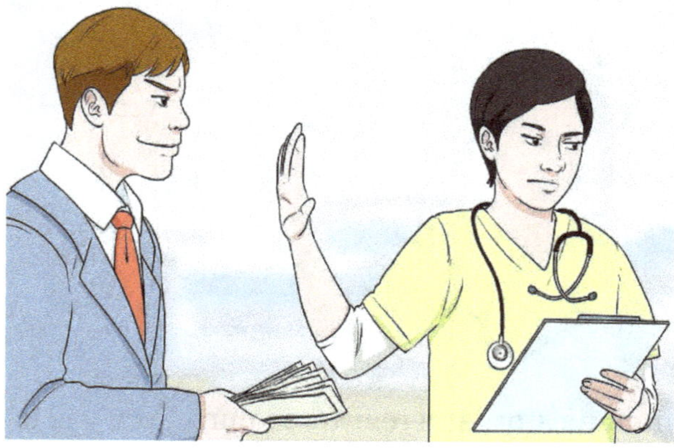

3. Make objectivity a top priority. After consolidating and analyzing a case's relevant information, a nursing consultant must be able and willing to leave their biases and opinions out of a case. Objectivity is vital skill in the field of consulting, and monitoring your own perceptions of a case will allow you to see the facts, rather than be powered by your emotions.

- By practicing in the field for years, a nursing consultant will allow their expertise and knowledge to drive their decision making process while consulting, not their own biases.

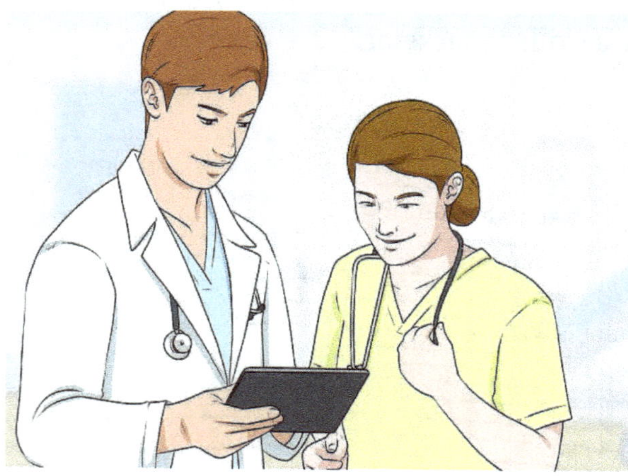

4. Focus on becoming a strong networker. Nursing consultants act as liaisons between health care professionals, attorneys, and clients. It is vital to network within both the healthcare field and the legal field in order to connect the two adequately. Focusing on making strong, trustworthy connections is an important aspect of being a consultant.

- While practicing as a registered nurse, make strong, long-lasting connections with other people in the field. These connections will become necessary once you become a consultant.

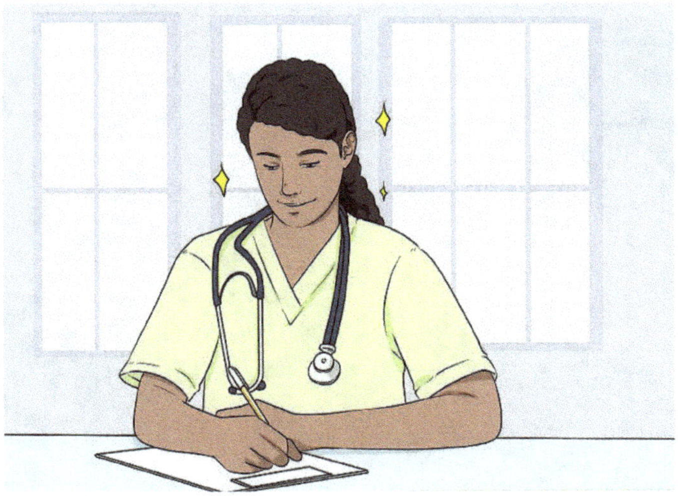

5. Act as a strong and confident advisor. As a nursing consultant, you must use your expertise in the field to provide confident, bold advising during a case. Whether you are working independently or for a firm, providing your objective outlook on a case with conviction will be an important skill to have and will come with adequate experience.

Part 3

Deciding where to Work

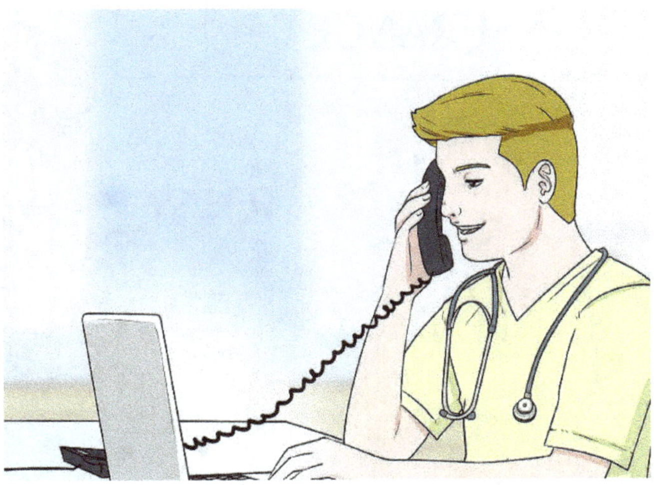

1. Practice independently as a nurse consultant. There are many paths when deciding where to work as a nursing consultant, but it is common for nursing consultants to begin their own independent practice part time while continuing their clinical practice. An independent practice will provide you with a flexible schedule and, as your practice grows, you can start to focus and orient your independent practice into a full time career.

- This is a good avenue for a self-motivated nursing consultant with the financial resources and business sense necessary to run their own business.

- Nursing consultants working independently will have to pay for their own overhead costs that are associated with starting a small business.

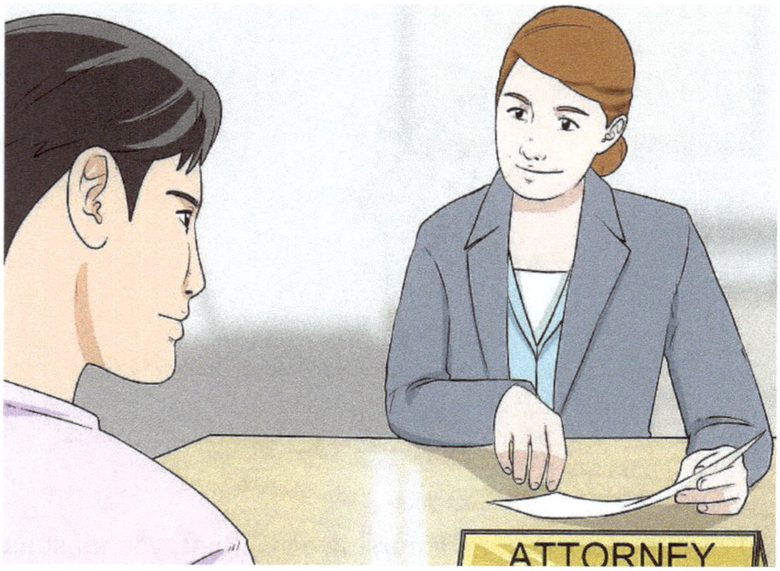

2. Provide expertise for a law firm. Working as a nursing consultant for a law firm will often be a full time position and will consist of assisting attorneys in cases involving health care and medical issues, such as malpractice. Common practices within law firms include summarizing medical records, conducting medical literature searches, and locating and communicating with expert witnesses.

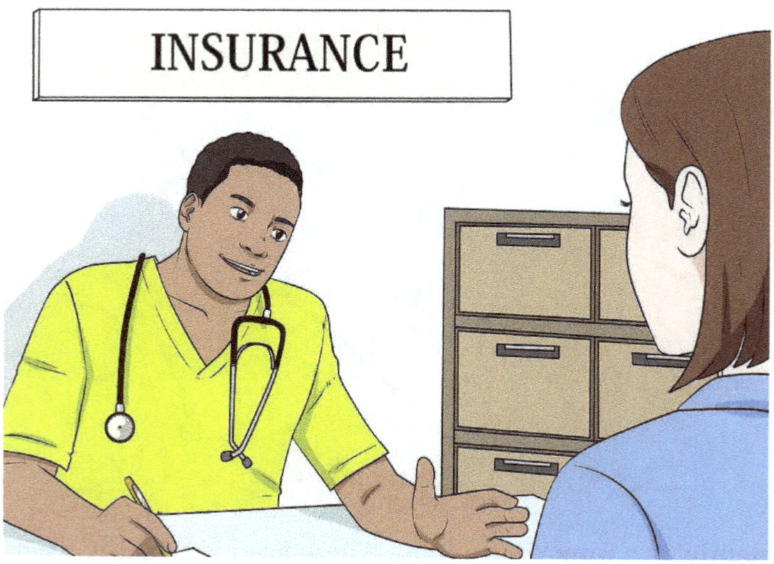

3. Work within an insurance firm. Accident, life, and health insurance companies will often hire nursing consultants to serve as case managers. The duties of nursing consultants within an insurance firm differ greatly from the duties necessary in independent practices and law firms. Rather than doing consultant work on legal cases, you will often work for accident, life, and health insurance companies as a case manager, a utilization review specialists, a medical bill auditor, or as a policy development coordinator and claims adjuster.

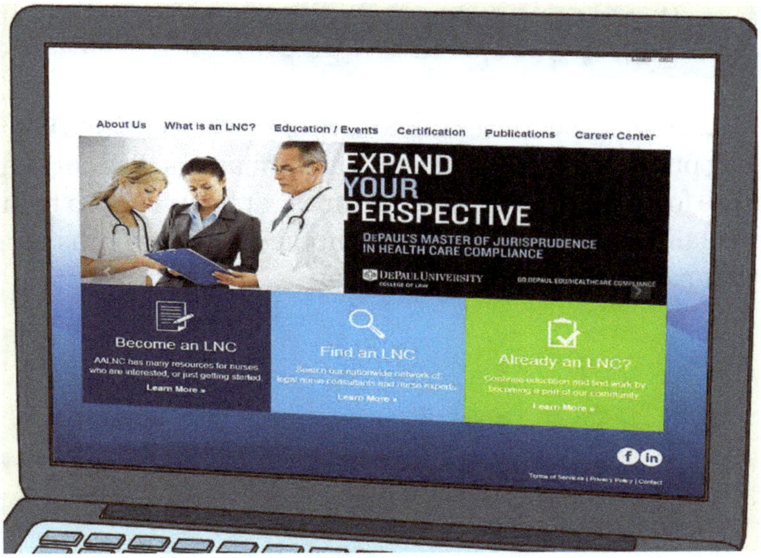

4. Go to work for the government or a corporation. Less common nursing consultant settings include governmental agencies, federal or state patient safety organizations, and business and industry settings. All of these paths will vary in terms of work provided and pay, but are all valid work settings for nursing consultants.

- To find out more about which field you should go into.

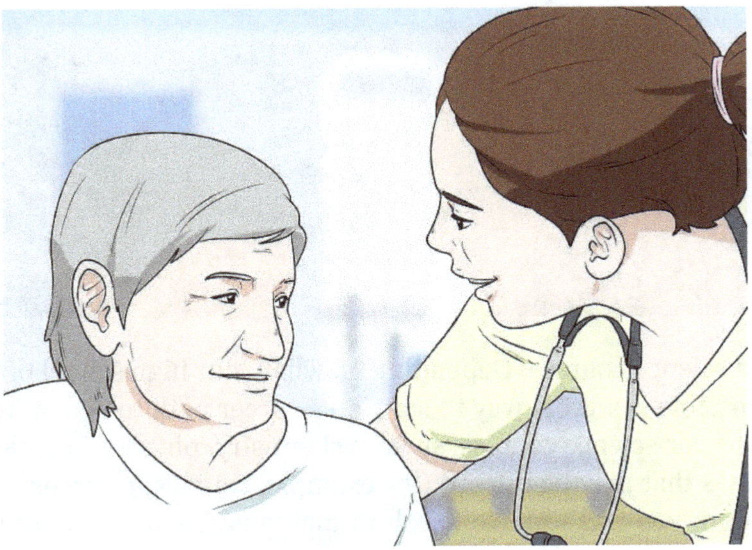

5. Take your expertise into the healthcare field. By working within healthcare systems, hospital, ambulatory care centers and clinics, you will review medical records, conduct patient and employee interviews, prepare reports pertaining to adverse patient outcomes, and participate in meetings regarding the facility's liability exposure. Many healthcare risk management programs in hospitals will hire nurse consultants to assist them in legal matters.

- Nurse consultants that work within healthcare facilities may also work in the area of corporate compliance. This work ensures the facility complies with various state and federal standards.

How to become a Neonatal Nurse

A neonatal nurse is a nurse who specializes in the care of newborn infants who are born with various problems including prematurity, birth defects, malformations, and surgical problems. Neonatal nurses generally care for these infants from the time that they are born to the time that they are released from the hospital. These nurses work with mothers and newborns on a daily basis and are an incredibly important part of our healthcare system.

Part 1

Preparing yourself in High School

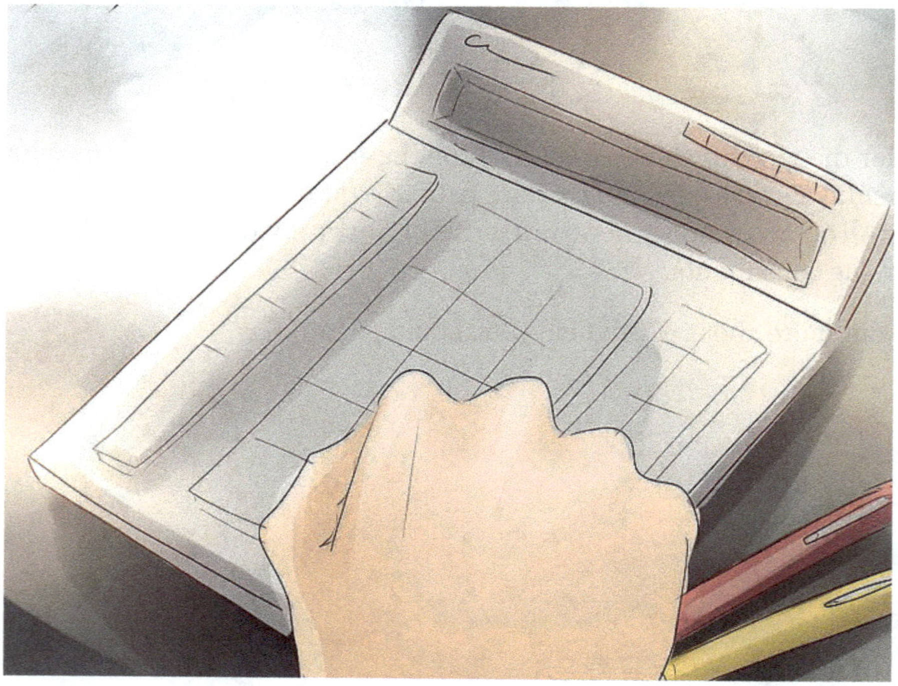

1. Enroll in math and science courses. Depending on what your high school offers, taking as many science courses as possible is a great way to start on a career path to becoming a neonatal nurse. You will want to take basic science courses, such as chemistry, physics, and biology, as well as any elective science courses that may be offered (for example, courses in forensics or anatomy would be helpful). In addition, you will want to enroll in mathematics courses, particularly in subjects such as algebra and calculus. Having a strong background in math and science will make you a more attractive candidate for college-level nursing programs.

- In addition to math and science courses, you should include English and language arts, psychology, and foreign language classes in your coursework if possible. All of these classes offer skills that you will require as a neonatal nurse.
- Take Advanced Placement (AP) courses if offered. These courses can help set you apart as a particularly high-achieving student and can propel you on the right trajectory to becoming a neonatal nurse when you begin college.

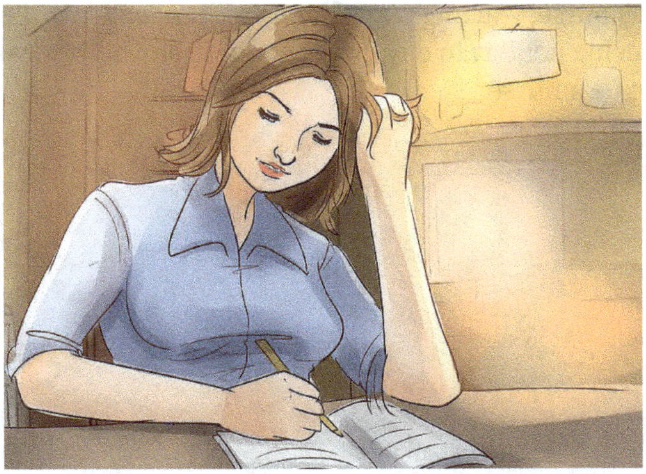

2. Work hard in the classroom. Admission into college-level nursing programs is very competitive, and your grade point average (GPA) will be important. If you are struggling in any of your courses, talk with your teacher or an adviser to prevent getting a poor grade that may affect your chances of getting into a competitive nursing program.

- In addition to having a high GPA, you should look to perform well on your college entrance exams (such as the SAT or ACT). A good score on these entrance exams can help you obtain a place in a great nursing program.

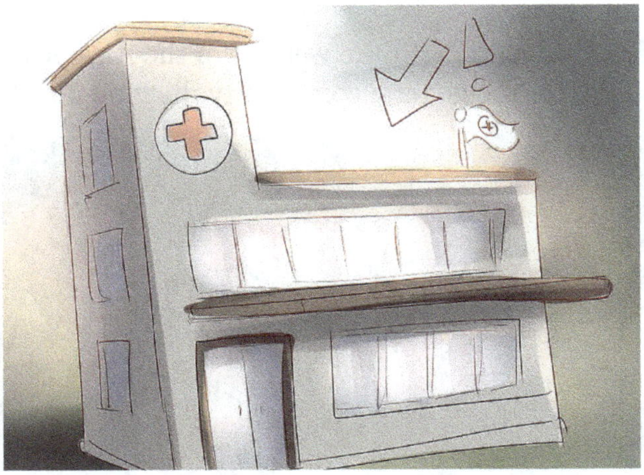

3. Volunteer at a local hospital. Volunteering is a great way to give back to your community and it is a great activity to include on a resume when applying to nursing programs. Volunteering in a healthcare setting shows that you have exposure to the demands of working in a healthcare profession and shows that you are caring and dedicated to helping ill people feel better.

- In order to find volunteer opportunities, check with your local hospital to see if they offer a summer volunteer program for high school student. In order to find a program near you, do an online search for "volunteer opportunities in hospital" and you will find many opportunities. Alternatively, visit your local hospital and inquire about any opportunities they may have.
- While you are volunteering, talk to nurses and to neonatal nurses in particular. They may be able to offer advice or insight into their careers that is hard to match. If you develop a

relationship with a nurse, you might ask her if you can "shadow" her for a day. By following her around and seeing her day to day duties and responsibilities, you will have a better idea of what it takes to be a nurse.

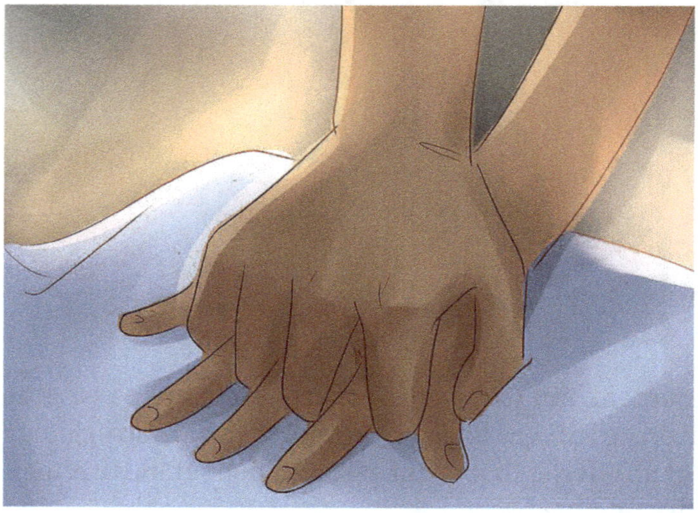

4. Take a first aid or CPR class. Your school may offer these classes as part of their curriculum, or you may have to seek them out from a local community center. Taking one of these classes will demonstrate that you have experience with health-related skills and will show your motivation to become a nurse.

- To find a first aid or CPR class, visit the website of the American Heart Association. They list options for courses for the general community that you may be interested in.

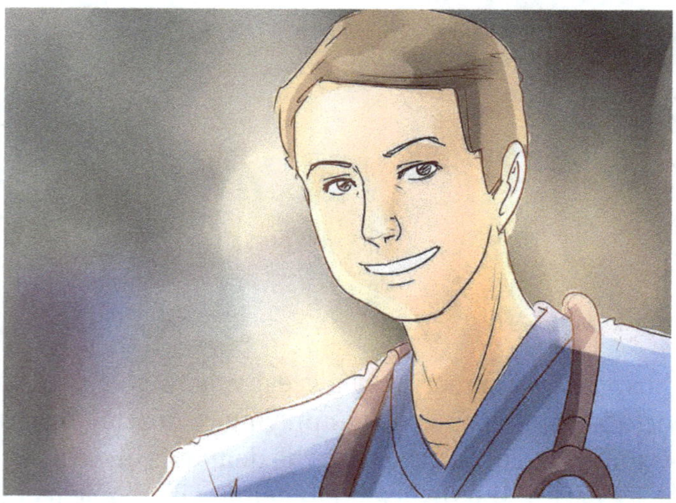

5. Attend nursing camp. If possible, you may want to look into attending nursing camp during one of your summers in high school. You can do an online search to see if there is a program that you can attend that's near you. For example, Seattle Children's Hospital offers a summer nursing camp to expose high school students to the role of a nurse in various clinical settings.

- Some nursing camps require you to apply. You will want to find out the entry requirements for a camp you may be interested in attending as early as possible.

Part 2

Pursuing Neonatal Nursing in College and Beyond

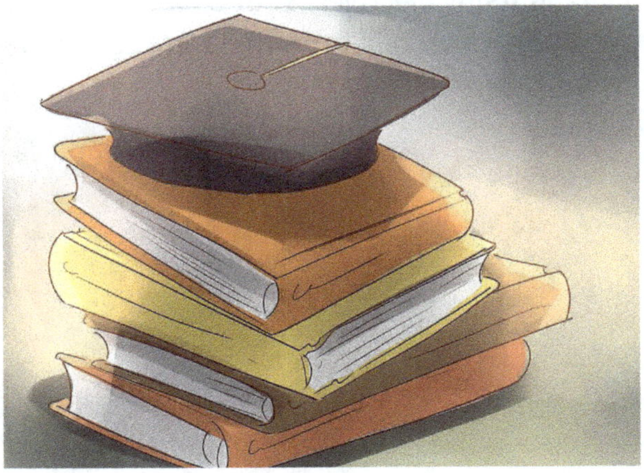

1. Enroll in an undergraduate education. You will want to enroll in a college or university where you can get a four-year undergraduate Bachelor of Science degree. Preferably, you will go to a university where you can receive a bachelor of science in nursing (BSN, BScN) degree.

- Within a BSN program, you will complete your general education courses and also have training in math and science requirements that will be integral to your future career as a neonatal nurse. These courses include statistics, microbiology, anatomy, and physiology.
- Do an online search for colleges and universities that you may be interested in that have BSN programs. If you are having trouble locating programs, speak with a guidance counselor or other teacher who can help you find a program that would be appropriate for you.
- Often times, states have universities and colleges that offer nursing programs. In-state tuition costs are less expensive than out of state programs, and public university is less costly then private.
- It is also essential you confirm that the program is accredited through a national organization.

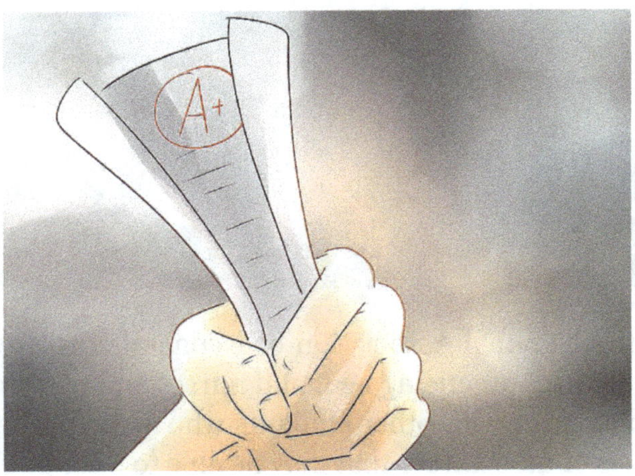

2. Keep up your grades. You will need to complete all the courses in your BSN program and keep your grade point average as high as possible. In order to get into a graduate nursing program

(which you will need for your training in a neonatal specialty), many programs will require at least a 3.3 GPA (on a 4.0 scale) as well as a grade of B or better in all science and nursing courses.

- If possible, take neonatal nursing electives. Your college advisor may be able to recommend some relevant electives, or you can talk to certified neonatal nurses to find out what kind of classes they would recommend that you take.

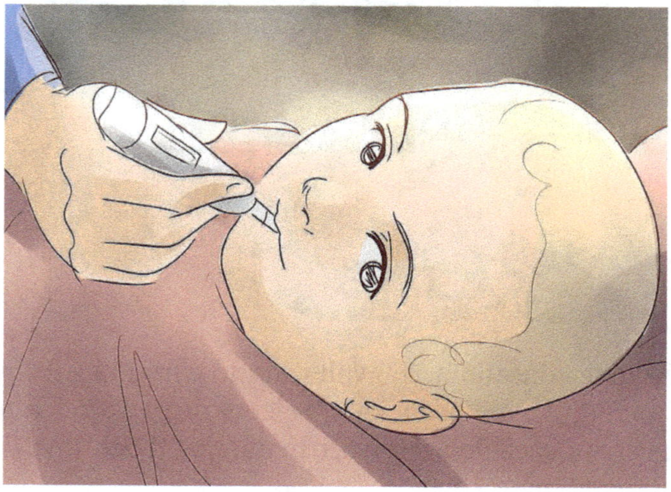

3. Obtain relevant work experience. In addition to having good grades, you will need relevant work experience. Many potential employers will want you to have experience in particular working with ill infants. This work experience will be critical for building up your resume. Try to get as much experience as possible working in a hospital setting, whether through internships set up by your college or university or by volunteering or shadowing neonatal nurses at a local hospital.

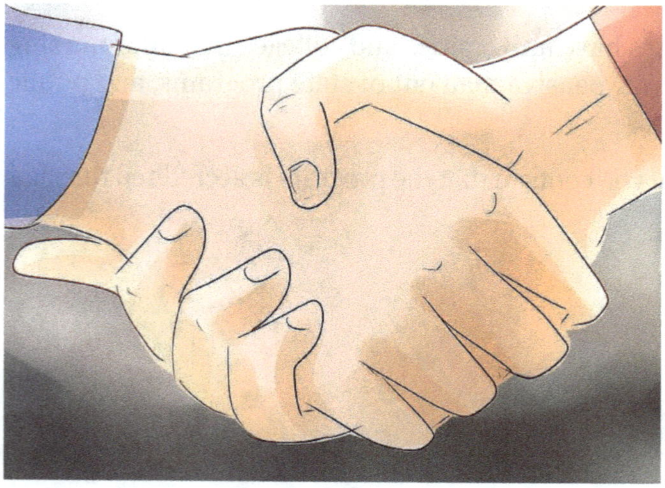

4. Become a member of the National Association of Neonatal Nurses (NANN). Membership in NANN can help you connect with practicing neonatal nurses and network with potential employers. This is a great way to connect with other students who aspire to become neonatal nurses as well as nurses in later stages of their career that may be able to offer guidance and advice.

- To join NANN. You are able to join online, by email, by mailing a membership application, or by calling NANN Member Services.

- When applying, you will be asked some basic demographic questions, including your academic credentials, your position, your work setting, and your employment status.
- If you are a member of the National Student Nurses' Association (NSNA), you can join NANN at a discounted rate of $45.

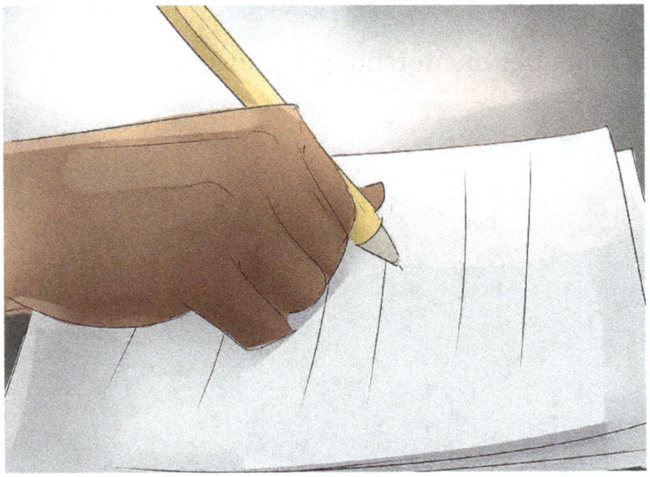

5. Pass the NCLEX exam. After graduating with your BSN, you will want to look into sitting for the NCLEX-RN exam. This exam is a comprehensive test that must be passed before you can earn your license. Passing this exam will enable you to practice in your state (and some states have licensing agreements with other states) by giving you a state license.

- Visit the NCLEX website to find out what you have to do to apply and register for the NCLEX. You will need to be declared eligible to test by the board of nursing/regulatory body. You can find all the necessary details on the NCLEX website.

Part 3

Continuing your Education

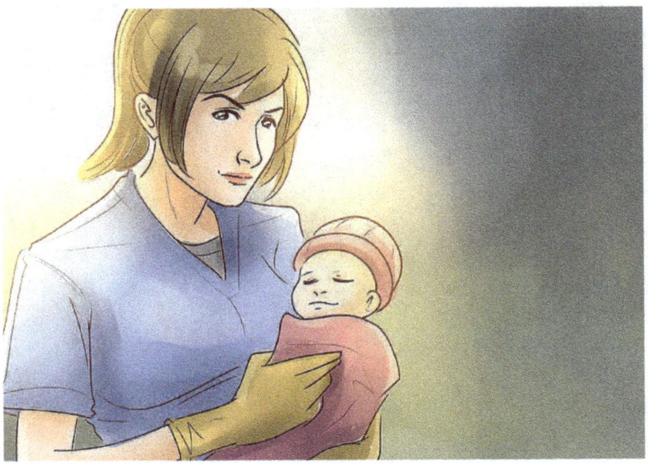

1. Find a job in a hospital with a NICU. After you become a registered nurse by passing your NCLEX exam, you will want to find a nursing job in a hospital that has a NICU. This will give you

the opportunity to get experience with ill newborns and enable you to start developing the skills that you need for a successful career in neonatal nursing.

- Many NICUs will hire graduate nurses who have an interest in neonatal intensive care. Look for a hospital that will give you the opportunity to work in a NICU as you begin your nursing career.
- Look for hospitals that offer mentorship programs.

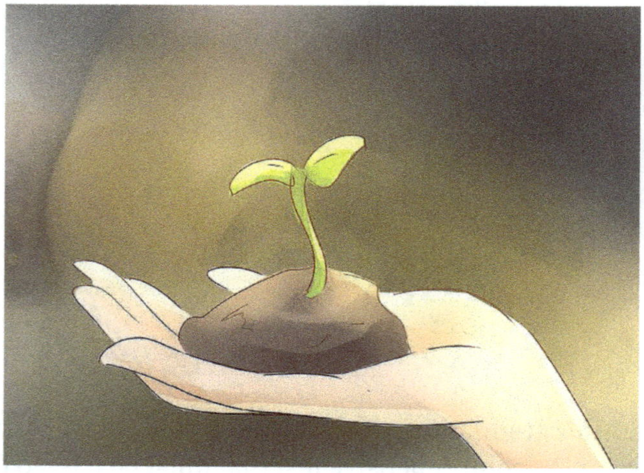

2. Grow your career. Many neonatal nurses start out working as staff nurses who care for ill newborns in hospitals. An average day can consist of assisting new moms with breastfeeding, delivering preterm infants, and caring for ill full-term infants. As you become more experienced in your neonatal nursing career you can grow your career by becoming a neonatal nurse practitioner (NNP).

- Look to practice nursing in a NICU (preferably a Level III NICU, which is geared to take care of the most seriously ill and/or preterm infants) as a staff nurse before applying to graduate school. This will give you essential experience that you need for your graduate school application.

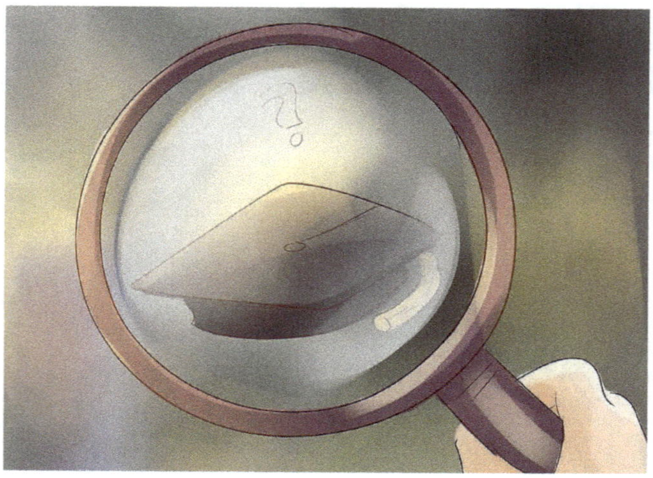

3. Look for graduate degree programs. To become a NNP (an advanced practice nurse who works with other staff to provide critical care to infants in the NICU), you will also need a Master of

Science in Nursing (MSN) degree or a Doctor of Nursing Practice Degree in Neonatal Nursing. These programs will prepare you to work with critically ill newborns and working in delivery rooms.

- Many nursing schools will offer a MSN degree through a two-year Advanced Practice Neonatal Nursing (APNN program). Enrolling in this type of program will get you ready to become licensed as a nurse practitioner or as a clinical nurse specialist.

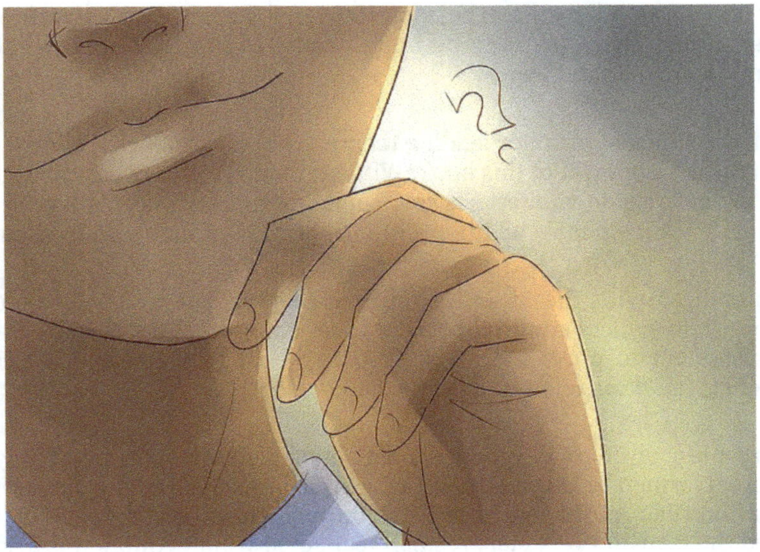

4. Choose your desired level. There are three different levels in the neonatal nursing specialty. The levels vary in their demands and in the level of intensive responsibilities. You should carefully reflect on what type of setting you want to work in and consider if your desire is to work with critically ill infants. Regardless of your level of nursing, you will make a difference in the lives of the infants that you care for.

- Level I nurses care for healthy infants. While still intense and demanding, this is the least demanding level of neonatal nursing.
- Level II nurses care for sick and premature babies that are in need of constant attention. They frequently work in the Neonatal Intensive Care Unit (NICU).
- Level III nurses work in the NICU and monitor the most seriously ill and premature infants. In addition to caring for these infants (usually around the clock), they also are responsible for teaching parents how to properly care for their sick babies.

Permissions

All chapters in this book are published with permission under the Creative Commons Attribution Share Alike License or equivalent. Every chapter published in this book has been scrutinized by our experts. Their significance has been extensively debated. The topics covered herein carry significant information for a comprehensive understanding. They may even be implemented as practical applications or may be referred to as a beginning point for further studies.

We would like to thank the editorial team for lending their expertise to make the book truly unique. They have played a crucial role in the development of this book. Without their invaluable contributions this book wouldn't have been possible. They have made vital efforts to compile up to date information on the varied aspects of this subject to make this book a valuable addition to the collection of many professionals and students.

This book was conceptualized with the vision of imparting up-to-date and integrated information in this field. To ensure the same, a matchless editorial board was set up. Every individual on the board went through rigorous rounds of assessment to prove their worth. After which they invested a large part of their time researching and compiling the most relevant data for our readers.

The editorial board has been involved in producing this book since its inception. They have spent rigorous hours researching and exploring the diverse topics which have resulted in the successful publishing of this book. They have passed on their knowledge of decades through this book. To expedite this challenging task, the publisher supported the team at every step. A small team of assistant editors was also appointed to further simplify the editing procedure and attain best results for the readers.

Apart from the editorial board, the designing team has also invested a significant amount of their time in understanding the subject and creating the most relevant covers. They scrutinized every image to scout for the most suitable representation of the subject and create an appropriate cover for the book.

The publishing team has been an ardent support to the editorial, designing and production team. Their endless efforts to recruit the best for this project, has resulted in the accomplishment of this book. They are a veteran in the field of academics and their pool of knowledge is as vast as their experience in printing. Their expertise and guidance has proved useful at every step. Their uncompromising quality standards have made this book an exceptional effort. Their encouragement from time to time has been an inspiration for everyone.

The publisher and the editorial board hope that this book will prove to be a valuable piece of knowledge for students, practitioners and scholars across the globe.

Index

A

Admission, 19, 29, 49, 59, 62, 204, 221

Appointments, 6, 19, 103, 204

Axillary, 137, 139-140

B

Bedding, 158-160, 162-163

Bedpan, 164-173, 175-176

Bedrail, 162

Bedspread, 159, 162-163

Blanket, 159-160, 162-163, 165, 167

Blood, 5, 26, 99, 127-130, 132-137, 144-149, 159, 177, 211

Blood Pressure, 26, 99, 127-130, 132-137, 177, 211

C

Caffeine, 128

Clinics, 7, 15, 24, 34, 186, 209, 219

Compassion, 26, 29, 78-80, 96, 164, 211

Critical Thinking, 26, 29-30, 54, 57, 73, 77, 211

D

Diabetes, 23, 26-27, 148, 150, 208, 211

Diagnose, 1, 19, 34, 73, 201, 204

Diastolic, 127, 133-136

Discharged, 25, 28, 210

Draw Sheet, 160-161

E

Ekgs, 26, 211

Emergency Room, 3, 33, 79, 185

Emesis, 159

Emotional Intelligence, 110, 113-114, 116

Emotions, 38, 78-79, 99, 110-119, 122-125, 216

Empathy, 26, 29, 79, 96, 114, 118-126, 211

Eq, 110-113, 115-118

F

Fluid Balance Charts, 6

Food Charts, 6

G

Gloves, 157, 160, 162-163, 165, 171-172, 176

Glucometer, 144-150

Glucose, 144-146, 149

H

Healthcare, 7-8, 12, 18, 22-26, 29, 32-34, 37, 41-43, 57, 60, 148, 187, 192-193, 200, 204, 207, 209, 211-212, 216, 219-221

Hearing Test, 178

Heartbeat, 128, 130, 133

Hospitals, 7, 10-11, 15, 22, 24, 30, 32, 34, 41-43, 54, 60, 69, 186, 188, 193, 195, 200, 207, 209, 219, 226

Hypertension, 135-137

I

Icu, 185, 187

Immunizations, 25, 64, 211

Infants, 137, 195, 220, 224, 226-227

Injury, 2, 24-25, 27-28, 164, 168, 199, 210, 215

Insulin, 144

Internships, 200, 224

L

Linens, 54, 158-162, 174

Lpn, 3, 7-10, 18, 41, 54-55, 187

M

Maternity Nurse, 183, 187, 192, 194

Medical Terminology, 83

Medication, 25, 28-29, 34, 74, 87, 103-104, 127, 135, 137, 144, 188, 201, 210

Mental Health, 3, 16, 23, 34, 98, 101, 200-203, 208

Mentorship, 226

Mucus, 5, 175

N

Neonatal Nurse, 183, 220, 223, 226

Notes, 6, 45, 48, 50, 73

Nurse Anesthetist, 18, 34, 183, 185-186

Nurse Education, 1

Nurse Practitioner, 18-20, 22-23, 25-26, 34, 188, 198, 200, 204-211, 226-227

Nursing Homes, 7, 15, 24, 34, 38, 42, 209

Nursing School, 7, 11, 40-41, 43-55, 57-59, 61-67, 69, 71, 189-190, 192, 196, 200

O

Observations, 6

Open-minded, 113

Operating Room, 79, 187, 189

P

Patience, 26, 29, 38, 105, 108-110, 164, 211

Pediatric Nurse, 183, 194-196, 198-200

Petroleum Jelly, 142

Pharmacist, 104

Physical Examinations, 25, 28, 210-211

Physicians, 1, 24, 27, 104, 183, 186, 193, 209-210

Pill Box, 103

Plan of Care, 1

Premature, 227

Prn Analgesic, 158

Psychiatric Nurse, 183, 200-201

Q

Quality of Life, 1-2, 72, 93, 126

R

Rectum, 141-142, 174

Referrals, 6, 19, 29, 204

Registered Nurse, 3, 9, 19-21, 23, 27, 30-31, 33-34, 41, 103, 184, 187, 197, 201, 204-206, 208, 213-215, 217, 225

Rounds, 6

Rubbing Alcohol, 138, 142, 144, 146

S

Self Awareness, 116

Self Management, 116

Senior Center, 101

Smoking, 128

Snell Test, 178

Social Work, 6

Sponge Bath, 150

Stethoscope, 130-132, 181

Stool, 5, 159

Stress, 27, 39-40, 47-48, 50, 75, 77, 81, 89, 94, 97, 110-111, 117, 128-129, 199, 212

Systolic, 127, 133-136

T

Therapists, 1, 4, 25, 28, 210

Thermometer, 137-144

Thyroid Gland, 180

Toileting, 6, 170

Turning Charts, 6

U

Urine, 5, 159

W

Ward, 5-6, 38, 102, 189

X

X-rays, 26, 211

www.ingramcontent.com/pod-product-compliance
Lightning Source LLC
LaVergne TN
LVHW080708210926
848485LV00003B/432
* 9 7 8 1 6 3 9 8 7 0 0 5 9 *